NURSING CONCEPTS AND PROCESSES

NURSING CONCEPTS AND PROCESSES

Carolyn Chambers Clark, EdD, RN
Formerly Instructor of Nursing,
Bergen Community College, Paramus, New Jersey

Carolyn Chambers Clark

Consulting Editor — Betty Dean, EdD, RN
ADN Series Editor — Angela R. Emmi, BSNEd, MS, RN
Technical Reviewer — Catherine H. White, MS, RN

DELMAR PUBLISHERS • ALBANY, NEW YORK 12205
A DIVISION OF LITTON EDUCATIONAL PUBLISHING, INC.

This book is dedicated to a teacher
who influenced my career choice —
Eugenia Schoen — and to my husband,
William F. Clark, who supports my
self-actualization endeavors.

DELMAR PUBLISHERS
COPYRIGHT ©1977
BY LITTON EDUCATIONAL PUBLISHING, INC.

10 9 8 7 6 5 4 3 2 1

LIBRARY OF CONGRESS CATALOG CARD NUMBER: 76-14095

Printed in the United States of America
Published Simultaneously in Canada by
Delmar Publishers, A Division of
Van Nostrand Reinhold, Ltd.

FOREWORD

The Delmar series in Associate Degree Nursing is designed for use primarily by students at two-year colleges. However, because each text was designed to meet specific instructional goals common to all, it is felt the texts will be valuable to students in any nursing program. The underlying themes of the series include: (1) the health-illness continuum, (2) developmental stages, and (3) integrated content. Each text is designed to involve the student in a total learning experience. Student objectives are listed for each chapter to guide learning and promote mastery of the content. Activities and discussion topics are suggested. Multiple-choice, matching, and essay-type questions test student achievement. An extensive glossary and bibliography are provided for each chapter for reference and reinforcement of subject content.

To verify the technical content and evaluate student opinions, portions of each title are classroom tested in AD nursing programs. All of the authors are actively involved in the instruction of ADN students and hold a master's degree in nursing or higher. The editors are former instructors and hold academic degrees in nursing and/or nursing education.

Nursing Concepts and Processes was prepared by Carolyn Chambers Clark.

Carolyn Chambers Clark, R.N., received her baccalaureate in nursing from the University of Wisconsin in 1964. She received her master's degree in psychiatric nursing from Rutgers, the State University, in 1966. Ms. Clark taught nursing for two and one-half years at Bergen Community College in Paramus, New Jersey. She received her doctorate in Physical and Mental Illness Nursing Instruction from Columbia University in 1975.

Dr. Clark is currently employed as Adjunct Assistant Professor of Group Dynamics for Nurses at Pace University, Westchester, Pleasantville, New York. She also maintains a private nursing practice in individual and family mental-health counseling. She is on the faculty of the Clinical Specialists Society of the New Jersey State Nurses Association in Psychiatric Nursing. In addition, Dr. Clark runs workshops that seek to teach nurses ways to implement mental-health concepts in their relationships with individual and groups of patients and peers. She was director for several workshops in nursing at the Downstate Medical Center in Brooklyn, New York for April and May of 1976.

Dr. Clark's special interests include the promotion of simulation/gaming as an educational technique in nursing, and the study of the effects of interpersonal intervention with clients who have long-term physical illness processes.

Carolyn Chambers Clark is the author of many articles dealing with various aspects of psychiatric nursing which have been published in several nursing magazines. She has been the speaker for self-help and chronic-illness groups regarding mental health. In October 1975, she presented a paper on simulation/gaming as an instructional method in nursing to the national conference of the North American Simulation and Gaming Association.

Dr. Clark is a member of the American Nurses Association, the North American Simulation and Gaming Association, and the Clinical Specialists Society of New Jersey Nurses Association. She is a Certified Clinical Specialist in Mental Health Counseling, Rockland County, New York.

Delmar publications for technical and professional nurses are:

Nursing Perspectives and Issues — Gloria M. Grippando, EdD, RN

Drug Interactions — Joseph R. DiPalma, M.D.

Basic Readings in Drug Therapy — Joseph R. DiPalma, M.D. and Morton J. Rodman, PhD.

More Readings in Drug Therapy — Morton J. Rodman, PhD. and Joseph R. DiPalma, M.D.

How to Read an ECG — Herbert H. Butler, M.D.

— Angela R. Emmi

PREFACE

Nursing Concepts and Processes has been developed for use throughout the theoretical and clinical nursing experience. The text may be used to complement or supplement areas of instruction which are currently under study; because of its flexibility, there is no need to follow the chapters in sequence. Themes which are interwoven throughout the book include the health-illness continuum, the developmental stages, and the integration of medical-surgical and psychiatric-mental health principles. An effort has been made to examine each concept or process through consideration of its meaning, the manner in which strengths or difficulties are assessed, and the nursing interventions that have been found helpful. For purposes of uniformity and clarity, the nurse is referred to as *she* and the patient as *he.*

Nursing Concepts and Processes is divided into five sections. Although the subject matter is not restricted and can be used throughout the program, the following guidelines may be utilized in planning instruction.

Section One on Health Care Relationships introduces the student to roles and relationships. It can be used in the beginning nursing course; the chapters on anxiety, and structuring the relationships in mental health and illness can be reviewed as the clinical assignments vary.

Section Two on Health-Illness Relationships will be useful whenever the clinical experience contains elements of health, illness, crisis, pain, or grief. Health-illness is viewed as a continuum, with crisis being seen as a point where coping efforts do not permit adaptation. Pain is examined from several viewpoints, and both physical and interpersonal interventions are summarized. Grief is presented as a normal reaction to loss. The two chapters on grief will be especially helpful for students working with patients who are dying or who have lost a significant other person, a body part, or the security of a comfortable environment.

Section Three, the Observation-Perception-Communication Process will probably be used most frequently by students in the first nursing course. The student may wish to review this section prior to the clinical experience which will involve use of the nursing interview. Nursing process and nursing care plans are included in this section as observation, perception, and communication are primary tools used in nursing assessment and intervention.

Section Four, Coping with Illness, introduces the beginning student to therapeutic and nontherapeutic factors which must be considered. Obviously, the student may refer to this section throughout the nursing program. The effects and ways to cope with stress, the influence of body image, mind and body relationships, stages of illness and the sick role are presented.

Section Five contains basic and more advanced information about the learning process. The beginning student may be assigned to read the chapter on nursing conferences quite early in his or her career in order to understand and participate more effectively in clinical and in teacher-student evaluation conferences. Chapter 28 can be assigned when the student is about to begin teaching patients. The last two chapters deal with student involvement with groups, both as participant and as leader. These chapters are especially useful to those who will be teaching patient groups, participating in staff meetings, or observing groups of patients involved in a project or activity.

Portions of *Nursing Concepts and Processes* were pretested with associate degree nursing students. Special features which may be of interest to the instructor or student are:

- Behavioral objectives listed at the beginning of each chapter alert the reader to upcoming content.

- Review questions at the end can be used to test the objectives.

- Sections and chapters are short and clearly titled to permit students to readily refer to appropriate material and to digest small amounts of information at one time.

- Chapter summaries help the reader to review important points.

- Activities and Discussion Topics at the end of each chapter can help students implement theory through specific actions. These activities can form the base for discussion or seminar presentations.

- Tables and charts are used extensively to summarize and reinforce what has been covered.

- An extensive glossary and bibliography is provided for each chapter.

CONTENTS

SECTION 1
HEALTH
CARE
RELATIONSHIPS

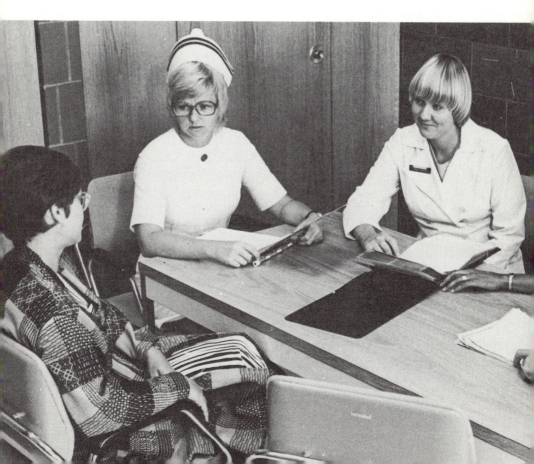

chapter 1
THE HEALTH TEAM
AND NURSING ROLES

STUDENT OBJECTIVES

- Define health team.

- Identify the relationship between the health team and the nursing team.

- List three reasons why nursing roles are changing.

- Identify seven roles which the nurse may assume.

The nurse and the patient do not form an isolated unit although both are involved in promoting the health of the patient. It is necessary to work with others to achieve this goal.

Nurses come in contact with other health personnel while caring for the patient. They join other health personnel to plan care and coordinate activities of other health personnel in order to insure minimal stress to the patient.

MEMBERS OF THE HEALTH TEAM

The *health team* is composed of all personnel who are concerned with promoting the health of people. Members of the health team may vary, depending on the situation. The nurse, physician, dietician, social worker and chaplain may work with one patient. The physical therapist, psychiatric-mental health nurse, and rehabilitation counselor may join the health team in caring for another. Figure 1-1, page 2, shows some possible members of the health team.

Currently, patients are interested in being included in health care planning. In fact, institutions who receive federal support for patient care are expected

1

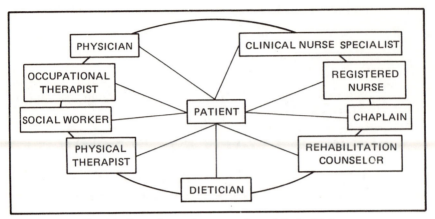

Fig. 1-1 The patient and some members of the health team

to include consumers as well as health care personnel in decisions about health care.

At times, health personnel are reluctant to include the patient as part of the health team. Decisions about patient care may be made without finding out what the patient wants. The patient probably has a good idea of how he would like to feel, and ways the personnel can help to achieve this feeling. As the member of the health team who often works most closely with the patient, the nurse is in an excellent position to encourage the patient to make his needs known to the health team.

In many health care institutions, the control of health care decisions is in the hands of physicians. Services to patients may not be distributed equally. There may be little interchange of information between doctors and nurses, between different health care agencies, and between health personnel and the patient and his or her family.

Although there is resistance in many settings, nurses are attempting to open up communication channels with doctors and other health team members. The nurse can bring an especially important component to health care delivery. Nurses are more concerned with the total person; doctors tend to focus on the illness or particular disease presented by the patient. Also, the education of nurses emphasizes the use of communication skills that promote constructive interaction between various health team members and health care facilities.

MEMBERS OF THE NURSING TEAM

The *nursing team* is a subsystem of the health team. Often, the nursing team consists of a registered nurse, a licensed practical nurse, and nursing aides or assistants. The functions of nursing team members may differ depending on the health care agency in which they are employed.

The registered nurse is usually responsible for supervising and coordinating the work of other nursing team members. Registered nurses are being increasingly encouraged to receive their education in an academic setting. Currently, nurses can prepare to be registered nurses in a college setting through either an associate degree or baccalaureate degree program.

On some patient care units, a registered nurse called the clinical nurse specialist is assigned on a full-time, part-time, or consultative basis. The clinical nurse specialist has a master's degree in a clinical specialty such as cardiovascular nursing or psychiatric-mental health nursing. Functions of the clinical nurse specialist may vary but can include teaching new methods of patient care to nursing team members, giving direct care to patients, and doing nursing research.

As head of the nursing team, the registered nurse is the role model who demonstrates to other health and nursing team members what nursing is all about. *Nursing* may be defined as an interpersonal process where people are assisted to their highest level of wellness. Nursing also includes a scientific aspect. Part of the science of nursing is the administration of care which is based on scientific principles derived from physical and natural sciences. Nursing practice is based on knowledge and theory that allows for the development and testing of *hypotheses* (reasonable assumptions) about approaches to patient care. Developing hypotheses and testing them is an important part of the science of nursing. When the nurse develops a new method of meeting patient needs, the rest of the nursing team can be guided toward testing and gathering information about the new method.

Nurses are particularly concerned with *continuity of care* which refers to the attempt to provide high level care for the patient at all times; this includes care from the patient's entry into a health care delivery system through discharge or transfer to another agency or facility. Continuity of care implies that there is clear and open communication between health team members of all agencies concerned with care for the patient. Generally speaking, continuity of care is the ideal rather than the attained goal at the present time.

The licensed practical nurse (or licensed vocational nurse) is another member of the nursing team and is often referred to as an LPN or LVN. Practical nursing programs are about one year in length. LPNs do many basic nursing procedures; they perform more advanced procedures under the supervision of a registered nurse or physician.

Other members of the nursing team are nursing aides, nursing assistants, and orderlies. These nursing team members assist the registered nurse with a wide variety of tasks. In some agencies, nursing aides primarily perform housekeeping

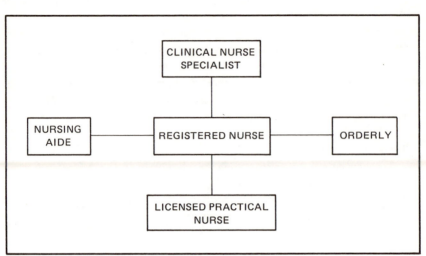

Fig. 1-2 **Some nursing team members**

tasks. In other agencies, nursing aides assist with or even provide a large percentage of patient care. Figure 1-2 shows some nursing team members.

NURSING ROLES

Nursing roles are in a period of transition. All nurses are taught a body of knowledge and skills that allow them to assist patients to meet basic needs. These needs include sleep, oxygen, food, and communication with other people.

All nurses are beginning to expand their roles. *Expanded roles* occur when nurses look for or are asked to assume tasks that formerly were completed by other health personnel. The physical examination is an example of a task formerly done only by physicians but now is being done by nurses who are specially prepared. Nursing roles may also expand when patients ask for or seem to need certain types of care and the nurse steps in to provide it. For example, counseling the patient through the use of communication skills is a function that nurses are using more extensively in their expanding roles.

Nursing roles will continue to be influenced by the way nurses define their functions. These roles will also be influenced by sociocultural changes such as national health insurance, and increase in the needs of the young and the elderly. Also, the average length of hospitalization time is decreasing. Treatment of the more acute patient conditions is being done in the hospital setting; long-term care is more likely to be given in nursing homes, extended care facilities, and in the community through visiting nurse services. All of these influence nursing functions.

Since nursing functions are changing, there are a number of roles which the nurse must assume. Current nursing roles include those of stranger, substitute person, technician, teacher, leader, counselor, liaison, coordinator, and patient advocate.

The Role of Stranger

When meeting a patient or family for the first time, the nurse is in the role of stranger. Since both nurse and patient are apt to be anxious in this new situation, it is important that the nurse carefully choose her words. Clear communication is essential; only those things which the patient is meant to hear should be stated. Simple statements about the setting and the purpose of the interaction may help to establish rapport and decrease the feelings of strangeness.

Substitute Person

Many patients have a need to cast the nurse in the role of some other significant person in the patient's life. The patient may view and react toward the nurse as if the nurse were a mother, sister, wife, or even a favorite teacher. Instead of relating to the nurse as a specific person, the patient may treat the nurse as someone else.

The actions of the nurse can promote or decrease the tendency for the patient to treat the nurse as a substitute person. If the nurse acts motherly, treats the patient as a child, and does not allow him to make any decisions, the patient is more apt to cast the nurse in the substitute role of a mother. The nurse can do much to increase awareness by helping the patient to see how the nurse is similar to and different from the other person. For example, if the patient says "You remind me of my wife," the nurse could reply, "In what way?"

By being herself, the nurse can help the patient realize that people are different. Being yourself includes knowing who you are and how you react to others. Nurses who are not aware of themselves are more likely to react as a substitute person for patients; they may also be inclined to cast a patient in the role of substitute person.

When patients are quite ill, they may require care that is similar to that which is given by a mother. The patient will be more likely to move to a more independent state if the nurse accepts and performs the necessary skills. The nurse who thinks that a dependent, helpless patient is repulsive or "cute" is not likely to inspire growth and more mature behavior in the patient.

The nurse may also be cast as a substitute person by the doctor or vice versa. The doctor may treat the nurse as a sister or mother and the nurse may look to the doctor as an authoritative father. Many nurses are currently trying to establish more equal peer relationships with doctors where joint collaboration can lead to improved patient care.

Technician

The technician role of the nurse includes the smooth and calm administration of medications, treatments, and all nursing procedures; it covers the technical aspect of nursing. As with other roles, the technician role has its place in nursing. However, the nurse must guard against becoming technically efficient but indifferent to the patient's response. Nurses who can move easily between roles, depending on the patient's need at the moment, are the most effective nurses.

Teacher

As the maintenance of good health and the prevention of illness increase in importance, the teaching role of the nurse is enhanced. In the teaching role, the nurse gives information that will assist the patient to higher levels of wellness. The information can be factual, such as, "An X ray will be taken of your left leg." The information can be interpersonal, such as, "I notice you tensed up just then." Through the teaching role, the nurse is able to help the patient deal with upcoming situations more effectively.

The nurse takes the teaching role when she helps the patient to assess and evaluate situations. Teaching is not merely transmitting facts established by a more knowledgeable authority. Teaching is helping the patient to assess, apply and evaluate new strategies in health and related fields.

Leader

Patients tend to look to the nurse as an authority who should have all the answers. The nurse assumes the role of an authoritarian or a democratic leader with patients and other personnel.

Authoritarian leaders are likely to tell others what to do, and to demand absolute obedience from their followers. In some nursing situations, it may be necessary for the nurse to direct the patient or nursing staff members. In these situations, the nurse may become authoritative. Authoritarian leaders evoke dependency because their followers are not allowed or encouraged to be independent.

Nurses can also be *democratic leaders.* Democratic leaders encourage others to be more independent. Nurses who are democratic leaders allow patients to take an active part in their own care. A primary goal in nursing is to establish democratic leadership where others are encouraged to be independent and participate in patient care to the fullest extent possible. Democratic nurse leaders teach patients and other nursing personnel to learn skills that enable them to become more independent.

Counselor

The nurse as counselor helps the patient to become aware of what is happening to him and to deal with his feelings. The counselor role is based on knowledge of communication skills and an ability to use them. The counseling process is concerned with patient communication and nurse responses. This means that the nurse relates to the patient helping him to deal with illness, hospitalization and discharge from the hospital or agency, health and/or death. Counseling helps the patient to be aware of his or her reactions so that the total illness or hospital experience can be integrated as a whole with other life experiences.

The nurse can guide the patient toward higher levels of wellness by accepting him as a person. Through demonstration and discussion, the nurse can help the patient to be a more effective communicator and to modify behavior so that more satisfaction occurs in interpersonal relationships with others.

Liaison Person

The nurse serves as liaison person when communicating information from one source to another. For example, the nurse may convey information between the patient and the health team; or, the nurse may deliver a message from one health team member to another health team member. In addition, liaison services between different health care units or agencies are sometimes necessary.

Coordinator

The nurse coordinates care for the patient. In the coordinator role, the nurse plans nursing care so as to provide the least amount of stress for the patient. For example, patients will not be subject to several consecutive procedures over a short period of time. Plans are made so that stressful treatments and taxing activities are well spaced and scheduled when the patient is rested, toileted, fed, and prepared for the upcoming situation.

There is another aspect to the nurse coordinator role; the nurse is often the person who meets the patient at the time of admission and works with the patient through discharge from the hospital, or transfer to another agency. As coordinator of care, the nurse plans with the other departments, agencies outside the hospital, and the family and friends to assure that the patient receives quality care.

Patient Advocate

In the role of patient advocate, the nurse makes sure the patient or client has sufficient information to make the necessary health care decisions. As patient advocate, the nurse also supports the patient's right to make these decisions.

Some groups in the health care system have tried to demonstrate their concern for the rights of patients. Nurses have been in the forefront of this demonstration. Playing the role of patient advocate may place the nurse in opposition to the doctor who may have strong feelings about what the patient is to be told and by whom. When the nurse assumes the patient advocate role, she must be prepared to work through opposition from other health team members and be sure that the patient will not be caught in the struggle.

The health care system is becoming increasingly complex, technical, and fragmented. In such a situation, it becomes more important that one professional group focus on the rights of the patient. The nurse is the logical person to assume the role of patient advocate. The nurse is with the patient throughout much of the patient's hospital stay or the client's association with an agency.

There is increased nursing interest in the patient's right to know about his condition, treatments, medications, and all alternative choices that are available. With the attempts to shift health care from an illness focus to a prevention base, there is a growing awareness that patients need to be informed about their care and be prepared to make constructive health decisions.

In the role of patient advocate, the nurse talks with the patient about medications ordered, the reason for taking them, what purposes the medications serve, and what possible helpful or adverse effects can be expected from taking the drugs. This kind of information may be best timed for discussion when the patient is feeling better. Time may be set aside for this discussion prior to discharge or transfer; this step is not left until the moment the patient leaves the hospital.

The nurse can help patients to become aware of how diet, medications, and treatments are related to each other and to patient medical disorders. Patients are also told what are normal expectations for growth and aging.

The doctor diagnoses the patient's condition. Once this is done, the nurse is the one who helps the patient to further clarify and understand what the diagnosis means to the patient. If the physician does not do this, the nurse supports the patient's right to ask the doctor for more information.

Nursing Roles	Examples of Behaviors
Stranger	Choosing words to say only what is meant when first meeting a patient or family.
Substitute person	Acting toward the patient or health team members as if they were a significant other person in the nurse's life.
Technician	Providing smooth, calm, efficient administration of medications, treatments, and procedures.
Teacher	Giving needed information to patients. Helping patients to assess, apply, and evaluate new health strategies.
Leader	Directing others' behavior. Encouraging others to be more independent and to share leader skills.
Counselor	Helping the patient to become aware of and deal with his feelings about what is happening to him.
Liaison	Giving and getting information from other health team members, and sharing this information with patients who are unable to speak for themselves.
Coordinator	Planning various aspects of health care so as to provide the least amount of stress for the patient.
Patient advocate	Making sure the patient has sufficient information to make decisions about health care. Supporting the patient's right to make these decisions.

Fig. 1-3 Current nursing roles

The patient also has a right to know the purpose of all treatments and procedures. Since the patient is paying for these tests or treatments, he has a right to know why it is necessary to have them, and to refuse them if he chooses to do so.

Unless legally committed through a court order, the patient also has a right to leave an institution with which he is dissatisfied. The nurse has a responsibility to be familiar with hospital policy and the legal issues involved with patient care.

Nurses who assume the patient advocate role must be prepared to deal with the effects of such behavior. Some patients may not be ready or willing to accept a more independent role in their health care decisions. Some nurses or other health team members may resent too much independent behavior in patients or nurses. CAUTION: As a student nurse, it is wise to discuss how to pursue this role with a nursing instructor before trying to be the patient's advocate. Figure 1-3 summarizes current nursing roles.

SUMMARY

The health team is composed of persons who are concerned with promoting the health of people. The nursing team is a subsystem of the health team and is often composed of registered nurses, licensed practical nurses, and nursing aides or assistants.

Nursing can be defined as an interpersonal process where people are assisted to their highest level of wellness. Although nursing roles are changing, there are a number of roles that nurses can assume. Current nursing roles include those of stranger, substitute person, technician, teacher, leader, counselor, liaison, coordinator, and patient advocate.

ACTIVITIES AND DISCUSSION TOPICS

- Find out as much as you can about the health team on the nursing care unit you are assigned to. Make arrangements to sit in on a health team meeting if possible.
- Talk with several patients about their views of the functions of health team members. Do the patients seem to understand the functions of each health team member? If not, what could you do to clarify their functions for the patients?
- Make arrangements to attend a nursing team conference. What can you learn about team functioning from attending such a meeting?
- Observe several nurses as they work. What percentage of their time does each spend in the stranger, substitute person, technician, teacher, leader, counselor, liaison, coordinator, and patient advocate role?
- Discuss the definition of nursing.

REVIEW

A. Briefly answer the questions.
1. Explain what is meant by *health team.*
2. List three reasons nursing roles are changing.

B. Select the item which best completes the statement.
1. The relationship between the health team and the nursing team may be described as:
   a. the health team is part of the nursing team.
   b. only nursing personnel serve on the health team.
   c. the nursing team is part of the health team.
   d. the health team and the nursing team are comprised of the same personnel.

2. When assuming the role of teacher, the nurse
    a. directs the behavior of others.
    b. plans care so as to provide the least amount of stress.
    c. supports the patient's right to make decisions.
    d. helps patient to assess, implement and evaluate new health strategies.

C. Study the examples of behavior. From the list of nursing roles select the one which is most appropriate.

Nursing roles:	Stranger	Teacher	Liaison person
	Substitute person	Leader	Coordinator
	Technician	Counselor	Patient advocate

1. Acting toward the patient as if he or she were someone personally involved in the nurse's life.

2. Giving and getting information from other health team members and sharing this information with the patient.

3. Helping the patient to deal with feelings about the illness.

4. Planning treatments so the patient will have a minimum of stress.

5. Administering a subcutaneous injection carefully and accurately.

6. Supporting the patient's right to make a decision based on sound findings.

chapter 2
THE PATIENT AND THE FAMILY

STUDENT OBJECTIVES

- Describe how the family functions as a unit or system.
- Identify possible problematic family situations.
- List the characteristics of effective family interaction.
- List five things a nurse would avoid when interacting with a family.

The patient is not an isolated person who comes to the hospital or agency for care. The patient is usually a member of a family unit. Even though the patient may be in the hospital, his position in the family unit continues to influence his behavior. Nurses who meet patients and their families can observe how one family member influences other family members.

Many circumstances arise where nurses come in contact with patients and their families. The nurse may talk with families who accompany a family member for treatment, observe and talk with families when they come to visit an ill family member, and console families when a member is critically ill or has been born with a birth defect. Teaching family members how to care for an ill family member in the hospital or in their home is another occasion for family-nurse contact. Nurses may observe, talk, and work with families in other circumstances. For this reason, it is important to learn the different ways that family members interact and relate with each other.

THE FAMILY UNIT

The family behaves as if it were a unit or system; a change in one part or person in the system can affect the family as a whole. The family acts as a unit in order to achieve a balance in relationships. Different events can create an imbalance in family relationships because they require the family to change or adapt. Changes which often occur are due to events outside the family unit; for example, financial depression or a war. Some changes occur in a patient's family such as sickness of a father or grandmother. Other changes are due to the entrance or exit of a family member. For example, family imbalance can occur when a grandfather comes to live with the family, or a daughter gets married, or a grandmother goes to a nursing home.

Some situations that create imbalance in the family are due to normal growth and development changes such as adolescence or menopause. Other reasons for imbalance are related to social or economic changes; for example, a child starts school, the family moves, a father loses a job or a mother begins to drink excessively. The nurse is alert to any changes which might require nursing intervention. Figure 2-1 illustrates several situations where imbalance of the family system could occur.

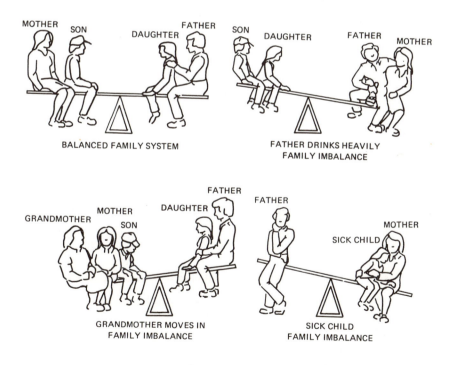

Fig. 2-1 The family is a system that can react to changes by adapting or becoming out of balance.

FAMILY INTERACTION AND SELF-ESTEEM

Years ago, the family performed many more tasks than it does today. Religious education for the most part is taught outside the home and education for future occupations has been taken over by institutions; formerly these were taught within the home and/or immediate community. At this time, the family provides the focus of emotional learning. As the size of the family shrinks, the intensity of its emotional reactions increases since there are fewer people with whom to interact; the family members may come to expect too much from each other.

People who have high self-esteem feel good about themselves and their ability to find satisfaction in life. People with low self-esteem do not trust other people, feel badly about their ability to find satisfaction, and may withdraw from or attack other people. In spite of having lost some functions, the family continues to be a major source of self-esteem. Self-esteem evolves from interaction with the family members. People who have not developed high self-esteem are not likely to be loving parents or spouses. These people can learn to feel better about themselves through satisfying relationships with a significant other person such as a nurse, teacher, husband or wife, psychotherapist or counselor, or member of the clergy.

Children who come from a family where parents continually criticize, withdraw, physically harm them, or do not set firm guidelines for behavior and stick to them, are likely to have low self-esteem.

FAMILY ROLES

Each member of the family is assigned one or more roles to play. Traditionally, the man was the breadwinner, and the woman the housekeeper and childraiser. However, in some parts of society these roles are changing; parents share or trade the roles of breadwinner and childraiser. In other cultural groups, the traditional male-female relationships continue.

Until recently, it was thought that female children acted a certain way because they were born with certain characteristics. It now seems clear that although there are physiological differences between male and female infants, boys and girls learn to behave in certain ways because they are treated differently by their parents and teachers. Girls are expected to look or behave well in order to be loved. Boys are loved for what they can do; they are expected to prove themselves in sports, and later, in the job market. Fortunately, there is a decided trend toward permitting girls and boys to achieve and prove themselves as individuals. Also, some parents are examining their behavior toward their children to determine how it affects the children's ability to achieve.

Some husbands and wives assumed roles in their earlier lives as children which they transfer to their marriages. For example, a man who has not separated emotionally from his mother may cast his wife in the role of mother. Women who have not given up emotional dependency on their fathers may cast their husbands in the father role. Cultural groups contribute to the furtherance of these roles where continued dependency on one parent or another is encouraged.

People also learn to play other roles in their own families; these may continue when individuals marry and raise children. Examples of such roles are helper, joker, and antagonizer.

When wives and husbands become parents, they teach their children how to relate to people and situations inside and outside the home. They do this through words and actions. If parents are disappointed in each other or feel upset, they will transmit these ideas to their children. As a result these children are cast in roles that do not allow for their greatest possible growth.

Children's Roles

Unfavorable roles which children are sometimes forced to assume are that of ally, messenger, peacemaker and problem child. A role that can stunt a child's emotional growth is that of an ally with one parent against the other. Here the child is expected to take sides. Another role that can stunt growth is the messenger role. In this case, parents talk to each other indirectly by having the child relay the messages. Peacemaker is another role that places undue responsibility on the child. In this role, the child is expected to resolve arguments between his parents.

Children can also be encouraged to take on the role of a problem child. In these families, parents often outwardly criticize the child for certain behaviors but indirectly allow or support the very behaviors they criticize. Permission to continue criticized behaviors can take many forms. One form is failure to follow through on threats. Another form is delayed punishment. A third form is indifference to or acceptance of the behavior at one time but not at another time, figure 2-2, page 16.

Other Family Influences. There are other things which may affect a child's behavior inside and outside of the family. These occurrences are the child's birth order, whether the child is a twin, whether the child is adopted, and whether the child or his parents are handicapped.

The firstborn child is like an only child — until the second child is born. According to Wrightsman, a social psychologist who has studied birth order,

Role	Stated or unstated example of role
Helper	"Let me do that for you."
Joker	"Don't worry about anything – have you heard the one about the traveling salesman?"
Antagonizer	"Bob has been picking on me all day – What are you going to do about it?"
Ally	"Sally, you can't trust men. See how your father embarrassed me?"
Messenger	"Daddy, mom wants you to turn off the ball game."
Peacemaker	"Mom and Dad stop arguing. I'll run the errand."
Problem child	Acts up because parents are unclear about what behavior is expected.

Fig. 2-2 Some family roles and expressions

firstborn children are often given more attention by their parents. Parents are likely to be more concerned and anxious about the child's behavior. Parents are also apt to be inconsistent in their treatment of a first child. Because of these early interactions with parents, firstborns are likely to be more dependent on others, more easily influenced by others, and more concerned with pleasing others than are laterborns. When they are in strange surroundings, being with others seems to calm firstborns; they report that they are less anxious. The nurse can perhaps use information about firstborn patients when planning nursing care for them.

Children who are born later usually benefit from the parents' experience with childraising. Also, they learn from *siblings* (brothers and sisters). Middle children may feel isolated or caught between their brothers and sisters.

The only child may experience feelings of loneliness more than the child who has brothers and sisters. The only child does not have the benefits of learning from siblings. Parents of an only child may focus more of their ambitious drives on that one child and may try to live out their own frustrated ambitions through the child. Since there are fewer family members, the only child may be forced to assume family roles for which he is not equipped.

Twins may have difficulty in being perceived as individuals by their parents and others. Twins are often quite close to one another and may have the same difficulty in viewing each other as a separate individual.

Adopted children may have unresolved feelings of being rejected or abandoned by their biological parents. Adults who were adopted as children will often seek out their biological parents. This seems to occur despite the fact that they had a loving relationship with the adoptive parents.

Children who are born with birth defects may be overprotected or under-protected by their parents. Parents who deny the strengths or healthy behaviors of their child may overprotect such children. Parents who deny the fact that their child has a disability may underprotect the child.

Sometimes parents have unresolved feelings of anger or guilt about having produced a defective child. For example, they may think their genes were to blame, or that they used poor judgment in having the child. Other parents may feel the birth defect was "God's punishment" or was due to poor health care given by doctors or nurses. When working with such children and their parents, the nurse must examine his or her own feelings, judgments, and attitudes. For example, does the nurse see a disability as more or less acceptable if it is due to genetic reasons, an attempt to abort the child, or improperly followed health directions?

Children of handicapped parents are apt to feel angry that their parents are not like other parents. These children may at the same time feel guilty that they feel angry. Their guilt may be related to the idea that it is not right to be angry with someone who is disabled. Children of handicapped or disabled parents may require mental health counseling if the parents have unresolved feelings about their ability to be adequate parents and transmit this insecurity. These children may also need counseling to assist them to deal with their own anger or guilt.

PROBLEMATIC FAMILY INTERACTIONS

Children compete with their parents and siblings for the attention and love of both parents. When a husband and wife are emotionally close to one another, a child may develop a feeling of being left out of family decisions.

When husband and wife are confident in their marital relationship, they can deal with the child's fears of being left out. Each can also allow a mother-child or a father-child relationship to develop. In fact, families seem to work best when the parents do have a different level of power and responsibility than their children have.

In problematic family relationships, responsibility is given beyond the child's maturity. Often he becomes afraid that he will affect and control what happens between his parents, when, in fact, he does not. Parents may turn to the nurse for support. The nurse can be helpful by pointing out that families do seem to work better when parents do not give children responsibility beyond their maturity. The nurse can also point out that as children grow they can gradually assume responsibility under parental guidance and supervision.

In families where self-esteem is low, family members develop strategies for coping. One strategy is to communicate a fear of being left out of family happenings. Family members demonstrate this fear by always wanting to be present when other family members talk. Fear of being left out may also be evident when one family member constantly interrupts another who is talking. Fear of being left out may even be expressed verbally; for example, a family member could say, "You always leave me out of things" or, "You never listen to what I say." In some families, indirect or unclear communication is used to camouflage areas of disagreement or difference.

Persons who have a low self-esteem frequently choose to marry persons who (they think) will make up for the qualities which are lacking. Once the marriage begins, the partner finds the other has many different characteristics. Being different can be threatening to someone with low self-esteem and can lead to disagreement between the marriage partners. If both spouses have low self-esteem and fear disagreement, communication becomes unclear and indirect. For example, instead of saying, "You don't hear me when I ask for something," a person with low self-esteem may say, "Nobody pays any attention to me." At this point, both partners are apt to feel even worse about themselves. The partner who heard the statement will probably feel frustrated because he or she does not know how to respond to the unclear, general statement and the person who made the statement will feel even more misunderstood because the partner does not understand or respond as expected.

Another strategy used by persons who have a low self-esteem is to pay no attention to whether others listen. For example, a family member may drone on and on, even though the other family members are bored and stopped listening; or, the person who spoke may clearly be misunderstood by others but makes no effort to clarify his or her message.

Still another tactic used by someone with low self-esteem is to get upset or angry at the way others respond to his verbal message. A person may say something which has a different meaning to the listener because of the facial expression or tone of voice. When the listener responds to the hidden meaning, the speaker may become upset; he was unaware he was sending more than one message.

Families with a high level of self-esteem realize that there will be arguments and disagreements. People with low self-esteem are especially fearful of disagreeing or arguing. They argue indirectly because they fear rejection or retaliation from others; they try to stop disagreements of any kind. Some families are able to disagree, but always seem to belittle others in the process.

Yet another device to increase one's own self-esteem is to view other family members as weak, asexual, or unable to function. Use of this tactic increases self-esteem somewhat because the person who sees others as weak and dependent on him feels more powerful. There are many ways to make members of the family dependent. Children or mates can be emotionally tied to other family members when, for example, limits for behavior are set inconsistently; what is said is not followed through with action; punishment is delayed; or some behaviors are treated with indifferent or preferential treatment.

In families where low self-esteem is prevalent, individuality is not encouraged and may be feared. Members try to increase their own self-esteem by not letting others be different; also they will not agree on what activities should be shared or done separately. Although these tactics are used to ward off low self-esteem, in the long run, they lead to even greater family difficulties.

EFFECTIVE FAMILY INTERACTION

Effective family interactions are direct communications that clearly ask for what is needed or desired. Effective family interactors ask for *feedback* or direct response from other listeners so the speaker will know what effect he has had on others.

In families where self-esteem is high, family members can disagree without belittling others. Family members who are confident about their relationships with others can allow two or more others to have special close relationships with each other. When interactions are effective, each member of the family respects the talents of the others, their characteristics, and their wishes. For effective family interactions, limits are clearly set on behavior and the limits are kept. In families where effective interaction occurs, all members are allowed to be different and to have separate interests as well as the opportunity to share family activities.

In families with LOW self-esteem:

- Children are given more or less responsibility than befits their age.
- Some family members feel left out of family activities.
- Communication is unclear, indirect, not listened to, or responded to inappropriately.
- Individual differences are seen as a threat.
- Disagreement is stopped or ends in belittling the other person.
- Some family members are treated as less healthy or capable of being independent than they are.

Fig. 2-3 Problematic family interactions

In families with HIGH self-esteem:

— Family members do not feel left out of family activities.

— Communication is clear, direct, and provides for feedback.

— Disagreement occurs without belittling others.

— Limits for family behaviors are clear and enforced.

— Being different is allowed and family members engage in separate activities as well as family activities.

— Family members are attentive to others' needs and desires.

— Family members are encouraged and guided to greater levels of independence.

— Everyone has their say, but decisions often rest with the parents or adult family members.

Fig. 2-4 Some characteristics of effective family interactions

Effective family interactions have other characteristics such as awareness of and attention to the needs of others. When the children are hurt or frightened they are given care and comfort. Husbands and wives show concern for one another. Children's statements are respected and not discounted because "He's only a child, and doesn't know." Family members do not take sides unless they are sure one member is teasing or tormenting another. No one tries to dominate any others or make them overly dependent. Each family member is allowed his say, even though decisions may often rest with the parents or adult family members.

THE NURSE AND THE FAMILY SYSTEM

Nurses who work with families may experience a strong desire to become part of the family system. Part of this pull may be due to the family itself. Some of the things the nurse may be asked to do directly or indirectly are to take sides on a family issue; to pay no attention to one or more family members; to punish a family member for being different; to treat a family member as a dependent person; and to participate in indirect or conflicting communication.

Part of the pull which may draw the nurse into a family system is related to her own family experiences especially if the nurse is quite involved in her own family unit. The family difficulties or involvements of the patient may remind the nurse of his or her family. Because of this, the nurse often is not aware of the fact that she can easily assume a nonuseful role in the patient's family system.

In general, the nurse can be most useful to a family if all family members are treated equally, differences are accepted, dependency is not encouraged and messages are direct and clearly stated. By following these actions, the nurse can make assessments and interventions that will assist the family to interact more effectively. The effects of the illness or change in family structure affects the whole family. This is one assessment the nurse can make. The person who has become ill or who has changed may make statements about the loss of inter-personal, economic, physical or intellectual ability. A patient often worries about how his condition will affect the financial and social relationships of the family. Family members may ask the nurse questions about the costs of hos-pitalization. She can provide whatever information is known, and then refer the family to other agencies and resources.

If the patient is a mother or wife, the household routine can be drastically disrupted by her hospital admission. It may be important to determine whether the family needs additional professional or volunteer help to provide for house-hold tasks. Not knowing how their family is managing without them can create added stress for hospitalized patients. The nurse can suggest a visiting nurse or homemaker service. She can also suggest the patient make a phone call home to see how the family is managing. When the family visits the hospital, a discussion can be held about family management.

If the ill person is an elder member of the family, there may be indications that the family fears he or she may die; the nurse can encourage the family to discuss their fears. Another common family concern is whether the elderly person may need to be transferred to a nursing home. Families often feel guilty about such decisions and may deny the need for such a transfer. The nurse can help the family discuss the pros and cons of such a decision. Such decisions are best made when the elderly patient is included. Although there may initially be more strong feelings expressed, clear communication at this point can decrease the possibility of unresolved family feelings when the patient is actually transferred.

A child who is ill, has a birth defect or a long-term illness may create feelings of anxiety and guilt in his parents. Because parents feel helpless, they may direct hostility or criticism toward the nurse. In assessing family reactions, the nurse always tries to remember that family hostility or criticism may be the only way they have to cope with feelings of helplessness. Although the nurse may feel upset by such hostility and criticism, she does not retaliate with anger since the family already is facing undue stress. Rather than suppressing these feelings, talking about it to another person not actively involved in the nurse-patient-family situation will give the nurse a better, healthier perspective.

The nurse is the most strategic person to help a family become more effective in their communication with one another. One way to do this is to restate and clarify how each family member views a situation. For example, the nurse might say, "Mr. Jones seems to be saying he's not ready to be discharged, while Mrs. Jones is getting ready for his homecoming."

The nurse can also be a family observer. In this role, a certain level of objectivity exists which the family members do not have. By quietly observing family interaction, the nurse can differentiate between messages that are clear and those that are not.

The nurse can participate in helping families to communicate by serving as a model for communication. In this role, the nurse demonstrates to family members how to communicate more effectively by being clear and direct in her own messages. One way to do this is by teaching them to check with one another to see if the message received had the same meaning as the one sent. For example, the nurse might say, "That sounded like you were kidding, Mr. Frost. I wonder if that's how you meant it?"

The beginning student nurse is not expected to be an excellent communicator. Family members, however, tend to copy or pay attention to what is said by the person who is giving care to the patient.

To be useful in this role, the nurse must be aware of his or her own prejudices and assumptions about families. When working with families, the nurse tries to convey to the family that each person's ideas are valued. Each family member is asked about thoughts and feelings; each family member must speak for himself. If a wife answers for her husband, or a mother speaks for her son, the nurse can turn to the husband or son to ask for their views.

Family members should be made aware of the fact that the actions of each one influence the behavior of the others. Families can be advised that each member is responsible for his or her own actions. Even use of physical force cannot guarantee that family members will act as others wish. For example, parents often think they can control their children's eating behavior. In fact, even if parents force feed their child, the child can reject this control by spitting up the food, or by stopping the parents' efforts in more indirect ways.

Parents may seek guidance for ways to deal with their children. They can be helped to understand their children by checking out parental assumptions about child behavior. Sometimes parents need to be reminded that it is very difficult to understand another's thoughts or feelings unless they are expressed. Asking children to describe or explain their behavior promotes better understanding. The nurse can support parental authority yet help parents see that as children grow they are better able to make decisions for themselves.

If parents ask for help with discipline, the nurse can find out about family rules and how they are enforced by asking questions such as, "How do you deal with discipline?" or "What's the worst thing Johnny could do?" The student

Assessment	Intervention
How has illness or change in the patient affected the family?	Give interpersonal, financial, or physical information to assist family.
	Direct family to appropriate resources to help restore family balance.
	Assist family to discuss pros and cons of health care decisions.
	Assist family to grieve over the loss or change.
	Do not retaliate if family members show their helplessness by attacking the nurse.
How effective is family communication?	Observe and report family interaction in an objective manner.
	Clarify and restate how each member views the situation.
	Teach family to be more effective in their communication.

Fig. 2-5 Nursing assessments and interventions with patients and their families

nurse should seek further help from more experienced nurses before attempting to deal with complex family problems, especially those dealing with discipline. Figure 2-5 summarizes some nursing assessments and interventions that may be used by the nurse. CAUTION: Family counseling requires further education, practice and supervision.

SUMMARY

The patient is not an isolated person. He is usually a member of a family unit that influences his behavior; this influence is still present even though he is hospitalized. Likewise, the patient influences the behavior of his family. Growth and development, social, economic, interpersonal or physical changes can lead to changes in the family system. When families do not adapt to these changes, a family imbalance can result.

The nurse must be alert to changes in the family system of the patient and the effect these changes can have on the patient. Being familiar with the family roles, the relationship between self-esteem and family interactions, and other influences on the family contribute to the nurse's effectiveness.

It may be difficult for the nurse to avoid being pulled into the patient's family system but it is imperative that she do so. Being useful to patients and their families includes making objective and appropriate family assessments and interventions.

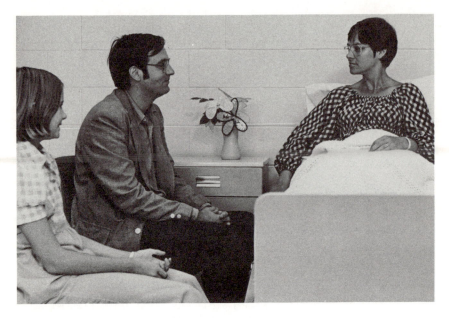

Fig. 2-6 Family interaction affects the patient's recovery.

ACTIVITIES AND DISCUSSION TOPICS

- Spend time in an emergency waiting room, clinic, or other health care unit where patients and their families may be available. Find out as much of the following information as you can. Compare your findings with interchanges in your own family.
  a. Who was present?
  b. What was the seating or standing arrangement?
  c. When was the tension level highest and lowest during the interaction?
  d. What family rules for acceptable and unacceptable behavior did you learn?
  e. Were there economic changes affecting this family?
  f. Were there interpersonal changes affecting this family?
  g. Were there physical changes due to illness or injury affecting this family?
  h. Were there major growth and development changes affecting this family?
  i. Were there social changes affecting this family?
  j. What seemed to be the effect of these changes on family relationships?
  k. How did the family attempt to cope with these changes?
  l. What roles did family members play?

    m. Did family members seem confident in their relationships with one another?

    n. Was communication clear and direct?

    o. Were family members receptive to feedback?

    p. Could family members disagree without belittling?

    q. Did family members treat each other as separate people with strengths as well as weaknesses?

    r. Were limits of behavior clear and enforced?

    s. Were family members allowed to be different?

    t. Was attention given to others' needs and desires?

    u. Did one family member dominate others?

    v. Did parents or children take sides?

    w. Did people interrupt one another?

    x. Who disrupted conversation?

    y. What occurred when there were silences?

REVIEW QUESTIONS

A.   Multiple Choice. Select the best answer.

    1. The statement that contains *only* problematic family situations is

        a. shows low self-esteem, gives indirect communication, allows others to be different.

        b. sets limits on others' behavior, disagrees without belittling, views others as weak or asexual.

        c. asks directly for what is needed, is receptive to feedback, does not let others be different.

        d. sets limits verbally but supports the behavior, fears being left out, belittles others when disagreeing.

    2. A situation that can create an imbalance in the family is

        a. adolescence.

        b. child starts school.

        c. father loses job.

        d. all of the above.

    3. People who have high self-esteem

        a. do not trust other people.

        b. may withdraw from other people.

        c. feel good about themselves.

        d. none of the above.

4. Families with a high level of self-esteem
   a. can expect complete harmony at all times.
   b. realize there will be arguments and disagreements.
   c. are fearful of disagreeing and arguing.
   d. argue indirectly.

5. Permission to continue critized behavior can be in the form of
   a. failure to follow through on threats.
   b. delayed punishment.
   c. acceptance of the behavior at one time but not at another time.
   d. all of the above.
   e. none of the above.

B. Match the items in Column II to the correct statement in Column I.

Column I	Column II
1. Role where child may be criticized for certain behaviors, but indirectly allowed or supported in continuing the behaviors.	a. ally
	b. messenger
	c. peacemaker
2. Role where the child carries messages between two parents who do not talk directly to one another.	d. problem child
	e. self-esteem
3. Role where the child is asked to take sides with one parent against the other parent.	
4. Role where the child is expected to solve arguments between his parents.	
5. How people feel about themselves and their ability to find satisfaction in life and their relationships with others.	

C. Briefly answer the following questions.

1. Explain how the family functions as a unit or system.

2. Name eight characteristics of effective family interactions.

3. What are the seven roles a family member may assume within the family?

4. State three ways the nurse can assist patients and their families with communication.

5. Name four factors that influence a child's behavior inside and outside the family.

6. List five things a nurse should avoid when interacting with a family.

chapter 3
STRUCTURING
THE NURSE-
PATIENT RELATIONSHIP

STUDENT OBJECTIVES

- Identify differences between a social and a professional relationship.
- List five goals of the orientation phase of the nurse-patient relationship.
- List two signs indicating that the nurse-patient relationship has entered the working phase.
- Identify effective actions in terminating or concluding the nurse-patient relationship.
- List three effective actions for dealing with patients who offer gifts.

Prior to entering a nursing program, the average student has had relationships that were largely social. Generally these relationships did not involve helping someone deal with problems. In a *social relationship*, conversations occur spontaneously and may cover a wide range of topics. The persons interact primarily for reasons of pleasure or companionship. It is not the intent of a social relationship to deal with one another's problems. If a silence occurs, there is a quick attempt to break it.

THE PROFESSIONAL RELATIONSHIP

The *professional relationship* is directed toward meeting the expressed or implied needs of the client. Silence often occurs in the nurse-patient relationship. Silence can be useful since it allows the patient to think over what has occurred and formulate what to say or do next.

The nurse-patient relationship is an example of a professional relationship in which the nurse, through special knowledge and skills, offers help to the patient or client. Unlike the social relationship, the nurse-patient relationship is directed toward a specific goal. Because of having attained special knowledge and skills, it is the nurse's responsibility to structure the relationship to meet the needs of the patient. This begins when the nurse first meets the patient. If the nurse presents herself to the patient by saying, "Hi. I'm Gerry Brown." the patient may think the nurse is there simply to chat. If the nurse says, "Mr. Jones, I'm Mr. Smith, a student nurse. I'll be working with you today until noon" the patient may have an entirely different perception of what the relationship will be.

The newness of the professional relationship may create some initial discomfort and even resistance. Such reactions are to be expected whenever a person, either a patient or a nurse, begins to form a new behavior pattern. As the person becomes more accustomed to acting in the new way, his discomfort will decrease. For this reason, it is important to continue to approach patients in a professional rather than a social manner. Both student and patient will become more comfortable as the new behavior pattern becomes more firmly established.

The nurse-patient relationship is divided into three phases which often overlap; the orientation phase, the working phase and the termination phase.

THE ORIENTATION PHASE

The first phase of the nurse-patient relationship is the *orientation phase.* Whenever meeting an assigned patient for the first time, the nurse should give him certain basic information. The statements which should be given to the patient during the orientation phase include the following elements:

- Acknowledgment of the patient as a person.
- Name and title of the nurse.
- Time available for the relationship.
- Purpose of the relationship.
- Place of meeting.
- Choice of alternative actions.

Acknowledgment of the Patient. Calling the patient by name implies recognition; it is an acknowledgment that he is an individual. It is best to address the patient by title and last name (for example, Mr. Jones) unless the patient states that he prefers to be called by another name. The practice of calling patients "Grandma" or "Pops," or using their first name without prior consent is a dehumanizing procedure that does not acknowledge the patient as a person.

Name and Title of the Nurse. The patient sees many health workers in the hospital and learns what to expect from each one. When the nurse identifies herself by name and title, the patient can begin to have some understanding of what possible relationships might develop. To orient the patient, the student can say something like, "I'm Mrs. Smith, a student nurse." Use of the formal titles, "Mr., Miss, Mrs. or Ms.," communicates the message to the patient that this is a professional, not a social relationship. It also reminds the beginning student of the professional nature of the relationship. As the nurse becomes more accustomed to a professional role, the nurse may wish to re-evaluate the use of formal titles. If a rapport develops to the extent that the nurse feels more comfortable on a first name basis, the patient may be encouraged to address her by first name. As stated earlier, the patient should also be given the right to be addressed according to preference. Deciding how to address each other is part of the developing relationship; it should reflect respect for each other as unique persons.

Time Available for the Relationship. The amount of time which will be spent with the patient should be stated. The patient needs to know the time limits of the relationship; for example, "I'll be here today and tommorow from 8 a.m. to noon." This allows the patient to know when he can count on the nurse for assistance. Also, setting a time limit for a task encourages both participants to work harder to achieve the task within the time limit. However, there should not be any feeling of tension due to this time limit; both persons should be aware of flexibility in the event of unforeseen circumstances.

Purpose of the Relationship. When the nurse is clear and concise about the purpose of the relationship, there will be fewer patient demands for requests the nurse cannot fulfill. If the nurse is not clear and concise, there is a greater tendency for patients to view the nurse as messenger or family member. One way to state the purpose of the relationship is, "I'll be helping you with your morning care today." Another statement is, "I'll be working with you until three this afternoon."

Place of Meeting. If the patient is ambulatory, it is helpful to agree to meet in a certain place. For example, when the patient is to have a treatment in the treatment room, the nurse can ask the patient to meet her in that room. If the

Situation	Choices Available	Choices Not Available	Stating the Alternatives
Instructor asks student to walk with a patient, Mr. Soam.	Which direction to walk	To walk or not	"I'm going to walk down the hall with you, Mr. Soam. Which way would you like to walk?"
	Which side of the patient the nurse walks on		"Which side do you want me to walk on?"
	How fast to walk		"You decide how fast to walk."
	Who takes whose arm		"Would you like to take my arm, or shall I take yours?"
Head nurse asks student to offer fluids to Mrs. Jones, a patient with no fluid restrictions	Which fluids to offer Mrs. Jones	To drink or not	"It is important that you drink more fluid. What is your choice of drink?"
	Which fluid the patient chooses		"Which of these drinks would you like?"
	How often to offer the patient fluids		"I'll come back in an hour to help you choose another glass of fluid to drink."
	How many times to encourage Mrs. Jones to drink		"Take another sip of juice now."
Instructor assigns student to talk with any patient for five minutes	Which patient to ask	To talk with a patient or not	"I'd like to talk with you for five minutes. Is it O.K.?"
	Which patient agrees to talk		"What would you like to discuss?"
	Who chooses the topic of discussion		"Tell me about your hospital stay."
	What to do if patient stops talking		"I'll sit here 'til you decide what we'll talk about."
	Which topics to pursue		"You said you're confused; about what?"
	How to end the discussion		"The five minutes is over; I'm going to leave now."

Fig. 3-1 Examples of offering choice

nurse is teaching the patient, it may be suggested that the patient meet the nurse "in the conference room" or wherever the teaching will take place.

By defining the work area as "this table," "the solarium," or "your room," ambulatory patients are less likely to approach the nurse for assistance in inappropriate areas, such as the coffee shop. It is helpful to think of the relationship as "work" since it is a serious undertaking where the nurse offers the patient a professional service. If the patient remains in bed or in one room, it is not necessary to state the place of meeting since the nurse will come to the patient.

Choice of Alternatives. Promoting the patient's independent action is one of the goals in all areas of nursing. One way to promote independent action is to allow the patient to make a choice by stating the available alternatives. Some guidelines for offering a choice to the patient include the following:

1. Offer choice only if there is a real choice available.
2. Decide what the alternatives are before discussing them with the patient.
3. Tell the patient exactly what the alternatives are.

Figure 3-1 lists some situations involving choice which beginning students might encounter.

Pace the Information

It is often impossible to give all of the orientation information and choices at once. Indeed, too much information may be overwhelming to the patient; the nurse should give small amounts during the first part of the initial meeting with patient or client.

In some situations the nurse must attend to the problems of the patient first and delay giving the orientation material. Such situations are when the patient is in crisis or distress. For example, the patient is having difficulty breathing, is bleeding severely, is vomiting, needs a bedpan, fell out of bed, is crying, or is emotionally upset. Figure 3-2, page 32, depicts a situation where other needs take priority over orientation needs.

In any of the cited situations, it may be necessary for the nurse to leave the patient to get assistance or equipment. Before leaving the patient, the nurse needs to state two things: (1) what she is about to do, e.g., "I'm leaving the room now" and (2) when she will be back, e.g., "I'll be back in two minutes."

Listen Actively

An important part of any orientation is active listening. Active listening requires "reading between the lines" of any statements made by the patient to

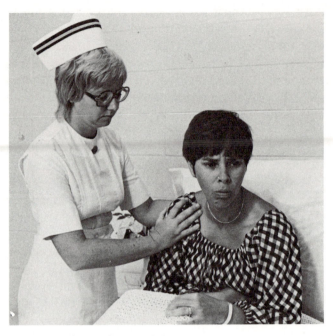

Fig. 3-2 At times, physical needs take priority over interpersonal needs; helping this coughing patient, for example.

gather information about his concerns. Nurse and patient get to know one another in the orientation phase. During this time, the patient might give the nurse clues which will show the need to modify the goals. If it becomes clear that the patient is opposed to the nurse's goals or purpose, this opposition must be dealt with immediately. (Specific techniques for dealing with patient opposition are examined in chapter 17.)

Answer Questions

Frequently patients have questions about their treatment or condition. Beginning students are often unable to answer questions asked by patients. Because of this, they may shy away from discussing the patient's concerns. One way to handle this dilemma is to tell the patient, "I don't know, but I will find out and tell you." Then, the student can leave the patient's room to find the answer; she may discuss it with a nursing instructor; ask a nurse; and read up on the treatment or condition. In this way, the student and the patient can learn more about the treatment or condition. It is always important to return to the patient with the promised information.

Anxiety and fear often underlie a patient's questions. A simple way to proceed is to state, "You seem concerned about your condition," and then wait for the patient to respond.

Try to answer all of the questions honestly without using technical words. Technical terms soon become part of the nurse's vocabulary but it should not be assumed that the patient understands such terms. Practice putting information gained from texts or in lectures into everyday language so the patient can understand.

Questions patients might ask can be divided into three general categories. One category includes questions patients ask about their condition and its effects; the second category includes questions about the patient's need for *dependency* (help from others) and the fear of being too dependent; the third category involves questions about hospital procedures, such as medicines and treatments, and about the schedule of events for the hospital day. Examples of questions patients might ask for information about their care can be found in figure 3-3, page 34. Think of how to respond to each question before a patient asks it. This method will decrease discomfort in the nurse when a patient does ask a difficult question.

Establish Consistency

Once the relationship has been structured according to the basic orientation information, it is important that the nurse maintain consistency by following through. If the nurse promised to be with the patient until noon, the nurse should be available until noon. By establishing this consistency, the patient can begin to trust the nurse. Trust is established not so much by words, but through actions which are consistent with the words.

THE WORKING PHASE

If the nurse-patient relationship is brief or if the patient or nurse is unable to progress to the working relationship, this phase may be very brief or even nonexistent. The *working phase* is the middle phase of the nurse-patient relationship; it involves giving the patient direction and assistance. If the patient and nurse enter this phase, the following goals can be pursued:

- Direct the patient to fill in areas of information that are unclear or missing.

  Examples: Gathering information about the patient's ability to assist with a bedbath.

  Assisting the patient to convey more information about attempted suicide.

Patients' Questions About Their Condition and Its Effects	Patients' Questions About Being Helped and Being Dependent	Patients' Questions About Hospital Procedures
"Am I dying?" "Am I getting better?" "What did the doctor mean?" "How do I know I'm better?" "When will I be well enough to go home?" "When can my family and friends visit me?" "Will my family abandon me?" "Will there be enough money to pay for this?" "Will I be scarred?" "Will I have to change my life-style now?" "Will I be able to stand the waiting to hear from the doctor?"	"How often will you be here?" "Do I have to move myself in bed?" "Will you turn me often enough?" "Do I walk alone, or will you help me?" "How long do I have to stay here?" "Am I a burden?" "How do I ask for a bedpan?" "Will I be left alone for long periods of time?" "Will I be bored?" "Will you help me if I can't sleep?" "Will I fall out of bed?"	"What is the procedure like?" "What is the pill for?" "Why do I have to follow this procedure?" "How long will the procedure last?" "How long will I have to take the pill?" "How often will I have to take the medicine?" "What does the medicine taste like?" "Is the procedure painful?" "How long will it last?" "What happens after the procedure?" "Will it be too noisy to sleep?" "When are meals served?" "When does the doctor come?" "When can I shower?" "Where are my belongings kept?"

Fig. 3-3 Questions patients may ask about their care

Helping the patient decide how to ask the doctor about being discharged.

- Assist the patient to cope with whatever is problematic in his illness experience.

    Examples: Exploring alternate ways to conserve patient energy for active exercises.
    Discussing more effective ways to deal with anger.
    Assisting the patient to verbalize feelings about being in a nursing home.

Signs that the working phase has been entered are apparent when the patient accepts the limits of the relationship and waits expectantly for the nurse.

Accepting Limits

In many nurse-patient relationships, the patient will continually test the limits of the relationship to see if the nurse really means what was promised. Testing behaviors could include requesting medication when there is none due, asking the nurse to stay longer than the stated amount of time, asking the nurse to take the patient to restricted areas or to provide experiences which are restricted. Two examples of restricted areas or experiences are helping the patient out of bed when on bedrest or giving extra food when the patient is on a low calorie diet. To maintain consistency, the nurse must maintain the limits originally set during the orientation phase. When the patient no longer tries to test the limits of the relationship, patient and nurse have entered the working phase.

Waiting Expectantly

By awaiting the nurse's arrival, the patient demonstrates increased investment and involvement in the relationship. More subtle signs that the patient is actively involved in the working phase include cooperation with nursing care efforts and significant give-and-take in both verbal and nonverbal interactions. Cooperation in itself is not necessarily a sign of the working relationship since many patients appear to cooperate superficially out of anxiety or fear. A patient may show distinct signs of entering the working phase of the nurse-patient relationship, figure 3-4.

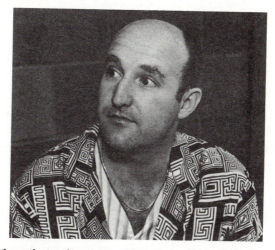

Fig. 3-4 When the patient waits expectantly for the nurse to arrive, the working phase of the relationship has been reached.

CONCLUDING OR TERMINATION PHASE

The final phase of the nurse-patient relationship is the *termination phase*; the relationship is brought to a conclusion. Ending a relationship can result in sad, glad, or frustrated feelings in both patient and nurse. Other common responses to the termination include anger, guilt, satisfaction, relief, and anxiety. The nurse is in a good position to demonstrate a healthy way to separate from relationships. By stating the termination date with the orientation material and by allowing time to summarize and evaluate the relationship, the nurse can promote an effective conclusion to the relationship.

Preparing for the Termination

Building the idea of ending the relationship into the orientation phase helps the patient to realize that the relationship will end eventually. Delaying the preparation for the end of the relationship can produce overreactions or unresolved feelings on the final day of a long and satisfying relationship. Often the nurse does not bring up the topic of termination because of her own unresolved feelings about separating from others. This reaction is especially prevalent in relationships where the nurse sees similarities between the patient and other people she has known. In the case of students, any thoughts and feelings of not wanting to end a relationship and uneasiness or distress as the termination date approaches should be discussed with the nursing instructor. It is important to sort out feelings about ending the relationship before beginning to work with the patient. When this sorting process occurs, not only is the nurse better able to help the patient but she also develops a greater self-awareness.

Summarizing and Evaluating the Relationship

The longer the relationship has been, the more time should be allowed to summarize and evaluate the relationship. Even in short relationships, five or ten minutes should be set aside to summarize and evaluate the relationship. Both nurse and patient summarize and evaluate what has transpired. To set the tone, the nurse might begin by stating observations and evaluations about the relationship. Figure 3-5 lists examples of questions the nurse might ask to help the patient and the nurse summarize the relationship.

The more intense the relationship, the more frequently the patient should be reminded of the date the relationship will end. For example, the nurse can say, "I'll be here three more days." Another way to remind the patient is to say, "I won't see you after Friday. On that day I'll be working on another unit in

Ways to Help the Patient Summarize and Evaluate the Relationship	Ways the Nurse Can Summarize and Evaluate the Relationship
"How would you summarize our work together?"	"I'd like to talk about our relationship. At first it was difficult for us to talk and work together, but now I'm sad that our relationship is ending. What do you feel?"
"How would you evaluate the care I've given you?"	
"What are your thoughts about how we've spent our time together?"	"It's been helpful to me to work with you and iron out how we could best spend our time together. What do you think about what I said?"
"What has been helpful about our relationship?"	
"If you could change something about our relationship, what would it be?"	"I expected it to be difficult working with you since you were so sick, but it's been a good experience. How has it been for you?"
"What did you dislike about our relationship?"	
"Let's summarize what we've done together; you start."	"I got angry at first because you wanted me to do things your way. I'm glad we worked it out. Now I feel satisfied about how we worked together. Were you angry with me too?"
"What did you expect our work together would be like?"	
"Was our relationship what you expected?"	
"What one thing did you expect from our relationship that didn't happen?"	"I think you expected me to know how to help you and were surprised I asked for your ideas. Were you surprised?"
"What can you tell me so I can help other patients with your condition?"	
"What was the most difficult about our work together?"	
"What are your thoughts about my leaving?"	
"What do you feel now that our relationship is over?"	

Fig. 3-5 Summarizing and evaluating the nurse-patient relationship.

the hospital." The word *termination* should in most instances not be used with patients as (1) it is a technical word and (2) the patient might have a different understanding of the word. To some people, the word *termination* means death.

Sometimes on the last day of a relationship, the patient behaves like he did on the first day of the nurse-patient relationship. For example, the patient may be distant, seem unaware of the nurse's presence, or be unusually dependent and ask for many things. Another common patient response is to attempt to continue the relationship by asking the nurse to write or visit him. Even though the patient may seem to plead for a continuance of the relationship, it is important to terminate it completely. If the relationship is continued merely to lessen the nurse's guilt feelings, the nurse will come to resent this imposition more and more as time passes. Likewise, giving the patient a noncommittal answer such as "We'll see, maybe I'll write" is not a suggested intervention. This type of response leaves the matter unresolved and does not help the patient toward a healthy separation. If the patient continues to press for a continued relationship, it is best to ask him to share his feelings. An important thought to keep in mind is that initiating new relationships and letting go of completed ones are growth experiences for both patient and nurse, even though such experiences may be uncomfortable.

Patients will often bring up new problems just as the nurse is leaving for the day or is concluding their relationship. Minor concerns can be dealt with at these times. Becoming involved in major problems is not useful for the patient or the nurse. Instead, the nurse reminds the patient that she is leaving now and that she will tell the nurse who will be working with him about his problem. The patient is also reminded to mention his problem to the new nurse. This must be said with firmness and the nurse must be convinced this is the appropriate response, otherwise, the patient will continue to test the nurse. Generally, when the nurse communicates that there is no choice involved in this issue, the patient will accept the limits as set. If the nurse promises the patient that she will share his problem or concern with the next nurse, it is important that she keeps her promise.

When the patient and nurse are allowed to summarize and evaluate the relationship, there will be a decreased need on the part of both to continue the relationship. Prior to the last meeting with the patient, the nurse should sort out her own thoughts and feelings about the relationship. This will focus the efforts on the task at hand, termination of the relationship; many patients may not be able to verbalize their thoughts and feelings about it but the nurse must offer them the opportunity. Merely by offering the opportunity, the nurse communicates that such thoughts and feelings are important and acceptable.

GIFTS

Despite rules to the contrary, patients may offer a gift to the nurse. The nurse should try to examine both the patient's motivation in offering the gift and her feelings about receiving the gift. Some patients think it is important to "pay off" the nurse; others are unable to verbalize their approval and so give a gift. Some patients think it is expected that they give a gift.

It is important for students to examine their feelings about accepting a gift before finding themselves in such a situation. They could be motivated to accept because of fear of disapproval, feelings of warmth and tenderness toward the patient, or fear of hurting the patient's feelings. Each of these nurse motivations should be examined in light of the patient's needs.

It is recommended that the nurse ask the patient to comment on the gift. For example, the nurse could say, "Why did you decide to give me a gift?" or "Tell me about choosing this gift." Figure 3-6 shows a nurse and patient verbalizing about a gift. Very expensive gifts or gifts that are given with implied conditions should definitely not be accepted. There are two situations where it would be more acceptable for the nurse to accept a gift; (1) the patient has been unable to give, or has an especially great need to give at this time, (2) nurse and patient have worked together on a project — such as an art activity — and the patient wishes the nurse to have the product as a remembrance of the joint effort. Experiences involving gifts should be discussed at student conferences and shared with fellow students.

SUMMARY

The nurse-patient relationship is a professional one where the nurse guides the relationship toward common goals. The relationship has three phases which may overlap: orientation, working, and termination. During the orientation phase, the nurse acquaints the patient with the nurse, the purpose, and the limits of the relationship.

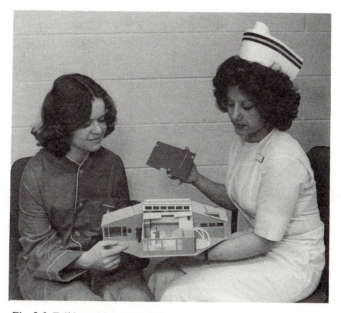

Fig. 3-6 Talking with a patient about a gift can be a useful experience.

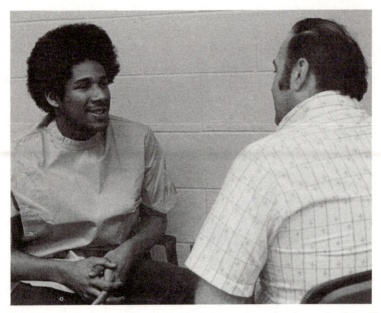

Fig. 3-7 The nurse-patient relationship is directed toward meeting the needs of the client.

During the working phase, the patient becomes a more active partner in the relationship. Signs that the working relationship has begun include decreased testing behavior and increased involvement with the nurse.

The termination phase can be a growth experience for both the nurse and the patient if the nurse begins termination during the orientation phase and if she allows time for an evaluation and summary of the relationship by both patient and nurse.

ACTIVITIES AND DISCUSSION TOPICS

- Introduce yourself to one patient as you would to a new friend. Find another patient and introduce yourself as a professional nurse. Include orientation information. Evaluate your thoughts and feelings in each situation. Write down reasons you might have felt as you did.

- Choose a nursing student; practice giving the orientation material to the other student. Then switch roles and play the patient while the other student gives the orienting information. Discuss together how it felt to play the nurse and how it felt to play the patient. Think of short, concise ways to state the information needed to orient the patient; they should be consistent with your style of speaking.

- Compile a list of feelings and thoughts people might have in reaction to ending a relationship.
- Think of what to do if the following patients offered you a gift on your last day with them:
  a. A patient you disliked.
  b. A patient you liked.
  c. A patient who reminded you of your boyfriend, girlfriend, husband, wife, sister, or parent.
  d. A patient who said he was "paying you off."
  e. A patient who had never been able to give a gift before.

REVIEW

A. Multiple Choice. Select the best answer. Some questions have more than one answer.

1. A professional relationship differs from a social relationship in that a
    a. professional relationship covers a wide range of topics while a social relationship focuses on only one topic.
    b. professional relationship is goal directed while a social relationship occurs spontaneously.
    c. social relationship is a give-and-take relationship while a professional relationship is distant and uncaring.
    d. professional relationship is directed toward meeting the needs of the patient while a social relationship is primarily for pleasure and companionship.

2. Terminating the nurse-patient relationship can be handled effectively if the nurse
    a. tells the patient she will come back to visit.
    b. allows ten minutes on the last day for the patient to evaluate and summarize the relationship.
    c. encourages the patient to bring up new problems and concerns for discussion.
    d. evaluates her own thoughts and feelings about ending the relationship.

3. Orientation information is best presented to the patient
    a. when the nurse first meets the patient.
    b. when the patient asks for orientation information.
    c. all at one time on the first day of the nurse-patient meeting.
    d. in small amounts towards the beginning of the first nurse-patient meeting.

4. The nurse maintains consistency of the nurse-patient relationship by

   a. sticking to the limits originally set in the orientation phase.
   b. conveying information to the doctor exactly as the patient stated it.
   c. staying longer than the stated time to show the patient he is special.
   d. calling the patient by his first name.

5. A professional relationship often creates some initial discomfort and resistance because

   a. it is not really necessary as the nurse and patient may be together for only a short time.
   b. it is difficult for people to begin new behavior patterns.
   c. it creates an indifferent attitude between nurse and patient.
   d. it interferes with the self-expression of each nurse to deal with each patient individually.

6. On the first day in the clinical area, a student is assigned to observe and talk with patients in a nursing home. A patient asks, "What is this pink tablet for?" The best nursing response would be

   a. "That is for pain."
   b. "I don't know. What does it taste like?"
   c. "I don't know. I'll check with my instructor and come back when I find out."
   d. "I don't know. I'm a new student nurse and this is my first day here."

B. Briefly answer the following questions.

1. Name five factors which should be included in basic information given during the orientation phase.

2. What are the two signs that indicate the working phase of a relationship has been entered?

3. Name three guidelines to help the nurse deal with the patients who offer gifts.

C.   Match the items in Column II with the correct statement in Column I.

Column I

1.   directed toward meeting the expressed or implied needs of the client.

2.   middle phase of the nurse-patient relationship where patient fills in unclear or missing information and the patient is helped to cope with his problems.

3.   "reading between the lines" of the patient's statements to gather information about the patient's concerns.

4.   concluding phase of the nurse-patient relationship where relationship is evaluated and summarized.

5.   occurs spontaneously; primarily for pleasure and companionship.

6.   a professional goal-directed relationship that is structured to meet the needs of a patient.

7.   first phase of the nurse-patient relationship where patient receives basic information.

Column II

a. active listening
b. nurse-patient relationship
c. orientation phase
d. professional relationship
e. social relationship
f. termination phase
g. working phase

chapter 4
ANXIETY IN THE NURSE-PATIENT RELATIONSHIP

STUDENT OBJECTIVES

- List four sources of anxiety.
- Differentiate between fear and anxiety.
- Identify cues used to assess each level of anxiety.
- State nursing interventions useful for each level of anxiety.

Anxiety is a vague feeling of discomfort that is experienced at some time by all people. Anxiety is useful when the feeling protects the person from a threatening situation or warns the person of danger.

SOURCES OF ANXIETY

Anxiety is probably first learned in interpersonal situations. For example, the infant may first encounter anxiety nonverbally when held by an anxious mother. As the child grows, anxiety may occur in embarrassing or unfamiliar situations and when dignity is threatened.

In adulthood, anxiety continues to be sensed nonverbally. If one person in a situation is highly anxious, the other person may also become anxious.

Unmet needs also lead to anxiety. Needs create tension. When internal tension increases, the person usually begins to search for ways to decrease the tension. Internal tension from unmet needs can sometimes lead to anxiety. Most of the time, however, internal tension leads to a change in the person's behavior, such as eating when hungry or seeking out people when loneliness is experienced. Anxiety can also occur when biological needs are not met.

People experience anxiety when they expect one thing to happen and something completely different happens. For example, when the student expects the nursing instructor to be cold and indifferent and the instructor is warm and caring, the student may feel anxious. People experience anxiety when they have a need to be recognized as having status or prestige and others treat them too familiarly. For example, some patients may feel anxious when called by their first name rather than by Mr. or Mrs. People experience anxiety when they receive disapproval from a person they consider significant. In the hospital, the nurse may be a significant person to many patients; when disapproval is conveyed to the patient, the nurse can increase his anxiety.

People also experience anxiety when others do not respect or recognize them; some patients put on their call light many times as a way to gain recognition from the nurse. People who are unable to perform as they would like to perform may experience anxiety. For example, patients who are weak and depend on the nurse for assistance, or who must learn new and difficult procedures, feel anxious about their ability to perform effectively, figure 4-1.

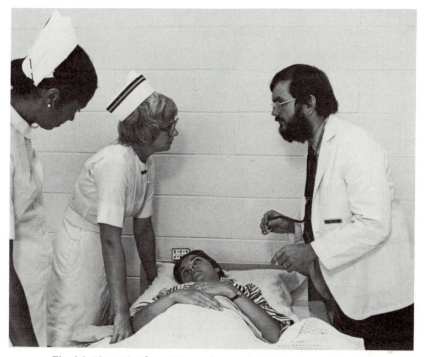

Fig. 4-1 The patient's anxiety can increase in the hospital environment.

Hospital experiences provoke anxiety because the patient is cut off from familiar surroundings and from the people who usually provide support. Being hospitalized is not the only situation that can create anxiety. It is likely to occur whenever a person is unable to escape from a threatening situation. Being hospitalized is seen as an inescapable situation by those who are acutely ill or weak. It is threatening to patients because the hospital is a place where many things that happen are foreign or unknown to the patient. Unfamiliar surroundings, people, and hospital procedure and routine all contribute to patient anxiety. While the patient is hospitalized, he may experience additional anxiety about pain, death, and actual or imagined losses such as disfigurement, loss of strength, loss of love and caring, and loss of the ability to return to a previous life-style. Several of these sources of anxiety can weigh on a patient at one time.

The nurse must also contend with her own sources of anxiety. Some sources of anxiety for the nurse may be:

- inability to spend enough time with patients.

- inability to decrease patient pain.

- inability to perform nursing procedures smoothly and efficiently.

- unmet expectations that the patient will be grateful or cooperative.

- failure of a patient to respond to treatment.

- death of a patient.

- angry or derogatory remarks made by a patient.

FEAR AND ANXIETY

Usually, *fear* is thought to occur when the person can identify the source of his upset feeling. For example, a man who steps off a curb and sees a car approaching at sixty miles per hour probably feels fear. *Anxiety* is thought to occur when the source of the feeling is less clear. For example, anxiety is often experienced when a person is not sure what will happen in a given situation.

Fear and anxiety often occur in combination. The patient who sees an unfamiliar nurse approaching with an injection may fear the pain of the needle. The patient may also feel anxious about relating to the nurse and how the interchange will be resolved. Some thoughts that might create anxiety for the patient in this situation are: Will I cry? Will the nurse be gentle? Will the nurse hit a nerve? Will the nurse approve of my behavior? The patient may have little awareness of these thoughts and may only experience an unexplained feeling of discomfort. This unexplained feeling of discomfort is anxiety.

LEVELS OF ANXIETY

People can shift from one level of anxiety to another level from minute to minute. For purposes of discussing nursing assessment, anxiety will be presented as if unexplained discomfort could be clearly broken down into categories. This is not always so. The student will soon learn to tell when most patients are comfortable, and when most patients are near panic. Some patients are so adept at covering up their feelings that they may not display outward signs of anxiety. For this reason, the nurse learns both psychological (interpersonal) and physiological signs of anxiety. Other patients, chiefly psychiatric patients, may only show they are anxious by their disconnected and distorted speech patterns.

Mild Anxiety

Mild anxiety is a constructive level of anxiety. If people had no anxiety at all, they would be apathetic and uninterested in their environment. Mild anxiety encourages the person to be alert to and interested in what happens in the immediate environment. The person who is mildly anxious is able to see, hear, feel, taste, touch, and evaluate incoming sensory information clearly. Communication with others is open and direct. People with mild anxiety are able to experience a oneness with their internal and external environment and are open to learning.

It is important for the nurse to realize that zero anxiety is not an optimal learning condition for the patient. Rather, a mild amount of anxiety in the patient may be the most constructive level for the nurse-patient relationship. Striving to decrease the anxiety to a mild level — not eliminate it completely — is often the goal in nurse-patient relationships.

There are physiological signs the nurse can use to assess anxiety. People who are mildly anxious have appropriate muscle tone. They are neither so relaxed that they are unable to sit up nor so tense that constriction of blood vessels occurs. Pulse, respiration, and blood pressure are strong and regular in rhythm. Speech is unhurried and clear. Figure 4-2, page 48, shows a person who is probably mildly anxious.

Moderate Anxiety

In moderate anxiety, the person is less open to all that is occurring within and around him. Perception may be more focused on a particular task. There is little awareness of things that happen which are not related to the task at hand.

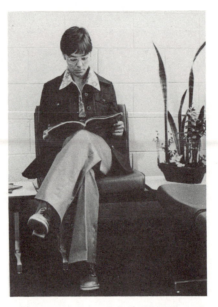

Fig. 4-2 Learning occurs during mild anxiety.

However, learning can still occur in moderate anxiety. Moderate anxiety may even be best for learning difficult tasks or developing capabilities.

In moderate anxiety, physiological changes occur. Slight perspiration of the palms of the hands or axillae (underarms) may be evident. Pulse and respiration may increase. Muscle tension increases. Increased muscle tension can result in "butterflies" in the stomach, diarrhea, frequent urination, tension headaches, or fatigue. All of these are signals that the person is preparing to fight or flee from the threat he perceives. Signals such as diarrhea may not clearly differentiate whether the person is experiencing moderate or severe anxiety. Communication patterns and vital signs are probably the clearest indicators of anxiety level. Changes in speech patterns may occur; the individual may speak more slowly or more quickly than usual.

Severe Anxiety

Somewhere between moderate and severe anxiety, people start to pay attention to only parts of experiences; they do not pay attention to those parts that threaten them, figure 4-3. Even though this *selective inattention* occurs, the person can still be helped to notice threatening parts of experiences if they are pointed out.

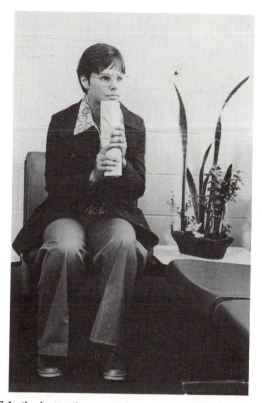

Fig. 4-3 Selective inattention occurs between moderate and severe anxiety.

In severe anxiety, the person may not pay attention to whole experiences or episodes. Entire interpersonal exchanges, hospital admissions, or other life experiences may be placed out of awareness by people who are severely threatened. Learning does not occur in severe anxiety and repetitive, automatic behaviors can be noted. Attention span is short. Severely anxious people focus on one small detail of an experience, or on scattered details of several experiences. Communications from severely anxious patients may seem confused and be difficult to understand.

Severe anxiety can be assessed in some other ways. Patients who are severely anxious may perspire profusely. There may be a further increase in pulse, and a rise in blood pressure. Respirations can become shallow and rapid. The patient's lips and mouth may be quite dry. Speech may become rapid, constant, loud, high-pitched, hesitant, or stammering. Muscular tension is further increased, and patients may have rigid postures, tremors, shivers, or clenched fists.

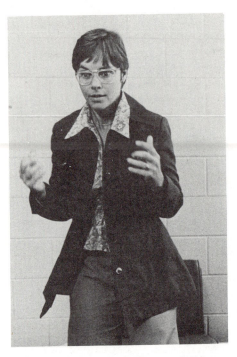

Fig. 4-4 In panic, the person may feel terror;
perception of others is completely disrupted.

Panic

An even higher level of anxiety is panic. People who experience panic may focus on a small detail of an experience and blow it up out of proportion. They may attempt to communicate but others can rarely understand what is being conveyed. The person in panic probably experiences terror and feelings of unreality. Long periods of panic can be so overwhelming that physiological functioning can become completely paralyzed. Panic places such stress on the person that prolonged panic could lead to death.

CONVERTING ANXIETY

Because anxiety is so uncomfortable, people often convert the energy available from anxiety into more comfortable behaviors and thereby obtain some relief. There are several ways to do this, some are constructive and some are not.

One way often used to convert anxiety is to become angry. Many times when people are angry they attack others because they themselves feel threatened.

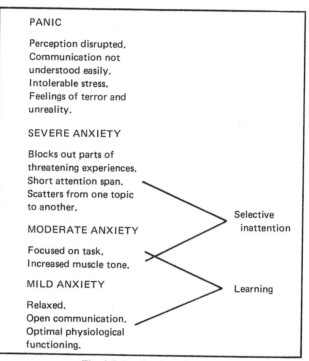

Fig. 4-5 Levels of anxiety

Arguments are often based on feelings of being threatened, disapproved of, or ignored by another person. If patients and nurses were more aware of their own feelings, they could recognize the feeling of being threatened and be less likely to argue destructively or "fly off the handle."

Another nonconstructive way to convert anxiety is to withdraw. Patients in hospitals often use this method because they feel that a showing of anger would be punished. Instead, they make few complaints, stay in their rooms, and interact infrequently with other people. Patients who are withdrawing are often left alone and thought to be convalescing well when, in fact, they may be quite anxious. Nurses also use withdrawal to convert their anxiety into more comfortable behaviors. Staying in the nursing station, transferring "difficult" patients, or calling in "sick" frequently are attempts to withdraw from uncomfortable situations.

Still another method for dealing with anxiety is somatization. *Somatization* is converting emotional energy into physical symptoms. Patients who are anxious may show their anxiety through increased blood pressure, tension headaches, diarrhea, fatigue, or other physical symptoms. Nurses use some of the same bodily symptoms to convert anxiety into more comfortable reactions. People who use somatization as a way of dealing with anxiety may do so automatically, and may not be aware of anxious feelings at all.

The most constructive way to convert anxiety is to try to analyze and learn from the experience that provoked the anxiety. However, people who are in severe anxiety or panic cannot learn from the experiences until their anxiety has been reduced.

NURSING INTERVENTION

In general, the goal for the nurse is to help the anxious patient learn from anxiety-provoking situations. The nurse does this by developing skill in identifying situations that create anxiety for the patient and by using the energy of the anxiety to help the patient explore and deal with upsetting situations. In this way, the disorganizing effects of anxiety are harnessed to produce an organizing effect.

If the nurse simply tries to reassure the patient not to worry or that everything will be all right, the patient will feel misunderstood. If the patient is not allowed to express feelings, these feelings will not be integrated with the whole hospital experience and his anxiety will not decrease. The nurse can help the patient to deal with immediate needs by helping him to deal constructively and openly with his anxiety.

Mild and Moderate Anxiety

Hildegard Peplau, an authority on nursing intervention in anxiety, recommends five steps to help the patient integrate anxiety-provoking situations and learn how to deal more effectively with anxiety. These steps can only be used when the patient is mildly or moderately anxious. Only then can the patient learn from his anxious experiences.

The first step is to help the patient become aware he is anxious. Observe the patient for signs of anger, restlessness, decreased eye contact, stammering, and so on. In some patients, signs of anxiety will be clear. In other patients, the nurse will have to know the patient quite well before observing signs of anxiety. Withdrawal or a change in the vital signs may be the best clues the nurse has to recognize the anxiety. Once the nurse has observed anxious behaviors, she helps the patient to actually name the feeling by asking, "Are you nervous now?" or "Are you tense right now?" or "Are you upset?" By giving the unexplained discomfort a name, the patient and nurse can then begin to discuss the feeling.

The second step in nursing intervention is to help the patient become aware of how the anxiety is relieved. The nurse might say, "What do you do to feel less tense?" or "What helps when you're anxious?"

The third step is to find out what happened just before the patient felt anxious. This will help the patient to see that anxiety does not occur without reason, but rather occurs when one feels threatened. The nurse might apply this step by asking, "What happened just before you felt upset?" or "Let's try to figure out what preceded your tension."

The fourth step is to help the patient understand the entire situation surrounding the anxious feeling. To do this, the nurse asks for a description of the incident. For example, if the patient tells the nurse, "I felt tense when the doctor was here," the nurse might ask some or all of the following questions:

"When was the doctor here?"
"Who else was there?"
"What exactly happened?"
"What did the doctor say?"
"What did you say then?"
"What did you think when the doctor said that?"
"What did you feel then?"
"What did you do?"

The final step in helping the patient deal with anxiety is to have him talk about other situations where he felt anxious. In this step, the nurse helps the patient to describe and explore each anxiety-provoking situation in minute detail (as in step four).

Student nurses may only reach step one or two with a patient. Yet, it is important to help the patient to begin the process. Later, some other student or nurse may then be able to assist the patient to complete further steps toward understanding the entire situation.

Severe Anxiety and Panic

When the patient is at the severe or panic level of anxiety, the nurse intervenes in other ways; nursing intervention is not directed at helping the patient to learn from the anxiety-provoking experience. The nurse does not ask the patient to describe or explore his feelings in minute or complex detail.

When the patient is in severe anxiety or panic, the nurse can intervene by remaining physically present and by decreasing sensory input. At such high levels of anxiety, the presence of a calm, reassuring figure may be the patient's only beneficial resource. During the disorganizing experience of high anxiety levels, the nurse often serves the same function for the patient as a mother does for a frightened infant.

Another intervention for patients with high levels of anxiety is to decrease sensory input. This decrease includes removing the patient from an overstimulating environment, and not bombarding him or her with questions or comments. Directions and information are conveyed in phrases of three or four words. Only one phrase is used at a time. Examples of statements to be used with patients in high levels of anxiety are:

"Sit down."

"I'll stay with you."

"I'm a nurse."

"Come with me."

"You're in the hospital."

"I want to help."

Staying with the patient and giving him small bits of information at a time usually decreases the patient's anxiety. Once anxiety has decreased, the nurse can begin to use the five steps recommended by Dr. Peplau.

Intervening effectively with anxious patients often requires that the nurse examine her own feelings. It is important to be aware of high anxiety because nurses can convey these feelings and increase patient anxiety. Nurses who work in psychiatric or mental health settings frequently undergo self-awareness procedures such as psychotherapy in order to derive the most effective use of themselves with their patients.

WHEN TIME IS LIMITED

When the nurse has only a short period of time to spend with an anxious patient, there are some other nursing inteventions that are especially helpful. The nurse can decrease anxiety by providing information about upcoming treatments; this decreases the number of unknown factors for the patient. By allowing the patient to participate in his own care, the nurse decreases anxiety by decreasing the patient's sense of being powerless; he feels he has some control over the situation. Telling the patient about others such as chaplains, social workers, or mental health nurses who are available to discuss feelings with the patient is another way in which the nurse may help to decrease patient anxiety. By showing interest in the patient and avoiding any show of disapproval or depersonalization, the nurse can diminish the probability of patient anxiety.

Level of Anxiety	Intervention	Sample Behavior
Mild or moderate	Help patient to name unexplained discomfort, "anxiety."	"Are you anxious now?"
	Help patient learn how anxiety is relieved.	"What helps when you're anxious?"
	Explore what happened just before anxiety occurred.	"What was going on just before you felt anxious?"
	Assist patient to connect all aspects of the anxiety-provoking experience. Assist patient to explore other anxiety-provoking situations.	"When was this?" "Who was there?" "What was said?" "What did you think at that moment?" "What were you feeling?" "What did you do?"
Severe and panic	Provide physical presence.	Stay with the patient.
	Decrease sensory input	Use infrequent, three or four word phrases. Remove patient from stimulating environment.
	Examine own feelings	Talk with instructor, therapist, supervisor, or more experienced nurse about own anxiety while with patients.

Fig. 4-6 **Nursing interventions for different levels of anxiety**

Unfamiliar nursing skills should be practiced prior to patient care as nursing students decrease patient anxiety when they are giving a confident performance of care. Planning physical activities and exercises for the patient helps to relieve muscular tension in anxious patients. Breathing and relaxation exercises can be taught to the patient by the nurse or physical therapist. By providing diversional activities, the nurse can sometimes assist the anxious patient to dwell less on himself. The nurse can work with the occupational therapist to plan diversional activities for patients.

SUMMARY

Anxiety is a vague feeling of discomfort that is experienced by all people at some time during their life. Hospital experiences can provoke anxiety. Any experience that is unfamiliar, unknown, disapproving, depersonalizing, or guilt-inducing can produce anxiety in patients and nurses.

Anxiety differs from fear. Fear has an easily identifiable source. Anxiety is often unexplained or vague in its origin. The nurse learns psychological and physiological indications of anxiety for mild, moderate, severe and panic levels. Since it is such an uncomfortable experience, anxiety is frequently converted into anger, withdrawal, physical symptoms, or learning experiences.

In mild and moderate anxiety, the nurse assists the patient to learn from his anxious experiences. In severe anxiety and panic, the nurse reduces sensory input, orients the patient to his environment, and directs his actions while remaining physically present.

When the nurse has limited time available to help anxious patients, she can provide information for the patient; and an opportunity for the patient to be more actively involved in his own care planning; she can recommend other personnel who might talk with the patient. Never does the nurse treat the patient impersonally, disapprove of his status or minimize his expressed concerns. It is also important for the nurse to display confidence while doing nursing care. Another way to help anxious patients is to plan physical and diversional activities for them.

ACTIVITIES AND DISCUSSION TOPICS

- Talk with several patients, observing their signs of anxiety. Keep track of your own anxious experiences for a week. Then answer the following questions about the patients and yourself:

   1. Did anxiety occur in unfamiliar surroundings?
      What were the surroundings?

   2. Did anxiety occur when the person was cut off from supportive people?
      What were the circumstances?

   3. Did anxiety occur when needs were not met?
      What were the needs?

   4. Did anxiety occur when expectations were not met?
      What exactly happened?

   5. Did anxiety occur when recognition was not given?
      How did it happen?

   6. Did anxiety occur due to disapproval from significant people?
      What happened?

   7. Did anxiety occur due to inability to perform effectively?
      What were the circumstances?

8. Did anxiety occur due to pain, death, or actual or imagined losses?
   What exactly happened?

9. Did anxiety occur at the same time as fear?
   How could you tell the difference?

10. What level of anxiety was present?
    What were the signs?

11. Was anxiety converted to anger, withdrawal, physical symptoms or learning?
    How did you know?

12. What interventions would have been useful for that level of anxiety?
    What prevented you from intervening?

REVIEW

A. Multiple Choice. Select the best answer.

1. The difference between fear and anxiety is
   a. fear has an unexplained source, while anxiety does not.
   b. anxiety has an unexplained source, while fear does not.
   c. fear is due to a threat to self-esteem while anxiety is not.
   d. anxiety occurs out of awareness, while fear does not.

2. The optimal learning condition for a patient is
   a. zero anxiety.   c. modern anxiety.
   b. mild anxiety.   d. moderate stress.

3. When a person is not sure what will happen in a given situation he often experiences
   a. panic.   c. anxiety.
   b. fear.   d. calmness.

4. Converting emotional energy into physical symptoms is called
   a. withdrawal.   c. intervention.
   b. depersonalization.   d. somatization.

5. When patients pay attention to only parts of their experiences and block out the parts that threaten them it is called
   a. confusion.   c. depersonalization.
   b. selective inattention.   d. apathy.

B. Match the levels of anxiety in Column II to the patient cues in Column I by selecting the correct letter.

Column I

1. Alert to occurrences in internal and external environment, open to learning, stable vital signs.

2. One small detail is blown out of proportion, communication is very difficult to understand, possible paralyzing of physiological functions.

3. Perception focused on the task at hand, learning occurs, some increase in muscle tone.

4. Threatening experiences placed out of awareness, short attention span, focus on one small detail of an experience or on scattered details of several experiences.

Column II

a. mild anxiety
b. moderate anxiety
c. panic
d. severe anxiety

C. Briefly answer the following questions.

1. List four sources of anxiety.

2. What are the four levels of anxiety?

3. State two nursing interventions for the patient who is experiencing severe anxiety or panic.

4. List five steps to help the mild or moderately anxious patient learn to deal more effectively with anxiety.

chapter 5
THE NURSE-PATIENT RELATIONSHIP IN MENTAL ILLNESS

STUDENT OBJECTIVES

- Describe four approaches to treatment of mental illness.
- List three differences between the general hospital patient and the psychiatric patient.
- State five common nurse reactions to psychiatric patients.
- Name at least four common goals of the nurse and patient.

In defining mental illness, there is no one model upon which all agree. However, several frameworks or models do exist that are used to understand and approach patients who are having difficulty in their relationships with others. These models include the:

- medical model
- social model
- psychological model
- behaviorist model

The *medical model* approach is influenced by the biological and physiological concepts of the body; mental illness is considered a disease like any other disease. In the medical model approach, treatment is accomplished through the use of drugs and physical therapies such as electroconvulsive treatment. The symptoms of the individual are the focus of treatment.

The *social model* approach focuses on the individual and his relationships with others. Family and community relationships are included in assessment and treatment. Treatment includes changing the social groups or systems within which the individual lives. In the social model approach the nurse is aware of how being poor or old can influence whether a person is hospitalized or not, and what type of care is provided.

The *psychological model* approach is based on Sigmund Freud's idea that all behavior is meaningful and understandable. Treatment is based on helping the patient understand and deal more effectively with his thoughts and feelings. In this framework, the patient's mental illness is his unsatisfying way of relating to others. People with mental or interpersonal difficulties are not seen as basically different from other people. There may be a difference in the degree or rigidity of behavior, but not in the type of behavior. In this model, no one is completely healthy or unhealthy mentally. All persons are thought to share common feelings and reactions to human situations. This view sees people as becoming less mentally healthy based on past relationships which were of an unsatisfying nature; it is felt that these interpersonal relationships can be influenced and altered by a satisfying relationship with another caring person. A major focus in the treatment is the relationship between the nurse and the patient. This therapeutic relationship helps the patient to experience, remember, and learn about past and present experiences that he has previously avoided.

In the *behaviorist model* approach, unsatisfying or annoying behavior is thought to occur because it is immediately reinforced or rewarded. The focus of treatment is on rewarding effective or satisfying behaviors, and not rewarding or responding to unsatisfying or annoying behaviors.

The nurse will find that, in her dealings with patients, some or all of these approaches may be used. The model or approach selected will depend on the treatment setting and the patient's needs at the moment. Being able to use various approaches will increase the effectiveness of the nurse as she moves along the mental health to mental illness continuum and encounters various situations. Figure 5-1 summarizes concepts of mental illness.

PATIENT DIFFERENCES

Patients in a mental health or psychiatric setting may appear to be somewhat different from patients in a general hospital setting. The differences may be due to the way psychiatric patients feel about themselves and others. These patients usually have very low self-esteem. They feel badly about their inability to function and may distrust others. They communicate their low self-esteem in a number of ways. One way is through their statements about the care they receive.

Concept or Model	Definition	Treatment
Medical model	Mental illness is a disease.	Drugs and physical therapies.
Social model	Mental illness evolves through relationships with family and community.	Change social groups or systems.
Psychological model	Mental illness is the patient's unsatisfying way of relating to others.	Therapeutic relationship helps the patient to experience, remember, and learn about past and present experiences that were previously avoided.
Behaviorist model	Mental illness is learned, ineffective or unsatisfying behavior.	Reward effective or satisfying behaviors; do not reward or respond to unsatisfying or annoying behaviors.

Fig. 5-1 Concepts of mental illness

Patient Statements About Care

Patients may convey their fright or anxiety in many ways; sometimes they may express it as the main complaint. A patient may say, "I was scared to come here" or "I get nervous and that's why I'm here." These patients may show a more obvious response to hospitalization than general hospital patients. Psychiatric patients may feel that the hospital is a safe, protective place, or they may feel they are in the hospital against their will. For example, a patient might remark, "I came here to rest and unwind" or "I don't belong here; my parents railroaded me in here." Extreme reactions to being hospitalized are not unusual.

Patients who have been in a psychiatric setting before may make statements about their expectations for this hospitalization. The patient's expectations for treatment at this time may be affected by past hospital experiences. For example, the patient may say, "When I was here before, one of the patients slugged me" or "I feel like I'm a failure because I had to come back."[1]

Some common responses patients have made to the question, "How do you wish to be treated while hospitalized" are: (1) to be given more human contact, (2) to be taken seriously, (3) to be respected, (4) to have promises kept.

Although not all patients can express these wishes directly, more verbal patients may state these requests as:

- "Talk to me."
- "Don't treat me like a case."
- "When you give me a shot, tell me what it is you're giving."
- "Don't make fun or joke with me; I'm serious."
- "It never occurs to some nurses that I might be scared of this place."
- "Don't tell me you'll talk to me later if you aren't planning to."

Patients who have low self-esteem are concerned about how others will view them. For this reason, confidentiality is of great importance when working with patients in a mental health or psychiatric setting. Patients are often fearful of how information they give out will be used. For example, the patient may say, "How are you going to use what I told you?" or "Will this get back to my doctor?" The nurse recognizes the patient's desire for confidentiality and tells the patient exactly who the information will be shared with. The nurse then follows through with what she said.

The nurse can use statements made by the patient to provide him with more effective care:

(1) The patient's statements can be used to assess his degree of anxiety or fear.

(2) The nurse can consider that a patient's feelings of relief about being hospitalized does not mean the patient is lazy or trying to get care when he is not entitled to it. The hospital may be viewed as a protective place because the patient's home situation was so difficult. Other patients may have mixed feelings about being hospitalized, and yet will talk only about being "railroaded."

(3) The patient's statements about prior hospitalizations can be used to assess the expectations for this hospitalization.

(4) The patient can be approached by the nurse to engage in nurse-patient discussions, even though outwardly the patient may not seem to want such contact.

The nurse must also be careful not to make jokes about the patient or his behavior. Few psychiatric patients have a sense of humor. As they become healthier, their sense of humor may improve. Actions and statements that may appear silly, hard to understand, or laughable to the nurse, may be the only way the patient is able to communicate at the moment; it may all be very serious to him.

Respecting the patient includes such things as telling him about upcoming procedures and treatments and responding to him as an individual. Keeping promises is important because it helps to establish trust of others. This is especially important for a patient who thinks others are untrustworthy.

Other Differences

Unlike the general hospital patient, the psychiatric patient does not always understand what the problem is or what must be done to regain health. Some patients are unclear about their thoughts, feelings, body boundaries, and ability to affect others. They are also unclear as to whether anyone does or can care about them, and whether others are trustworthy. These patients may have strong feelings of inferiority and a tendency to distort what they see, hear, or feel.

It is assumed that all human beings want and need human contact. Many times, psychiatric patients seem to want to be left alone when in fact they need and want human contact. Because of these mixed feelings about relating or not relating, they may be quite uncertain and easily embarrassed when approached by the nurse. Some patients may then try to withdraw from the nurse, berate her, or refuse to talk; some may talk or move constantly, or communicate in indirect ways that are difficult to understand. General hospital patients may be better able to communicate in more socially acceptable ways. Psychiatric patients may need or desire human contact more than others, yet have difficulty in reaching out for it because of their mixed feelings. Figure 5-2 contrasts general hospital and psychiatric patient differences.

THE PSYCHIATRIC PATIENT MAY BE MORE CONCERNED ABOUT:

- trusting self and others
- responses to hospitalization
- human contact
- respect
- having promises kept
- confidentiality
- why he needs treatment
- being inferior

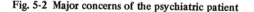

Fig. 5-2 Major concerns of the psychiatric patient

REACTIONS TO MENTAL HEALTH-PSYCHIATRIC NURSING

As members of society, nurses share many of the views held by others in that society. Myths include the idea that people with interpersonal difficulties are crazy, bad, dangerous, or funny. These myths occur despite the fact that:

- No patient is ever completely out of contact with reality at all times.
- Patients often act as they do, not because they are bad but because they have had difficult or faulty learning experiences with other people.
- Many psychiatric patients are less dangerous than other people because the patients tend to withdraw when upset.

In addition to feeling fearful or judgmental about psychiatric patients, the nurse may have other reactions. A common reaction of the nurse who has never been on a psychiatric unit is anxiety about what to expect. Prior to the first experience on a psychiatric unit, the student may have dreams or thoughts about locked doors, keys, bars on windows, and noisy and aggressive patients. However, unless assigned to work on a highly active unit, the student or beginning psychiatric nurse will find that patients will probably be more withdrawn than aggressive. It is impossible to predict exactly what the nurse will find on a mental health or psychiatric unit. It is useful to discuss fears with an instructor or psychiatric head nurse before going to the ward. The nurse's expectations will probably be influenced by myths of the society.

Thinking about future talks with a psychiatric patient often makes the inexperienced nurse feel frightened and inadequate to the task. A common expression is, "If only I had something to do with my hands — some physical care to give — I would feel better." Although nursing in mental health and mental illness does not exclude physical care, the main focus is on the relationship with the patient. Anxiety and fear are expected because the nurse will have to deal with an unknown situation. Also, the nurse has probably been influenced by societal myths.

The nurse who has not been involved in the care of the mentally ill may believe that she may be useless to patients, appear like a beginner, or may harm the patient by wrong statements or actions. Fears of harming the patient are common. Generally, one or two statements cannot significantly harm a patient. If the nurse is conveying concern and interest to the patient, misstated phrases or awkward silences will probably be of little importance. Many patients will be too anxious to notice that the nurse is a beginner. On many psychiatric units, patients are hungry for interpersonal contact, and the nurse's very concern and physical presence can be helpful. A goal the nurse can strive for is to be concerned and interested in the patient, and to develop communication skills.

Putting the two together takes time and practice but can be developed with persistence.

The nurse may fear that the patient will not talk to her. However, patients often make an attempt to be verbal; they know the student is there to talk with them and may be on their best behavior to make the student feel comfortable. Some patients are less verbal and will talk less often. In these cases, the nurse can learn a lot about nonverbal communication and how to relate with nonverbal people. Not talking is also a form of communication; silences need not always be filled by the nurse or patient. A relationship with a nonverbal patient can be an exciting, if frustrating, experience.

In medical or surgical areas, the nurse always reads the patient's chart prior to giving care. In some mental health nursing experiences, it is thought best not to read the patient's chart. This is done for several reasons. Each two-person relationship is different. The way the patient relates to a particular nurse may be different from the way the patient relates with the person who wrote on the chart. Also, a large part of the nurse-patient relationship is getting to know the patient. This is accomplished through the application of communication skills and the passage of time. Patients sometimes even resent the nurse knowing more than they are ready to reveal.

It may be useful for the nurse to examine her reasons for wanting to read the patient's chart. It may be that the nurse is anxious and will feel more in control of the situation if she knows more about the patient. It has been noted that experienced practitioners observe how the patient relates to them and often find this kind of information of more use than the summary of facts and observations that can be found on the chart.

Concern that the mental illness of the patient will affect her own mental health is another reaction of a student or newly assigned psychiatric nurse. It may be felt that an intense relationship with a patient will lead to finding unhealthy behaviors in oneself. All people share common reactions, thoughts, and feelings because they are human. Having far out thoughts or feelings is not a sign of mental illness. Not being able to function in activities of daily life is a better indicator of mental health and illness. When working with psychiatric patients, the nurse is constantly assessing the patient's healthy and unhealthy behaviors. Because the patient is hospitalized, there may be a tendency for the nurse to forget that much of the patient's behavior is healthy. Seeing similarities in patient reactions to events and nurse's reactions is not a sign the nurse is becoming less healthy. Rather, noticing such similarities is a human response to the healthy and unhealthy aspects of patient behavior.

At first, the nurse may fear harming the patient or not being helpful to him. In time, the nurse may be concerned that the patient will demand too much.

```
┌─────────────────────────────────────────────────────────────────────────┐
│  COMMON NURSE RESPONSES TO WORKING WITH PSYCHIATRIC PATIENTS:             │
│    –  anxiety                                                             │
│    –  fear of being useless                                              │
│    –  fear of appearing like a beginner                                  │
│    –  fear of harming the patient                                        │
│    –  fear the patient will not talk                                     │
│    –  fear that the patient's mental health will affect the nurse's mental health │
│    –  patients are bad                                                    │
│    –  patients are crazy                                                  │
│    –  patients are dangerous                                             │
│    –  patients are funny                                                  │
└─────────────────────────────────────────────────────────────────────────┘
```

Fig. 5-3 Some nurse responses to psychiatric patients

Patients often do have expectations for a relationship which are beyond the role of the nurse. With guidance from a nursing instructor or supervisor comes an understanding that some of the patient's demands may be unrealistic. The nurse firmly sets proper limits on the relationship as a way of teaching the patient what expectations are realistic. Figure 5-3 lists some nurse responses to psychiatric patients.

COMMUNICATING WITH THE PATIENT

Much of mental health-psychiatric nursing is helping the patient to engage in an understandable interchange with the nurse. This interchange is not always verbal. Gestures, stances, movements, facial expressions, and rate of speech are just a few of the ways the patient and nurse convey meaning to one another. Being understood may be of great value to a patient who has felt out of touch with other people. When patient and nurse share a common meaning to a situation, an experience is shared that some patients have never enjoyed before. Each successful attempt to communicate with the nurse can build self-esteem and encourage the patient to relate with others.

The nurse's own anxiety and lack of experience in observation and the patient's lack of clarity in communicating may make it difficult for nurse and patient to understand each other. Psychiatric patients are apt to make statements that have a hidden as well as a surface meaning. For example, if the patient complains, "It's cold in here," the patient may be complaining of the nurse's indifference and distance as much as the temperature of the room.

If the patient does not talk a lot, the nurse may have difficulty staying with him in silence. Assessing the type of silence is crucial in a nurse-patient relationship. Only through knowing if the silence is anxious, angry, peaceful, or withdrawing can the nurse know whether to break the silence or not. For further information on silences, refer to chapter 16.

In a psychiatric setting, the nurse may encounter three different kinds of patient communication. One kind is mostly nonverbal. Another kind comes from the patient who talks so much and so fast that the nurse feels overwhelmed by the amount of information. The nurse may have difficulty deciding what to explore with the patient. A third kind occurs when the patient uses common words in unusual ways or invents new words without telling the nurse their meaning. Trying to understand and share experiences with patients who are nonverbal, verbally overwhelming, or who invent their own meanings or words may be a real challenge for the nurse.

The nurse must not act as if she understands the patient when she does not. Neither should she convey the impression that it is impossible to understand anything the patient is trying to say. When the patient is difficult to understand, it is better to ask, "Tell me what you mean in another way" or "Explain that to me."

Tone of voice and interested manner can convey to the patient that the nurse is trying to understand. Being persistent in attempting to establish a relationship with the patient can bring rewards after the patient accepts the fact that the nurse really is interested in communicating with him.

Timing nurse statements is another important communication tool used in the psychiatric setting. If the nurse can learn when to talk and when to remain silent, a flow of communication can develop. In general, the nurse uses communication skills to encourage the patient to do most of the talking. With nonverbal patients, the nurse may initiate conversation and try to engage the patient at his particular level of capability.

The major aid used in mental health-psychiatric nursing to help study and perfect communication skills is the *process recording.* A process recording is a word-for-word written report of the patient's verbal and nonverbal communication and the nurse's verbal and nonverbal communication in the sequence it occurred. Complete process recordings also include an analysis, an evaluation of nurse-patient interaction, and a restatement of the nurse's ineffective messages. Figure 5-4, page 68, shows a process recording with a nonverbal patient. Figure 5-5, page 69, shows a process recording with a verbal patient.

NURSING ASSESSMENT AND RELATIONSHIP GOALS

The general purpose of the nurse-patient relationship in psychiatric settings is to assist the patient to higher levels of emotional and interpersonal health.

Patient Communications	Evaluation	Nurse Communications	Evaluation	Restatement
Swinging legs. Mouth in chewing motion. Huffing and puffing.	Her mouth fascinates me. Does she have teeth or is she chewing her cheek?	Looking toward patient.		
"Excuse me." Goes to light another patient's cigarette from hers.	Anxious?	Sit waiting for her to return.	I feel silly, but want to communicate. I'll wait for her.	
Comes back, sits down and looks at me. Puffs on cigarette sucking on it hard.	Seems to not have heard me. She knows that it's time for medications. Could be a sign of a strength; responds to cues in her environment.	"You lit Mrs. King's cigarette."	Observation of an actual event O.K., but I probably was anxious about her not talking.	Could have remained silent.
"Gotta get my medication now." Gets up from chair and leaves.		I look around to see if anyone notices I'm just sitting here alone.	I really feel silly sitting here alone; guess it's not my usual social behavior and it makes me feel anxious.	

Fig. 5-4 A process recording with a nonverbal patient (read from left to right)

Patient Communications	Evaluation	Nurse Communications	Evaluation	Restatement
"My intestines fall out."	Patient seems to have a G-I disorder.	"How often?"	Was overwhelmed and thought the patient was describing a G-I disorder.	Entered into patient's delusion. Should have said, "I don't understand; please explain."
"My mother went with me to the doctor. Those guys had knives and the officer shot them."	Patient switches the topic; may be anxious. Unclear pronouns need clarification.	"When was this?"	I wanted to unravel this.	Question was O.K., but patient unable to answer. "Which guys?" "Who was shot?"
"I like my sister-in-law better than my mother."	Patient doesn't like her mother?	"You like your sister-in-law?"		
"My mother punched my sister-in-law when she ate those frankfurters."	I can't see the relationship between eating and getting punched.	"Did your sister-in-law say something to upset your mother?"	An assumption.	Could have said, "What happened just before your mother punched your sister-in-law?"
"After she died, her son threw her down the sewer."		Looked shocked.	I was shocked by what she said.	Could have tried to clarify this, e.g., "After who died?"

Fig. 5-5 A process recording with a verbal patient

The goals of each particular relationship may differ. One aspect of the relationship that will affect goals of the relationship is the way the patient came for help. People who are forced to come to the hospital or to relate with the nurse may have different goals than those who come willingly for help. The patient's perception of the problem will also affect the goals of the relationship. If the patient sees his problem as needing to get away from a nagging wife, goals for the relationship will be different than if the patient comes to the hospital because he fears he may harm someone.

An important part of defining goals for the relationship may include asking the patient what kind of help he would like. Some patients prefer to stay as they are; yet, nurses and doctors set goals and then may be frustrated when the patient does not change. For patients who are involved with their families, it may be important to find out if the family and patient have goals which are different from the health personnel's goals. In order for goals to be met, patient and nurse must agree on what those goals will be.

While talking with the patient, the nurse can get a sense of how the patient views himself. Learning to assess the patient's self-views can help the nurse to see why this patient might come for help at this time. Often, people who are looking for care, love, or protection will seek help when they lose people who have cared for, loved, or protected them. People who value being right or good may seek help when there is a threat to seeing themselves as good or right. People who are orderly, punctual and logical may seek help when there is a loss of ability to be orderly, punctual or logical.

Besides assessing interpersonal concerns, the nurse attends to the patient's physiological difficulties. Skin color, breathing, pain, appetite, and urinary and sexual functioning may reflect physiological or psychological difficulties.

The nurse also assesses the patient's strengths, which include the ability to succeed in academic, family, work, or recreational situations. Strengths can also include the ability to communicate, or to withhold information if the information may be detrimental to the patient. For example, when patients know that hallucinations or delusions are considered reasons for transfer to a long-term facility, they can demonstrate strength by not giving this information about themselves or others. The nurse should be alert to patient strengths that can protect him from stressful situations. In this way, the nurse and patient cooperate to increase healthy coping behaviors in the patient.

Nurse and patient work together to formulate goals for the relationship. To some extent, goals are closely related to why the patient came for treatment. Goals remind the nurse and patient of the limits of the relationship and what each can expect of the other. Patients who are hospitalized for short periods of time may have different goals than patients who are hospitalized for long periods of time. Being clear on the goals for the relationship decreases the possibility that the nurse will try to be all things to all patients. Such nurse expectations are unrealistic and do not encourage healthy behaviors.

Unlike nursing goals used in the general hospital setting, goals in the psychiatric setting may be tailored to the patient and nurse who are involved. When mental health-psychiatric goals are too general, it is impossible to tell when the goals have been achieved. The more clearly and specifically goals are stated, the easier it is to tell when they have been met.

The nurse makes every effort to set goals that will be the same or similar to those of the patient. If the nurse's goal is to help the patient understand his anger and the patient's goal is to get a weekend pass, the relationship may be fraught with conflict and frustration. The nurse adjusts her goals so they are more in line with the patient's. It is not the nurse's responsibility to change the patient's goals. Figure 5-6 lists some specific goals for the nurse-patient relationship.

NURSING CARE PLANS

In devising a nursing care plan for the psychiatric patient, the nurse attempts to define the problems the patient is having in adapting to interaction with others. The nurse can observe the patient's strengths and difficulties as he interacts with her. Some types of information the nurse can look for are: how the patient perceives himself and others, how clear and logical his communication is, how well he can meet his own needs, and what level of growth and development

---

Explore ways the patient is harmful to himself.

Examine how the patient perceives what happens to him.

Explore with the patient how his behavior leads to favorable reactions from others.

Describe the patient's strengths.

Discuss a ward event that was upsetting for the patient.

Discuss how to get a weekend pass.

Discuss how anxiety can lead to hallucinations or delusions.

Explore how the patient deals with anger in self and others.

Help the patient to decide what to say to ask for discharge.

Complete a task such as sitting together for one hour or attending a full session of activity therapy.

Talk about the purpose and effects of a prescribed medication.

Fig. 5-6 Some specific goals for the nurse and patient

he has attained. In the psychiatric setting, growth and development levels are not the same as those expected for the patient's chronological age. Some patients may not have achieved tasks expected at the lowest growth and development level because they have not learned to trust others.

Through interacting with the patient and watching him relate with others, the basics for a nursing care plan are developed. When devising nursing care plans, the nurse considers her own strengths and difficulties in working with patients. Not all nurses can work with all patient difficulties. Both patient and nurse frustration can be decreased when she is aware of the difficulties and how they can be best handled. It is also important to consider hospital regulations and personnel values since both influence the attainment of goals. Availability of family and community resources are also aspects to include when devising nursing care plans. Nursing care plans that do not fit with hospital regulations, personnel or family attitudes, or community resources are likely to be ineffective.

When planning nursing care, the nurse can list behaviors to be encouraged and discouraged and the appropriate interventions. For example, the nurse may decide to encourage the patient's statements of when he feels anxious. The interventions would be to ask the patient to tell the nurse when he feels anxious and to observe when the patient is anxious and ask whether the patient feels anxious.

After encouraging and discouraging patient behaviors the nurse evaluates the effect of her intervention. At this time, new behaviors to be discouraged or encouraged are added, or more effective interventions are planned. A partial nursing care plan for a psychiatric patient is illustrated in figure 5-7.

| Pt. Initials | Sex | Age | Occupation | Marital Status | Diet | Admitted: 10/20 | Diagnoses: |
| R. S. | MALE | 51 | TEACHER | DIVORCED | REG. | Discharged: | SCHIZOPHRENIA |

Need	Problem	Objective	Intervention	Rationale	Evaluation
INTERPERSONAL	ANXIETY	ASSIST PATIENT TO BECOME AWARE OF OWN ANXIETY	ASK PATIENT TO TELL NURSE WHEN HE FEELS ANXIOUS. ASK PATIENT, "ARE YOU ANXIOUS?" WHEN HE CHANGES TOPICS	BEING ABLE TO NAME THE FEELING IS A FIRST STEP TOWARD DEALING MORE EFFECTIVELY WITH ANXIETY	PATIENT ABLE TO NAME FEELING AS ANXIETY. PLAN TO DESCRIBE AND ANALYZE SIT- UATIONS THAT LEAD TO FEELING OF ANXIETY.

Fig. 5-7 A partial nursing care plan for a patient in a psychiatric setting

SUMMARY

In the treatment for mental illness, there is no one model upon which all agree. Nurses may use the medical, social, psychological, or behaviorist model in their work with psychiatric patients.

Patients in a mental health or psychiatric setting may be somewhat different from patients in a general hospital setting. Unlike the general hospital patient, the psychiatric patient is not clear about what the problem is or what he must do to get better.

As members of society, nurses hold views and myths that are prevalent in the society. Because of this, nurses may approach their first experience in a psychiatric setting with high levels of fear and anxiety.

A large part of mental health-psychiatric nursing is focused on the nurse-patient relationship. The nurse helps the patient to engage in an understandable interchange with her. The process recording is the main tool used to help the nurse communicate more effectively with the patient.

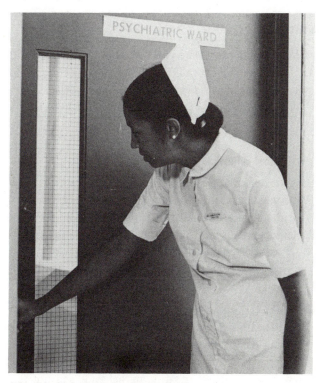

Fig. 5-8 Nurses may approach their first experience in a psychiatric setting with some anxiety.

Goals for the nurse-patient relationship are often specific to the patient and nurse involved. In defining goals, the nurse considers the patient's goals, how the patient came for help, what goals the patient's family may have, physiological signs and symptoms, and the patient's strengths. In devising a nursing care plan, the nurse assesses (1) how the patient perceives himself and others, (2) how clear and logical his communication is, (3) how well he meets his own needs, (4) what level of growth and development he has attained, and (5) the constraints of the work environment.

ACTIVITIES AND DISCUSSION TOPICS

- Talk with various members of the mental health-psychiatric team about which framework or model they use to understand and approach patients.

- Talk with several patients in a psychiatric setting about their goals for care. Find out what they think about care they are receiving. Would any of this information be useful to the health personnel working there? How could you communicate it so as not to offend personnel or overstep limits of confidentiality?

- Make a list of myths and fears you have about psychiatric patients. Talk with family members or friends about their views of psychiatric patients. What purpose could such views or myths serve for society?

REVIEW

A. Multiple Choice. Select the best answer.

1. The statement that best defines mental illness is:
   a. Mental illness is a disease like any other illness.
   b. Mental illness originates in family and community relationships.
   c. Mental illness is ineffective or unsatisfying behavior.
   d. There is no one model upon which all agree.

2. In the social model approach to mental illness, the focus of treatment is on
   a. the physical symptoms of the patient.
   b. the patient's relationships with others.
   c. helping the patient to understand and deal with his thoughts and feelings.
   d. rewarding effective or satisfying behavior and not responding to unsatisfying behavior.

3. The main focus of nursing care for the mentally ill is on
   a. physical care.
   b. the relationship with the patient.
   c. charting evaluations.
   d. involving the patient in creative activities.

4. An indicator of mental illness is
   a. not being able to function in activities of daily life.
   b. having "far out" thoughts or feelings.
   c. associating with another person who is mentally ill.
   d. none of the above.

5. In a psychiatric setting, the nurse may encounter patients who
   a. are nonverbal.
   b. are verbally overwhelming.
   c. invent their own meanings or words.
   d. all of the above.

B. Match the concepts of mental illness in Column II to the definitions in Column I.

Column I	Column II
1. a disease like any other disease	a. behaviorist model
2. originating in family and community relationships.	b. medical model
3. patient's unsatisfying way of relating to others.	c. psychological model
4. behaviors which are reinforced and so continue.	d. social model

C. Briefly answer the following questions.

1. What is a process recording and what does it include?

2. List three ways in which the psychiatric patient differs from the general hospital patient.

3. List five common fears or reactions to psychiatric nursing.

4. List four goals which may be shared by the nurse and patient in their relationship.

SECTION 2
HEALTH-
ILLNESS
RELATIONSHIPS

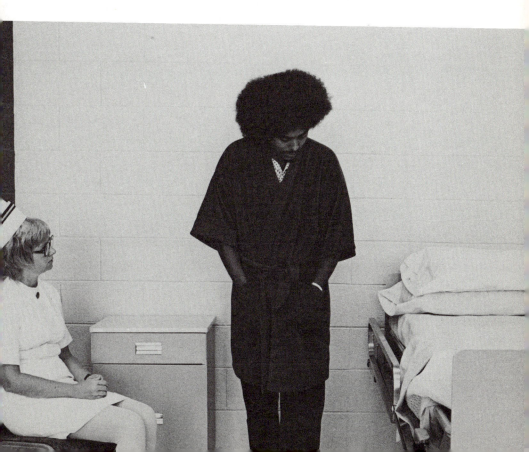

chapter 6
STABILITY

STUDENT OBJECTIVES

- Name four factors that can influence perception of health and illness.
- State the relationship between adaptation and needs.
- State the relationship between stress and a person's internal and external environment.
- Describe the relationship between competence and high level wellness.
- Name four ways the nurse assists the patient to high level wellness.

Nurses work with patients in various stages of health and illness. Because of this, it is important for the nurse to know factors that influence how health and illness are defined and how health and illness factors are related. This unit deals with factors that help individuals to be evaluated by themselves and others as "healthy" or "well." The factors explored in this unit include: perception of health and illness, adaptation, needs, stress, homeostasis, level of wellness, competence, and the nurse and level of wellness.

PERCEPTION OF HEALTH AND ILLNESS

All cultures have ways to evaluate health and illness; however, cultures do not agree on the definition of health and illness. The same symptoms can be called health by one culture and illness by another. For example, the sickle cell trait is not considered to be a sign of illness in the Mediterranean area because it decreases the chance of contracting malaria. In the United States, the sickle cell trait is considered illness because malaria is not a problem. Likewise, in some cultures the ability to "see things" others do not see is considered to be a special sign, a sign of priesthood. In the middle-class American culture, such behavior is called hallucination and may lead to psychiatric hospitalization.

People tend to interpret life experiences in ways that are meaningful to them. The definition of health and illness is also a search for meaning. In order to know what is meaningful to the patient, the nurse must have knowledge of his social class, ethnic, educational, and religious group. Membership in different groups provides the person with various ways of understanding and dealing with symptoms of illness. These learnings influence how the person views himself when ill, how he interprets pain, and what his attitudes toward health personnel will be.

For example, a laborer may describe himself as being ill if he cannot lift 50 pounds of equipment. A suburban housewife would use a different measure for her illness. Some ethnic groups are more likely to rely on folk medicine and family care than on help from doctors and nurses. Some groups associate illness with being bad or sinful. Some religious groups are convinced that body illness is a result of negative thinking and loss of faith. For these people to describe themselves as being ill is to risk loss of support from family and friends. Some people will *deny* (act as if an occurrence has not happened) or *suppress* (actively try not to think about) pain or symptoms. Denial or suppression are sometimes used by people when being ill does not fit with their concept of themselves as being "well." People with less formal education may not seek help because they lack knowledge of bureaucratic procedures or lack understanding of what a symptom might mean. Some people will not seek help due to fear of being humiliated or mistreated.

Because nurses work with people from cultures and subcultures different from their own, it is necessary to gather information about these critical differences. Figure 6-1 suggests some observations and questions the nurse can use to assess the patient's perception of health and illness.

There is no clear-cut dividing line between health and illness. What appears to be a state of health in one person may later prove to be *prodromal* (an early warning) to an illness process. For example, a heart attack may surprise some people because it occurred without any observable symptoms that prevented the usual daily activities. Nurses are often concerned with preventing future recurrences of unhealthy behaviors. To the lay or nonprofessional person, a person may be defined as "sick" when he cannot perform normal daily activities. Present behavior is the only consideration. To the nurse concerned with preventive health care, however, chronic and recurrent conditions are often viewed as more damaging than acute or emergency symptoms. Because of these

Areas to Assess	Further Observations	Questions to Ask
1. Perception of health-illness	1. What is the patient's understanding of the meaning of his/her symptoms?	1. "How do you know when you're healthy?" "How do you know when you're ill?" "What did you think was happening when you first noticed something was wrong?"
2. Perception of who will help	2. Who does the patient first turn to for help? Does the patient think nurses and doctors are to be trusted? Does the patient fear being "humiliated" by health personnel? Does the patient have difficulty understanding how to get help in the health system?"	2. "Who do you go to first for help when you're ill?" "Have you known anyone who distrusted doctors and nurses?" "Have you sometimes had trouble trusting doctors or nurses?" "Does it seem that some hospital policies or procedures are humiliating?" "Which ones?" "Is it hard to know how to get through the red tape here?"
3. Cultural and family influences on perception of health-illness	3. Has the patient learned certain ways to identify or give meaning to health and illness?	3. "How does your family feel about your condition?" "How do you feel about your condition?" "What do you do to relieve pain?" "What does your religious group think about your condition?" "What do you think caused your condition?"

Fig. 6-1 Perception of health-illness

differences in point of view, nurses should find ways to teach preventive health measures yet allow the patient to keep his cultural supports.

ADAPTATION AND NEEDS

The transition between health and illness is often vaguely perceived by the person affected. Health and illness are more accurately assessed when the person (and his internal environment) is examined in relation to the person's external environment of people and things. *Adaptation* is the way in which the person is able to regulate both his internal and external environment in a meaningful and successful way. Adaptation is a complex interaction of biological, psychological, social and cultural resources. Adaptive behavior is probably healthy behavior.

Some people may have an easier time adapting because they have more money, education, or power to regulate their external environment. Some people may receive more understanding and support from family and friends which can help in adaptation. For example, a blind child may be given less taxing chores by his family. This decrease in chores frees the child to either become more dependent on other people or to use the free time and energy improving other skills. In this example, the family relates with the individual child to provide several alternate ways of adaptation.

A basic motivation for people to seek a balanced state between the internal state of their bodies and their external environment is their needs. Needs can be classified into physiological, safety, interpersonal and self-actualizing categories. *Physiological needs* include the need for oxygen, food, water, sleep and activity. *Safety needs* include avoiding injury and repairing normal wear and tear as well as repairing abnormal tissue damage. Abnormal tissue damage could occur due to infection or other illness processes. Normal wear and tear includes processes that are always in operation to keep the body functioning as a whole organism.

Interpersonal needs include the need to feel loved; the need to belong and be part of a group; and the need to establish a consistent self-image in relation to other people. Interpersonal needs can only be met by being with other people.

Self-actualization needs are concerned with pursuing goals other than the basic physiological and interpersonal and safety needs. A goal toward self-actualization might be going to school in order to become a nurse. Self-actualization goals are ways to achieve the highest potential possible for the self. Each person has different potentials and interests; therefore, self-actualization needs may be different for each individual. Other examples of self-actualization goals could be: to be president of a country, win a Nobel Prize, write a book, earn a job promotion, knit a sweater, or plant a garden. A self-actualization goal can be anything that *optimizes* a person's potential; that is, develops potential to its most effective, fullest possible state.

There are a number of ways to classify human needs. One way is to try to cluster needs around the most essential need, oxygen. Without oxygen no life exists and so no other needs can be met. Figure 6-2 depicts needs clustered around the essential need, oxygen. In figure 6-3, the patient is meeting his basic need for sleep.

There is a tendency to consider physiological needs, such as those for food and fluid, more basic than interpersonal or self-actualization needs. However, each person establishes the priority given to each need. Many people give up sleep in order to be with other people; others diet to lose weight. A parent may forget the need for safety to save a drowning child.

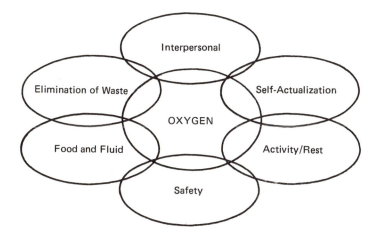

Fig. 6-2 Cluster of human needs

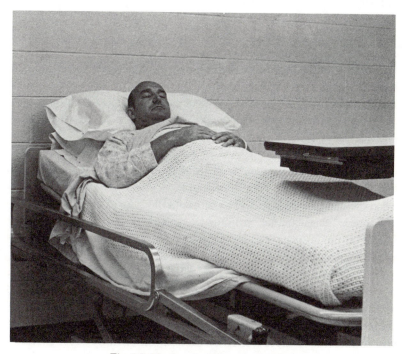

Fig. 6-3 Meeting the basic need for sleep.

Although everyone has the same needs, people vary in the way they attempt to satisfy them. Tension is created when meeting a need is threatened. The person then directs both external behavior and internal body processes toward reducing that tension. It is generally accepted that behavior is always considered to be meaningful because it is directed to meeting needs. People who have been successful in having their needs met are likely to be more patient and delay satisfaction.

When a person has learned to satisfy a need in a certain way, he will continue to try to use that approach because it has been successful. Changing the approach to meeting a need is usually due to one of the following reasons:

- Something changes, and the usual approach does not work anymore. (When the old approach no longer works, the person can experience enough discomfort to try a new approach.)

- A new approach is attractive because it promises greater satisfaction or reward.

- Other people or situations force the person to change.

The nurse's task is not to judge whether the patient's approach is right or wrong; it is to help the person to find different, more workable approaches.

STRESS AND THE ENVIRONMENT

People tend to try to achieve the highest level of wellness possible for them. This level is a function of the balance between internal and external environmental demands. All people have the same basic needs. However, some people have more alternatives in satisfying these needs. For example, an infant can only cry in order to be fed. The small child can walk over, tug on her mother's arm or even take the food. As the child gets older and acquires speech, asking for the specific food brings results. Soon the child helps herself to food she wants. Eventually the child is old enough to earn money and buy the food she wants.

Each of these attempts to achieve an adaptation, or to balance the demands of the internal and external environment, creates stress. *Stress* is a condition produced by the normal wear and tear of bodily processes. Examples of normal wear and tear are breathing, circulating the blood, and digesting food. Stress is also produced when a person is exposed to cold, an argument, a virus, an exam, or any of the countless demands of the environment. Each person tries to strike a balance through adaptation between these internal and external demands. *Stressors* are the cause of stress. Examples of stressors are cold, viruses, arguments, and exams. A direct correlation between the intensity of the stressor and the person's response to the stressor does not always exist. Some people use an

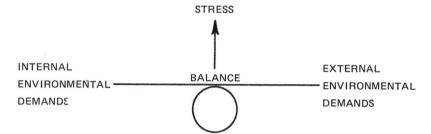

Fig. 6-4 **Stress results from attempts to balance internal and external environmental demands.**

excessive amount of adaptive behaviors or an insufficient amount of adaptive behaviors. People can produce even more stress by using too little or too much energy trying to adapt. Remember that stress is the result of attempting to balance environmental demands with adaptive capacities. Figure 6-4 depicts the relationship between stress and the person's internal and external environment.

Homeostasis is a term that describes a healthy, more or less stable state where there is no undue imbalance. Imbalance can occur due to many different stressors. For example, anxiety or lack of rest can affect homeostasis and create an undue imbalance. People are always trying to achieve homeostasis. Since living things are constantly interacting with their environment, it is not too useful to think of homeostasis as a point in time where everything is in a balanced state. Rather, try to think of homeostasis as a condition where there is no undue imbalance in the relationship between a person's internal and external environment. By this definition, *illness* is an imbalance that occurs when the person is unsuccessful in attempts to adapt to complex physical and emotional stressors in the environment. When stress levels become too high, and balance is not achieved, illness results. If people are able to change when the environment requires change, health can be achieved. If people are not able to change, illness results.

There can be positive as well as negative outcomes from an illness process. Although the illness can create an imbalance, people can learn new adaptive methods or develop untapped potentials during or after an illness. For example, persons who have become paralyzed due to an illness process have turned to develop artistic or verbal skills.

LEVEL OF WELLNESS

Until recently, health meant the absence of illness. As long as health is defined as the physical well-being of a person, level of wellness is fairly easy to

Body Rhythm	Questions
Activity/Rest	
Sleep	"How many hours do you usually sleep?" "What time do you usually go to bed?" "How long does it take to fall asleep?" "When do you nap?"
Activity	"When are you most active?" (morning, noon, night) "What activities do you do?" "When do you concentrate best?" "When are you most easily distracted?" (a.m. or p.m.)
Food and Fluid	
Appetite	"When do you get hunger pangs?" "When do you usually eat breakfast?" "When do you usually eat lunch?" "When do you usually eat supper?" "When do you have a snack?" "How much fluid do you drink each day?" "When do you drink fluids during the day?"
Weight	"What is your weight in the morning?" "What is your weight at night?"
Elimination of Waste	
Bowel Function	"When do you have a bowel movement?" (morning, noon, night, after coffee) "What is the nature of them?" (normal, loose, foul-smelling, normal odor, constipated, yellowish, nearly black)
Urinary Function	"How often do you urinate?" "What is the color of your urine?"
Interpersonal Mood	"When do you feel alert?" "When do you feel depressed?" "When do you feel happy?" "When do you feel foggy?" "When do you feel productive?" "When do you like being with others?" "When do you feel like being alone?" "When do you feel tired?" "When do you feel sensitive?"
Symptoms	"What symptoms do you have?" "At what time do you most notice this symptom?" "Do all of your symptoms occur at the same time?" If not, "When does each occur?"

Fig. 6-5 Questions about body rhythm

determine. When social and emotional well-being is included, the state of well-being becomes much more complex and difficult to assess.

Another factor is that a person's level of health changes week by week and even hour by hour. Each person establishes an individual pattern of activities or *body rhythm*. Body rhythm helps to explain why people are more susceptible to infection and emotional upset at certain times during the day. Body rhythm also explains why people perform at high or low levels at different times during the day. Body rhythm helps to maintain homeostasis. An upset in body rhythm often signals an undue imbalance. Upsets in body rhythms frequently signal an illness process. For example, changes in bowel habits, sleep, or emotional feeling can signal an illness process. Figure 6-5 shows some of the questions one may ask to determine body rhythms.

Since the interaction between illness and wellness factors is so complex, there are as yet no specific tools to measure the exact state of illness or wellness of a person. The best tool available is a combination of the person's expressed feelings and objective observations of the person's signs and symptoms.

The tools available to measure illness are not too accurate because different people may report feeling ill at different levels of illness. Learned social and cultural patterns for reporting pain and discomfort influence patients' reports. These patterns can change over a period of time. Even nurse attitudes and values are affected. As an example, there has been an increased interest in heart disease in the past few years. This interest is related to the increased interest in physical fitness and exercise. As more becomes known about heart disease, assessment tools may become more specific, and possibilities for earlier detection of illness will occur.

It is helpful to think of level of wellness as a continuum, with zero health equal to death, and perfect health equal to an unknown optimum level. Figure 6-6, page 88, depicts the relationship between zero health and peak wellness. In high level wellness, the individual is maximizing his potentials as well as maintaining a balance and purposeful direction with the environment. Each person could be located somewhere along the continuum from death to peak wellness. Due to nonspecific measures, it is only possible to locate four or five markers along the continuum at this time. These markers are death, illness, homeostasis, high level wellness, and peak wellness. The last mark, peak wellness, is an unobtainable ideal to strive toward.

In figure 6-6 homeostasis is the point where balance is attained. A person located at any marker to the left of homeostasis is in undue imbalance. A person located at any marker to the right of homeostasis is in balance. Homeostasis is the point in the figure where internal processes are in balance with external processes. *Internal environmental processes* include biochemical maintenance

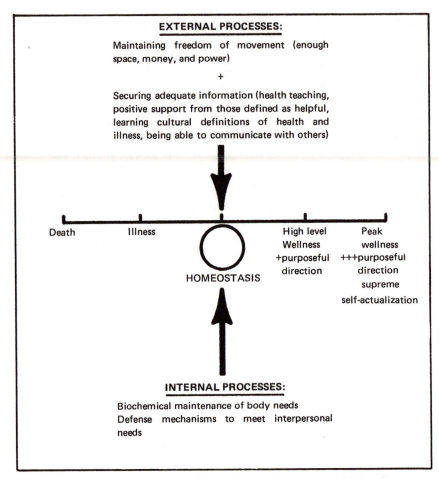

EXTERNAL PROCESSES:

Maintaining freedom of movement (enough space, money, and power)

+

Securing adequate information (health teaching, positive support from those defined as helpful, learning cultural definitions of health and illness, being able to communicate with others)

Death   Illness   HOMEOSTASIS   High level Wellness +purposeful direction   Peak wellness +++purposeful direction supreme self-actualization

INTERNAL PROCESSES:

Biochemical maintenance of body needs
Defense mechanisms to meet interpersonal needs

Fig. 6-6 Level of wellness is influenced by both external processes and internal processes.

of body processes as well as defense mechanisms to meet interpersonal needs.

External environmental processes include maintaining freedom of movement and securing adequate information about the environment. People maintain freedom of movement in many ways. Some of these ways include: securing enough space in an elevator, asking for a private room in a hospital, signing out of the hospital against medical advice, earning money to meet needs and so on. Securing adequate information includes gaining information through health teaching, getting positive support from those defined as helpful, learning cultural definitions of health and illness, and being able to communicate meaningfully with other human beings.

High level wellness means maintaining homeostasis as well as pursuing goals beyond the basic needs. High level wellness, therefore, includes meeting self-actualization needs. A person with high level wellness may have most of the following characteristics:

- A balanced, unified outlook on life.
- Ability to adapt in an efficient way to new problems.
- A liking of self and others.

COMPETENCE AND WELLNESS

There seems to be an inbuilt tendency for people to try to deal effectively with their environment. *Competence* means fitness or ability to deal with the environment. Even in the first year of life, the infant's play seems to be directed, selective, and persistent. Children soon want to "do it myself." These direct attempts to deal with the environment are high level wellness behaviors. As communication through language is learned, competence increases in the ability to deal with people and objects. Manipulation of objects, locomotion, language, and effective behavior in relation to other people increases each person's sense of competence.

People are prone from a very early developmental period to engage in *competence behaviors*. Any behavior that shows an attempt to control or master the environment is a competence behavior. The nurse needs to be involved in observing and supporting these competence behaviors.

THE NURSE AND LEVEL OF WELLNESS

The goal of the nurse is to assist the patient to adapt in a way that is effective, efficient, and self-actualizing. The nurse determines the existence of threats to one or more of the basic needs of the patient. These threats are then evaluated by how well the patient appears to be adapting to the threat. Certain symptoms are more likely to be evident when a specific need is threatened. The nurse also determines what needs the patient is able to meet without assistance; she gives support but is careful not to take away the patient's independence. In areas where the patient is having difficulty adapting, the nurse moves to meet these needs and/or teaches the patient more efficient ways to adapt.

Sometimes this goal toward wellness can be attained when the patient uses energy. At other times, it will be met only when the patient saves energy. For example, suppose a patient with a heart condition who needs to rest quietly in bed is strongly motivated to complete a business merger. If the patient does

Assessment Area	Observations	Examples of Maladaption
1. Do both patient and nurse give the same priority in ranking the patient's needs?	Does the patient place oxygen, elimination, food and fluid, self-actualization, inter-personal, activity/rest, or safety first?	Patient insists on doing office work in hospital. Places self-actualization and activity needs high on priority. Nurse refuses to allow patient to do work.
2. How many stressors must the patient cope with now?	Which of the following stressors are impinging on the patient? surgery, infection, allergic reaction, strong emotion, isolation from others, lack of appetite, weakened body organ, insomnia, excessive noise, new surroundings.	Too many stressors.
3. How has the patient coped with similar stressors before?	Which of the patient's usual coping actions. are possible now? cultural or religious support, avoidance, physical activity, work, yelling, crying, denying.	Patient unable to use usual coping actions.
4. Do both patient and nurse identify both internal and external demands?	What are the internal and external demands? Do patient or nurse act only on one kind of demand or the other?	Nurse identifies only internal demands. Nurse identifies only external demands. Patient identifies only internal demands. Patient identifies only external demands.
5. In what ways does hospitalization or treatment disrupt the patient's usual behavior?	What are the patient's usual patterns of eating, sleeping, interaction, elimination?	Patient is used to being highly mobile, but is now on bedrest. Patient is used to being independent, but is now dependent on the nurse. Patient is used to eating with others, but now is required to eat alone.

Fig. 6-7 Ways the nurse can assess adaptation efforts of the patient

1. How does the patient view the situation?

2. What are the external and internal environmental demands being placed on the patient?

3. How efficiently is the patient using his/her internal and external resources?

4. Does the patient use too little or too much energy in attempting to adapt?

5. Is the patient directing energy toward one goal or towards too many goals at once?

6. How can the patient environment be used more effectively to help the patient to adapt?

Fig. 6-8 Questions which may be asked to determine the patient's level of wellness.

not complete the merger, the patient may be subjected to untold stress because of decreased economic freedom, self-concept, and positive support from his peers; an inability to communicate the seriousness of this merger to other human beings (such as the nurse) adds to this stress. Suppose the nurse and doctor refuse to allow the patient one-half hour to complete the merger due to the stress it might place on the patient's heart. Would allowing the patient to complete the transaction be more stressful than preventing his participation in the event?

The nurse needs to ask, "Is the patient being assisted to a higher or lower level of wellness by my actions?" Remember, to reach a level of homeostasis the patient must be assisted to balance internal *and* external environmental processes. At times, nurses become too involved with internal environmental processes and forget that external processes may have a higher priority for the patient. Figure 6-7 shows ways the nurse can assess adaptation efforts of the patient.

To determine the patient's level of wellness, the nurse observes the consistency, orderliness, and direction of the patient's actions. The patient's actions then need to be compared with the level of wellness continuum. Some questions the nurse can ask about level of wellness are listed in figure 6-8.

SUMMARY

The nurse gains knowledge of the patient's social class, ethnic, educational and religious group in order to begin to understand the patient's perception of health and illness. People regulate both their internal and external environments and seek to achieve a balance (homeostasis) through adaptation. Needs can be divided into categories but it is always important to evaluate the patient's priority of needs before nursing intervention is chosen.

People learn a way to satisfy a need and then continue to repeat that learned approach until discomfort, reward, or force leads them to try different approaches. Stress results from both normal wear and tear of body processes and from external stressors.

Level of wellness is difficult to measure, but it is increasingly becoming the focus of nursing intervention. Health and illness can be thought of as a continuum from zero health to peak wellness. The nurse's goals are to evaluate how well the patient appears to be adapting, to support the areas where he is successful in coping and to assist him in achieving more efficient modes of adaptation.

ACTIVITIES AND DISCUSSION TOPICS

- Using figure 6-1, ask three persons to answer the questions in column three. Each person should be of a different social class, ethnic, religious and/or educational group.

- Think of situations that might influence a person's priority of needs. Make up a list of these situations and compare them with your classmates' lists.

- Compile a list of your own self-actualization goals.

- Think of situations where you have been forced to change behavior or have been rewarded for changing. Recall which needs you were attempting to satisfy.

- Evaluate your own level of wellness.

REVIEW

A. Multiple Choice. Select the best answer.

1. An example of an interpersonal need is the need to
    a. feel loved.
    b. sleep.
    c. avoid injury.
    d. pursue goals.

2. Another name for the biochemical maintenance of body processes and defense mechanisms to meet interpersonal needs is
    a. homeostasis.
    b. external environmental processes.
    c. body rhythm.
    d. internal environmental processes.

3. Cold, viruses, arguments and exams are examples of
   a. prodromes.   c. stressors.
   b. depression.   d. adaptation.

4. An imbalance that occurs when a person is unsuccessful in attempts to adapt to complex physical and emotional stressors in the environment is called
   a. illness.   c. suppression.
   b. homeostasis.   d. denial.

5. The ability to deal with the environment is called
   a. internal environmental processes.   c. competence.
   b. external environmental processes.   d. none of these.

B. Match the items in Column II to the correct definition in Column I.

Column I

1. the way in which a person is able to regulate both his internal and external environment in a meaningful and successful way.

2. a healthy, more or less stable state, where there is not undue imbalance in the relationship between a person's internal and external environment.

3. an individual's pattern of activities which helps to maintain health through regulating performance levels, susceptibility to infection, and emotional upset.

4. actively not thinking about a situation or occurrence.

5. a basic motivation for people to seek a balanced state between the internal state of their bodies and their external environment.

6. maintaining health as well as pursuing goals beyond the basic needs.

7. a condition produced by the normal wear and tear of bodily processes as well as by environmental demands.

Column II

a. adaptation
b. body rhythm
c. high level wellness
d. homeostasis
e. need
f. stress
g. suppression

C. Briefly answer the following questions.

1. Name the four factors that can influence perception of health and illness.

2. What are four ways the nurse assists the patient to high level wellness?

3. What is the relationship between competence and high level wellness?

4. What is the relationship between adaptation and needs?

5. State the relationship between stress and a person's internal and external environment.

chapter 7
CRISIS

STUDENT OBJECTIVES

- State what basic knowledge is required to recognize and treat a crisis.
- List three characteristics of a crisis.
- State three ways a crisis is perceived.
- Give an example of a developmental crisis for each growth and developmental period from infancy to adulthood.
- List ten examples of situational crises.
- Identify the sequence of responses in a crisis.

A *crisis* is an upset in the balanced or stable state for which usual methods of adaptation are not sufficient. Being confronted by the crisis requires new resources to adapt to the situation. These new resources may be internal competencies, such as new ways to think out a problem or they may be external social skills, such as phoning a suicide prevention center.

Crises are unusual or threatening situations that demand (1) a decrease in stressors or (2) a reallocation of energy. A person in a crisis is faced with new and often overwhelming adaptive tasks. These new task requirements offer potential for growth, or reorganization at a less healthy stable state. A crisis, then, can be a turning point; it is a time when important decisions are made.

Certain life events tend to precipitate a crisis. However, whether a crisis actually occurs depends on how a person perceives the events. The crisis, then, is not the event itself; it is the reaction of a person who is unable to cope with the event using his usual adaptive methods.

1. Are the usual methods of adaptation ineffective now?
2. Does the situation seem threatening or overwhelming?
3. Does the person perceive the event as a crisis?
4. Is the person experiencing a life event that tends to be crisis-producing?
5. What are the relationships among the crisis and the patient, his family, and his community?

Fig. 7-1 Considerations in defining a crisis

The nurse requires a basic knowledge in two general areas if she is to be able to recognize and treat a patient in a crisis state:

- An awareness of life events or stressors that tend to produce crises.
- The patient's perception of life events.

It must be remembered that the patient cannot be viewed as an isolated unit; he is part of a family and community. Figure 7-1 summarizes some beginning considerations in defining a crisis.

CHARACTERISTICS OF A CRISIS

A crisis tends to be self-limiting. It does not continue indefinitely. The individual's goal is always to return to the balanced state of homeostasis. People either solve the problems presented or they adapt to nonsolution. In either case, a new state of balance is reached.

A crisis demands a relatively immediate response because of its tendency to disturb homeostasis and to create confusion and uncertainty within the individual. Generally, people tend to dislike a state of confusion and uncertainty and seek to become more in control of their lives. For a certain period during a crisis, however, there is more openness to change and new information. This may be due to the fact that the usual resistances to change have been upset along with other homeostatic devices.

Because there is a temporary state of disorganization occurring, a person in a crisis is likely to remember old problems that are related to the present event. For example, if the present crisis stems from the loss of a body part, previous losses such as tooth extractions, a tonsillectomy, or even separation from loved ones are likely to be remembered by the patient because it stimulates memories of past unresolved problems. A crisis is a particularly crucial event.

A high level of anxiety often exists during the crisis. As the anxiety level increases, the person's ability to perceive what is happening becomes more and more limited. Although anxiety is most often associated with crisis, any strong *affect* (feeling) produces internal disorganization and decreased perception. Therefore, feelings of grief and shame can also be associated with a crisis.

Despite the length of the crisis, people follow a definite sequence in their response to it. It is possible that the nurse could come into contact with the person in a crisis at any step in the sequence. Steps in the sequence are:

(1) The encounter with the life event that is defined by the person as a threat, loss or challenge.

(2) Increase in stress as the person responds to having defined the event as a crisis.

(3) The attempt to use usual adaptive activities.

(4) The realization that usual adaptive activities do not restore homeostasis. Increased anxiety, confusion, internal disorganization and feelings of helplessness frequently result.

(5) A solution to the problem presented by the crisis, or the person's acceptance of nonsolution.

Whether an imbalanced state occurs and a crisis is defined seems to be dependent on the person's perception of the event, his perception of help or support from others, and his ability to cope, figure 7-2.

CRISIS PERCEPTION

Whether or not a person perceives an event as a crisis seems in part to be related to that person's sociocultural group. Since patients are part of a family and cultural group, the nurse needs to be familiar with some sociocultural aspects of crisis. The structure of the patient's community, as well as the community's system of customs, values, rewards and punishments may influence the patient's perception of a crisis.

A CRISIS:
- is self-limiting.
- disturbs homeostasis.
- is not responsive to usual adaptive activities.
- demands a relatively immediate response.
- produces openness to change.
- brings unresolved problems to foreground.
- is associated with increased affect.
- follows a definite sequence.

Fig. 7-2 Characteristics of a crisis

In addition to sociocultural influences on perception, there are also individual psychological perceptions of crisis. When an event is defined as a crisis, there are various ways to perceive it. If the crisis is perceived as a threat, high anxiety may be experienced, especially if the person experiences a threat to basic needs or to sense of self. For example, a person who is unable to breathe will probably experience high levels of anxiety because his basic need for oxygen is threatened.

A crisis can be perceived as a loss. A loss need not be actual; it can occur in anticipated thought. Also, the person who perceives an event as a loss may experience depression. For example, a person who is told he is to have surgical amputation of both legs may experience depression when he is told, or in the future after the amputation has taken place. A similar depressed response could occur even if the person only thinks he might lose both legs.

A crisis can also be perceived as a challenge. The person who perceives a crisis in this way is more prone to begin mobilizing energy toward problem-solving activities.

Whenever a stressful event occurs, the way the patient perceives that event can affect whether homeostasis will be upset or not. If the event is perceived as being related to stress, there is a greater chance that the person will reduce the stress effectively and restore homeostasis. If the event is distorted, the person may not recognize the relationship between the event and the stress; attempts to reduce stress may be ineffective. Sometimes attempts to reduce stress are ineffective because they are not directed at the appropriate source of stress. For example, a person who was driving a car in which a friend was killed may perceive the event in a number of ways. One way would be to assume that the driver is a bad person because the friend died. This perception of the event is likely to lead to a crisis because the driver is perceiving the event as a threat to her sense of self. This perception of the event is a distortion because being a bad driver does not mean one is a bad person. In addition, even this assumption is not an accurate picture because it is not clear whether the driver actually drove badly or not. Perhaps the error may have been due to another driver or to mechanical failure of the car.

Another perception of the same event is that the friend was killed by accident. Such a perception could also evoke a crisis but it might be the crisis of grief, which is more easily resolved. The driver could then direct energy toward grieving the death of the friend. Grieving is a much more goal-directed task than trying to change the self-image of "bad person."

Sometimes the successful completion of a task is perceived as a crisis. For example, a student who graduated from school as valedictorian could experience a deep depression because the graduation with honors had a special meaning to her. In understanding the perception of this event, it would be useful to find answers to the following questions:

- Does the student think she should be given this honor?

- What does graduation from school with honors mean to her now?

- What does she think it will mean in the future?

- How does she explain graduating with honors to herself?

Support Perception

Most people are inclined to depend on certain others for assurance of their worth and acceptability. These significant other people are often family members but can also be respected friends, teachers, or nurses. *Significant others*, then, are those who have an influence or effect on the self-image a person may have. When there are significant others available during a stressful situation, there is less likelihood that a crisis will develop. They can provide support during stressful situations by such behaviors as: listening, accepting the other's behavior, and helping to sort out the relationship between stressors and perception of stress.

Stable cultures or communities develop ways to help their members deal with crises. Interested, nonprofessional people are often available to help on an informal basis. However, in urban areas or rapidly changing communities these members of the local community may not be available to assist with the crisis. For this reason people who do not have community services available are more likely to turn to the nurse for help.

Traditionally, the family provides support during periods of crisis. People without families may find friends to provide this support. Since people are social beings, they look around them for feedback from other people. *Feedback* is the verbal or nonverbal response to another's behavior. When people receive feedback to their actions, they learn what is desirable or anticipated behavior.

Turning again to the student who perceived graduating with honors as a crisis, it would be of interest to find answers to the following questions related to her perception of support from others:

- How secure does she feel about relating to her classmates as valedictorian?

- To what degree do her classmates seem to support her?

- How does she stand with members of her family, now that she's graduating as valedictorian?

- Who can she talk to about her thoughts and feelings concerning graduation?

Coping Perception

People learn to cope with stressors by using methods that were successful in the past. For example, if a person learned that escaping from an unpleasant situation by going to bed had resulted in successful returns to homeostasis, that person might take to bed when under stress.

In a general way, coping devices include educational, work, political, and social skills. *Coping devices* are used by people when they perceive stress. Some people are aware of what they do to protect and maintain homeostasis; others react so automatically, due to habit, that they are not aware of their coping devices. People who are aware of their own coping devices are able to tell the nurse how they cope with stressors. Some common coping devices are thinking a problem out and talking it out with others. Other ways used to cope with stress are: crying, swearing, kicking a chair, arguing with others, blaming others, withdrawing from the situation, and taking drugs.

To return to the example of the student who perceived graduating with honors as a crisis, it would be important to find answers to the following questions about coping perception:

- How has she dealt with past crises?

- What does she usually do when depressed?

- Has she tried her usual ways to combat depression?

Figure 7-3 summarizes ways to evaluate the patient's perception of a crisis.

TYPES OF CRISES

There are two types of crises: developmental and situational. *Developmental crises* are turning points or periods of great change. Periods of great social, psychological and physiological change increase the possibility that a crisis will develop. These periods occur in the normal growth and development of all people. However, not all cultural groups define growth and development periods in the same manner. For example, other cultures do not consider entry into school and middle adulthood as crucial periods in the way that Americans do.

Hazardous situations that are not easily anticipated and for which a person is inadequately prepared are called *situational crises*. These situations do not necessarily occur as part of the normal growth and development sequence. Situational crises in the American culture, such as suicide or intake of hallucinogenic drugs, may not be defined as crises in some other cultures.

Perception of the Event	Perception of Interpersonal or Community Supports	Perception of Coping Devices
1. What is the event?	1. To what degree does the patient think others support her?	1. How has the patient dealt with past crises?
2. Why does the patient think the event is occurring?	2. What are the patient's feelings about relating to others?	2. What does the patient usually do when depressed (anxious, confused, challenged)?
3. What is the current meaning of the event to the patient?	3. How does the patient stand with her family about this event?	3. Has the patient tried her usual ways to combat depression (anxiety, confusion, success)?
4. What is the possible future meaning of the event to the patient?	4. Who can the patient share her feelings with about the event?	
5. How does the patient explain the event to herself?	5. Is the patient receiving consistent feedback to her actions?	
6. What is novel about this event that a crisis resulted?	6. What behaviors are valued and punished by the patient's family or friends?	
	7. Does the patient feel safe and valued or isolated and threatened?	

Fig. 7-3 Ways to evaluate perception of a crisis

Developmental Crises

Even within the middle-class American culture, there are different ways to mark off turning points in growth and development. The presentation in this chapter is a combination and adaptation of the theories of Harry Stack Sullivan, Erik Erikson, and Robert White.

Infancy. The first developmental crisis may occur during infancy. *Infancy* is the developmental period between birth and the first one and one-half to two years of life. During this time, the infant learns beginning trust. If there is no significant other person who relates to the infant in a warm, unconditional manner, trust cannot develop. The person who provides unconditional love does so whether the infant cries, is irritable, or whatever. *Unconditional love* is love that does not hinge on the infant's ability to please or reward the significant other person. Many infants who were raised in institutions were adequately cared for physically but died, seemingly, due to lack of interpersonal love and caring. In infancy, then, the lack of a significant person to provide necessary physical care and/or lack of unconditional love could be stressors that lead to a crisis.

Another task during infancy is learning to explore and manipulate the environment. The infant learns to cry, to invent words, to put objects in and take them out of his mouth, to use a cup and spoon, to learn about the permanency of objects, and to test the reaction of environmental objects (including people). Inability to complete these tasks or inability to maintain homeostasis could lay the foundation for a crisis.

Childhood. The next developmental period is *childhood* which occurs between the ages of one and one-half to six years. Childhood begins with the capacity for communicating with others through speech; it ends when the child begins to need association with peers. During this stage, the child learns to delay satisfaction of needs. That is, the child sees that others respond and meet his needs so there is less pressure to have immediate satisfaction. As communication methods and motor control improve, the child gains a sense of mastery over the environment. He increases control over his own body and learns new ways to gain assistance from others. This increased sense of mastery adds to the child's ability to delay satisfaction. Through interactions with others, an *autonomy* or *sense of self* emerges as the child begins to express who he is (*I, me*) what is his (*mine*) and that he has some control over what happens to him (*no*).

As the child moves into later childhood, he begins to learn more about physical, social, economic, and sex differences. An ever-increasing control over body and speech allow the child to expand imagination and to undertake tasks with a purpose. Adaptation is increased as the child has better locomotion and can move to correct homeostatic imbalances. Feelings are more differentiated also. In the young infant, only discomfort or anxiety were differentiated from rage. In childhood, feelings of *shame, guilt, anger* and *doubt* are differentiated. The feeling of shame begins to become associated with a sense of self-consciousness. For example, the child may feel shame when her mother says, "Anne, you have on two different colored socks." Guilt is a feeling the child can learn to experience in situations where others define her as incompetent. The child can also learn that although rage is not a socially acceptable feeling when others restrict her movements, anger is a more socially acceptable feeling. Doubt can be learned at the time the child assumes a questioning attitude about her behavior, and begins to delay immediate satisfaction of her needs. Developmental crises can develop in childhood when physiological, social, or psychological adaptation cannot or does not occur.

Juvenile Period. The *juvenile* period occurs between the ages of about six and nine years. Development of competence is especially important during this stage; it is the first time that others are more important than family. The child with many interpersonal difficulties now has a chance to work them out with a favorite teacher or pal of the same sex.

Children and parents can experience the child's entrance into school as a crisis. Juveniles begin to learn how to compete, compromise and cooperate. Because the juvenile must learn to function in more than just a family setting, the idea of *role* becomes more clear. The juvenile may notice that he acts one way in relation to his teacher, another in relation to his mother, and still another in relation to his friend; the roles of student, son, and friend become more differentiated at this time.

With the ability to concentrate for a longer period of time, the juvenile is more productive. He is able to create things such as paintings and carry out school assignments for written work. The juvenile can also express an even higher level of love than the unconditional love given to the infant. The juvenile can care for a pal and want that pal to be as satisfied and secure as he is.

Preadolescence. Overlapping the juvenile era is the *preadolescent* or prepuberty period. Between age nine and twelve some physiological sexual change is occurring. Peers of both sexes take on increased importance. Incidents which interfere with normal growth and development tasks appropriate to this level could precipitate a crisis.

The development of a continued sense of industry is taking place during this time also. The preadolescent focuses his efforts on producing in school and at home as a way of becoming more independent. These changes may be signalled through increased hostility, restlessness and irritability.

Adolescence. *Adolescence* is often associated with the physiological sex changes that occur between ages twelve and fourteen. These physiological changes can begin earlier in some cultural groups and later in others. Adolescence can also be defined as the time when strengths and limitations are evaluated. This is done through experimentation in social, sexual, educational, and work experiences. Due to rapid technological advances and lengthened educational experiences, adolescence frequently extends to age 21 and sometimes beyond that time.

During late adolescence, people learn to become interdependent with others. Before reaching this stage one or the other was allowed to be dependent or independent; however, there was resistance to the switch in roles, and frequently high anxiety accompanied such a switch. In *interdependence,* each person can rely on the other for certain aspects of the relationship.

Learning to delay satisfaction becomes more clearly understood in late adolescence. Hard work and dull tasks can be undertaken with patience; future satisfaction is kept in mind. Stressors which interfere with successful evaluation of strengths and limitations could cause a crisis.

Adulthood. The final developmental period is adulthood. The adult helps to establish and guide the next generation. This may be done within the family through procreation and socialization, or outside the family through teaching or working with another generation.

Recently, the idea of middle adulthood and its potential crises have become more important. Middle-class American culture is achievement oriented; therefore the issue of success creates a potential crisis for many people. The woman whose children are grown and have left home may feel useless; she may be confused as she assesses her limitations and strengths in areas other than as homemaker and mother. The man who has reached middle age may feel that he has not been successful in his chosen career. The aging process is more apparent in the middle years; persons who are very concerned about their physical appearance or activity level can experience a crisis as they perceive the limitations. In view of the fact that male and female roles are becoming less differentiated, success and achievement crisis may become more similar in the future.

Late adulthood is a time to reassess life experiences and work through feelings about death. Reminiscing about past experiences seems to be important at this time and is necessary for achieving the maximum level of wellness. Many adjustments to physical, social, and economic restrictions are necessary.

Retirement with subsequent feelings of uselessness, and a decrease in financial income can be crisis inducing. Some societies tend to institutionalize or isolate older members. Sensory and social deprivation could precipitate a crisis in these persons. Figure 7-4 summarizes information about potential crises at each developmental level. The age levels and tasks listed on the chart are for purposes of gross comparison only. Also, it is important to remember that even healthy people may pass through developmental levels without completely resolving the tasks appropriate to that age level. Most people continue to work on and resolve tasks appropriate to the earlier levels of development throughout their lives.

Situational Crises

There are three kinds of environmental situations that could be considered stressors for situational crises:

1. The loss of the source which satisfies a basic need.

2. The threat of losing this source of satisfaction.

3. A sudden challenge that overtaxes present resources.

Loss of a Basic Need Source. Stressors that are related to the loss of the source which satisfied a need could lead to a crisis. Examples of such stressors are:

- death or separation from a significant other person
- physical or emotional marital separation

Developmental Level	Approximate Age	Events which might Precipitate a Crisis
Infancy	Birth to 1 1/2 or 2 years	Lack of unconditional love. Lack of other's meeting basic needs. Lack of ability to make beginning environmental manipulations.
Childhood	1 1/2 to 6 years	Inability to influence others with verbal communication. Inability to delay satisfaction. Inability to increase motor control. Refusal of others to grant autonomy.
Juvenile	6 to 9 years	Entry into school. Inability to learn appropriate roles. Inability to produce objects assigned. Difficulties with pal relationship. Inability to compete, compromise, or cooperate. Blocks to increasing motor, social and/or physiological growth.
Preadolescent	9 to 12 years	Confusion about physiological (sex) changes. Blocks to becoming more independent. Blocks to producing socially and educationally.
Adolescence	12 to 21+ years	Blocks to evaluation of strengths and limitations of self and others. Difficulties with independence, dependency and interdependency. Confusion about the future.
Adulthood	21+ to death	Inability to produce children. Parenthood, especially firstborn. Blocks to communication with other age groups. Inability to achieve personal concept of success. Inability to adapt to success. Aging process. Blocks to reassessing life experiences. Inability to face death. Extreme physical, social or economic restrictions. Social or sensory deprivation.

Fig. 7-4 Potential crises

- divorce
- a jail term
- physical illness
- loss of a body part
- retirement
- sex difficulties
- school graduation.

Perception of the loss is an individual perception; thus, the loss of a fingertip or of a beloved pet could create a crisis response in some individuals.

Threat of Loss. Stressors that threaten to endanger satisfaction of a need can also precipitate a crisis. Such stressors could include thoughts or feelings that a significant other person will leave the individual, for example, die or seek a separation or divorce. Such misinterpretations are perhaps more characteristic of patients who need socioemotional support than is characteristic of patients who require physical nursing care. However, some patients who are admitted to hospitals for major or minor surgery frequently express fears of death and mutilation greater than would be expected. A patient who may be waiting for a diagnosis can experience severe anxiety; a crisis can result if the patient thinks the diagnosis will be especially devastating. Likewise, thoughts of being fired or that a family member is about to move out of the house could result in crisis. The person's perception of the event that is occurring or is about to occur signals whether there is a crisis.

Sudden Challenge. A sudden challenge that requires immediate adaptation without sufficient preparation or resources can lead to crises. Such challenges could include:

- unwanted pregnancies
- premature birth
- emergency hospitalization
- involuntary placement in a nursing home
- flood or other natural disaster
- holidays
- move to a new residence
- outstanding personal achievement

Combination of Stressors

Some situational crises could include aspects of the three stressors: actual loss, threatened loss, and sudden challenge. For example, although minor surgical procedures (such as setting a broken leg under anesthesia) rarely end in death, patients report fear of death, and may need to rise to the sudden challenge of awaking from an emergency surgical procedure. Also, holidays are especially critical events for those who no longer have a family and are depressed by remembering better times, figure 7-5. The first year anniversary after the death of a significant person may be especially difficult for survivors because they are reminded of their loss, especially if it is unresolved. Figure 7-6, page 108, summarizes some of the stressors that could precipitate a situational crisis.

THE NURSE IN CRISIS

When patients do not respond to the attempts to provide care, the nurse may be confronted by a potential crisis of her own. She may find herself

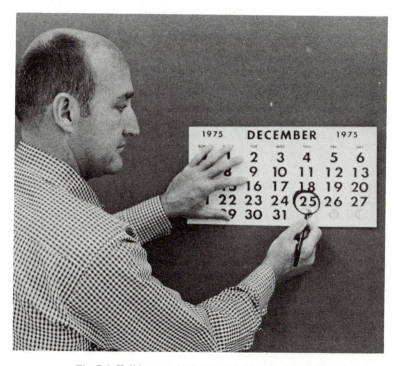

Fig. 7-5 Holidays can lead to a crisis for some people.

Types of Environmental Situations	Stressors
Loss of a basic need source	Death of a significant other.
	Marital difficulties (separation, divorce, non-support, alcoholism, drug addiction, sexual problems and infidelity).
	Jail term.
	Family member leaves household.
	Physical illness.
	Loss of body part due to surgery or injury.
	Unemployment.
	Retirement.
	Graduation.
	National disaster.
	Holidays.
Threat of loss of a basic need source	Fear that significant other will die.
	Thoughts of being abandoned by marital partner.
	Fear of being jailed.
	Thoughts that family member will leave household.
	Fear of physical illness.
	Fear of unemployment.
	Fear of loss of body part.
	Fear of retirement.
	Fear of graduation.
	Awaiting diagnosis.
Sudden challenge	Holidays.
	Unwanted pregnancy.
	Premature birth.
	Move to new residence.
	Physical injury.
	Emergency hospitalization or surgery.
	Involuntary placement in nursing home.
	Outstanding personal achievement.
	Natural disaster.
	New member in household.
	Suicide or homicide.

Fig. 7-6 Examples of stressors that can precipitate a situational crisis

following the same sequence of events that others experience in a crisis. The following is an example of such a possibility.

1. Encounters a patient who dies, or one who threatens the nurse or challenges her role.
2. Recognizes a crisis and experiences the increased stress.
3. Continues to use usual adaptive activities.
4. Anxiety increases.
5. Solves the problem or accepts nonsolution.

When the nurse becomes aware that she or another nurse is experiencing a crisis, behavior patterns which inhibit the nurse-patient relationship can be identified. In order to define the presence of or potential for a crisis, three areas must be examined by the nurse: (1) her perception of the patient situation, (2) her perception of support from others, and (3) her perception of coping devices.

Perception of the Patient Situation

If the nurse distorts the meaning of the patient's behavior or views the patient unrealistically, she may be at high risk for a crisis. This high risk can occur because the nurse will be responding to the patient on the basis of inaccurate perception.

Inaccurate perception can be due to several kinds of distortion. One kind of perceptual distortion is to describe and react to the patient on the basis of a single characteristic of that person; this is called *labelling* or *stereotyping*. For example, if a patient is being described as "He's a faker" or "She's always demanding things," the patient is being labelled or stereotyped.

Another inaccurate perception is failing to see all sides of an issue or situation. For example, if a nurse views a patient as being courageous and good, while the family is described as uncaring or interfering, it is quite possible that she is perceiving the situation inaccurately. Understanding of the family as well as the patient is the key to an accurate perception of the patient situation.

Perception of Support from Others

Students and graduates often indirectly ask for support from their peers, instructors, or supervisors. These requests may be conveyed by: repeated expressions of dissatisfaction with the patient's progress; undue concern for the patient; and threats of refusing to work with the patient any longer. Since the call for support is an indirect one, others may not recognize it and may fail to respond. The nurse in crisis may then perceive it as a lack of needed support from others.

Perception of Coping Devices

Nurses may or may not be aware of their usual coping devices. Coping devices which are often useful in nurse-patient situations may be maladaptive in other nursing situations. For example, patient teaching can be a useful way to assist the patient to attain high level wellness. If the patient does not cooperate with the teaching attempts, however, the nurse can experience increased levels of anxiety and subsequent crisis.

Another coping device used by nurses is to withdraw from an unusual or upsetting nurse-patient situation in order to seek out or think out different approaches. Leaving the suicidal or dying patient can lead to increased anxiety in both patient and nurse and to subsequent crisis.

Another coping device nurses use to cope with their stress is to assume the patient thinks and feels as the nurse does. This coping device is called *projection* because the nurse "projects" her thoughts and feelings to the patient. When the nurse uses projection, she assumes the patient is experiencing the same thoughts and feelings as the nurse. If the nurse attempts to convince the patient that she knows best — without first trying to understand the patient's thoughts and feelings — increased anxiety and frustration will be felt by the nurse when the patient does not follow the suggestions.

SUMMARY

A crisis is an upset in homeostasis that requires new resources or competencies. Certain life events are more likely to precipitate a crisis. Whether a crisis occurs or not depends on the person's perception of these events.

Crises are self-limiting; they disturb homeostasis, are not responsive to usual adaptive activities, demand a relatively immediate response, produce openness to change, bring unresolved problems to the foreground, are associated with increased affect, and follow a definite sequence. Perception of a crisis is related to responses from the person's sociocultural group and his view of the crisis as a threat, a loss, or a challenge.

Crises are of two general kinds: developmental and situational. Developmental crises occur during normal growth and development when there are periods of great social, psychological or physiological change. Situational crises are situations which are not easily anticipated and do not necessarily occur as part of the normal growth and development sequence.

The nurse can also experience a crisis when patients do not respond to the attempts to provide nursing care. Defining a crisis for the nurse includes the nurse's perception of the patient situation, perception of support from others, and perception of her own coping devices.

ACTIVITIES AND DISCUSSION TOPICS

- Make a chart of your own life event crises. On the left side of the chart, place the life event you defined as a crisis. On the right side of the chart write down whether you perceived the event as a threat, loss, or challenge.

- Make a list of your own coping devices. Try to improve the perception of your own coping devices by asking others for observations about your coping devices.

- Refer to figure 7-6. Add up the number of stressors you may be currently experiencing.

- Review the charts of several patients and add up the number of life events or stressors to which each is attempting to adapt.

- Contact the social sciences department of your college and talk with an instructor who has an interest in sociology or anthropology. Discuss cultural perceptions of health and illness. Try to become familiar with cultural perceptions of a number of different subcultural groups with whom you may have to work.

REVIEW

A. Multiple Choice. Select the best answer.

1. Crisis can be defined as
   a. a response which can occur as a result of being restricted or as a response to anxiety.
   b. a sense of questioning and delaying satisfaction.
   c. an upset in the balanced or stable state for which the usual methods of adaptation are not sufficient.
   d. a way of dealing with stressors ranging from internal thought responses to externally visible behavior.

2. Verbal or nonverbal communication in response to another's behavior is
   a. acceptance.   c. interdependent relationship.
   b. unconditional love.   d. feedback.

3. The juvenile era occurs between the ages of
   a. 1 and 6.   c. 12 and 14.
   b. 6 and 9.   d. 9 and 12.

4. Whether a crisis occurs or not depends on the person's
   a. life-style.   c. perception.
   b. income.   d. none of these.

B. Match the items in Column II to the correct statement in Column I.

Column I

1. the ability of each person in the relationship to allow the other to be dependent on the other for some aspects of the relationship.

2. describing and reacting to another on the basis of a single characteristic of that person.

3. ways of dealing with stressors ranging from internal thought responses to externally visible behaviors in a group.

4. periods of great social, psychological and physiological change that occur as part of the normal growth and development process.

5. assuming the other person has the same thoughts and feelings or is to blame for an unwanted occurrence.

6. hazardous situations that are not easily anticipated and for which the person is inadequately prepared.

Column II

a. coping devices
b. developmental crises
c. projection
d. situational crises
e. stereotyping
f. interdependent relationship

C. Briefly answer the following questions.

1. List three characteristics of a crisis.

2. What are the three ways a crisis is perceived?

3. Name the two areas in which basic knowledge is needed to be able to recognize and treat a crisis state.

4. Give an example of a developmental crisis for each growth and development period:
   Infancy:
   Childhood:
   Juvenile:
   Preadolescent:
   Adolescence:
   Adulthood:

5. List ten examples of situational crises.

D. People follow a definite sequence in their responses to a crisis. Number the following events in the sequence in which they occur.

Increased anxiety at realization that usual adaptive activities are ineffective.

Experiencing stress as the crisis is recognized.

Encountering event that is defined by the person as a threat, loss, or challenge.

Continuing to use usual adaptive activities.

Solving the problem or accepting nonsolution.

chapter 8
CRISIS ASSESSMENT
AND INTERVENTION

STUDENT OBJECTIVES

- State three reasons why the nurse is especially suited to assess and intervene with crises.

- Match crisis assessment areas with appropriate assessment questions for each area.

- Identify useful ways to communicate during a crisis.

- List three preventive measures for averting crisis.

- List two factors which block the nurse's efforts towards crisis intervention.

Certain characteristics make the nurse especially useful in crisis work. First, the nurse has a public image of skill and sensitivity to the needs of suffering people. Second, the nurse has a history of giving care to the whole person. Third, the nurse has frequent, regular, and intimate contact with patients and their families.

Because of these special chacteristics, the nurse is perhaps the best person on the health team to work with patients in crisis. Being readily accepted as a helping person by most people in crisis, the nurse is also usually the most available.

There is still another characteristic of nurses which allows them to be useful in dealing with crises. This characteristic is the nurse's education and experience in providing emotional support. *Emotional support* is the ability to convey an interested, nonjudgmental concern through remaining physically and emotionally present with the patient. This ability to remain physically present and keep calm when others might be upset makes the nurse indispensable in crisis situations. Since the ability to remain calm is often a learned response, new students should not expect to be able to deal with crisis situations without experience and supervision from more experienced nurses.

CRISIS ASSESSMENT

Crisis assessment involves evaluating the following areas:

- Communication and level of anxiety
- Coping devices
- Significant other people
- Suicide or homicide potential
- Perception of crisis significance
- Personal strengths

Focus on the Crisis

Since a crisis may be an overwhelming experience, people in crisis may have trouble focusing on it. Communication and level of anxiety are severely affected. Anxiety level may be high; as a result, communication is poor and the patient may jump from one topic to another (scattering) or blow one detail of a situation out of proportion (exaggeration).

A crisis can also be indicated by absence of the expected feeling or response. Withdrawing, showing no feeling, or becoming depressed in a situation that usually creates anxiety should be a signal to the nurse that a possible crisis exists. For example, patients who appear too calm prior to major surgery or who do not show any feeling when a loved one dies may be in crisis.

Coping Devices

Observing the patient's response to the nurse and others helps to reveal his usual coping devices. Blaming the nurse or others (projection), not talking or moving (withdrawal), and developing bodily symptoms (somatization) can be observed and noted as the nurse talks with the patient.

When the patient is ready, the nurse assesses the use of coping devices by asking the patient how he usually handles similar problems. The nurse must be careful not to force the patient to talk about coping devices if he is not willing to do so.

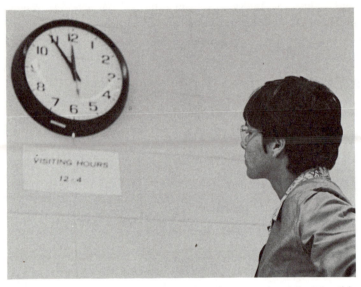

Fig. 8-1 Visits from family or friends can provide support for patients in crisis.

Significant Others

The nurse collects information about the patient's relationships with significant other people in the patient's life through observing and questioning. The nurse notices who accompanies the patient for care and who visits him. Also of value are discreet inquiries about whom the patient lives with, his family and friends, and the persons he can ask for assistance. She must be tactful and show genuine interest when collecting this information.

Suicide and Homicide Potential

People who feel inadequate to handle life stressors may turn to suicide as a way to deal with their hopelessness and despair. Suicide attempts may also be a cry for help when the person feels unable to communicate with significant other people.

The nurse may be familiar with the patient's past history and already know that he has made suicide attempts. It is not true that people who talk about suicide or attempt it often are not suicidal. Chances are that these people will succeed in killing themselves; if not on purpose, they may succeed by accident.

The nurse must be familiar with high risk groups. Suicide attempts are more likely to occur when a depression lifts because the person then has the energy necessary to carry out the decision. Statistics show that (1) females make more suicide attempts than men, (2) men are more often successful in their attempts since they are likely to use lethal methods such as guns, and (3) in Caucasians, the frequency of suicide increases with age, the reverse is true of the Negroid race. The use of alcohol and barbiturates are closely tied to suicide attempts.

Strong religious ties can decrease the potential for suicide since few, if any, religions look upon suicide favorably. People who live alone or have few significant others to count on are more likely to withdraw and see suicide as the only alternative to a hopeless situation. One of the reasons for suicide is lack of open communication with significant other people. The nurse can decrease this factor by keeping open communication with patients, especially those in crisis.

If the nurse feels that a patient may be thinking of killing himself or someone else, she should encourage the patient to discuss these matters. Homicidal potential can be handled in the same manner. Discussion can center around the following: is the patient thinking of killing someone? has he chosen the method, time, and place? if so, what are they? Once these thoughts and feelings are out in the open, they can be examined.

The new nurse may not feel comfortable or experienced enough to intervene in the suicidal or homicidal crisis. If so, it is wise to consult a more experienced nurse clinician or a clinical specialist in psychiatric mental health nursing. The

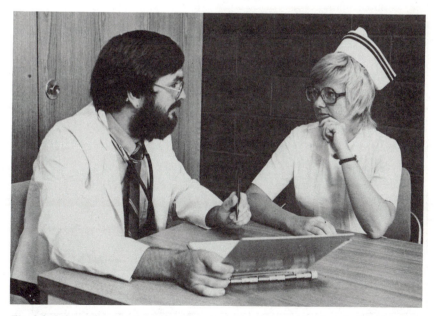

Fig. 8-2 Information about suicide attempts or thoughts must be shared with other health personnel.

preparation of a clinical specialist includes education and experience in crisis assessment and intervention. CAUTION: Suicidal and homicidal thoughts or feelings must be recorded in nursing notes *and* reported verbally to the nurse in charge. Suicide and homicide are emergency situations that require immediate intervention. The patient should be told that the nurse cannot keep this kind of information confidential and that it must be shared with the rest of the staff involved in caring for the patient.

There are a number of reasons why it is important to share the responsibility for the knowledge of suicidal or homicidal thoughts and feelings. The nurse's responsibility is to promote health. Also, the guilt that can result when only one person bears the responsibility — and a suicide or homicide does occur — can be overwhelming. By taking correct measures, the nurse avoids being overwhelmed so she can be effective in dealing with patients. This can be done through study and application of concepts which prepare her to meet situations

High Suicide Potential	Lower Suicide Potential
Specific suicide plan	No specific plan
Inability to see other alternatives	Can talk about other alternatives to suicide
Lack of communication with significant others	Good communication with significant others
History of lethal suicide attempts	No suicide attempts or only nonlethal attempts
Depression is lifting	In depression
Many stressors	Few stressors
Chronic, debilitating condition	No chronic condition
White persons over age 50	White persons under age 50
Black persons under age 50	Black persons over age 50
Males	Females
No religious ties	Strong religious ties
Wants to be reunited with dead significant other	Uses suicide as a cry for help
Reports constant pain	No reports of pain
Hears voices telling him/her to kill self	No voices
Takes hallucinatory drugs	Takes no hallucinatory drugs
Intake of alcohol, barbiturates or both	No alcohol intake No barbiturate intake

Fig. 8-3 Factors to consider in assessing suicide potential. The greater the number of high suicide factors, the higher the suicide potential.

that require intervention. Student nurses and new graduates should discuss suicidal or homicidal crises with more experienced staff members to determine what is the best way to intervene. Figure 8-3 summarizes information on the crisis of suicide.

Perception of Crisis Significance

Through observation and direct questioning, the nurse is able to learn about the patient's attitude toward the crisis and how it will affect his life. Has the crisis affected the patient's ability to move, walk or work? What activities are now affected by the crisis? How do the members of the family and the patient's friends feel about the crisis? CAUTION: The nurse does not bombard the patient with questions. She studies and practices verbal and nonverbal communication methods prior to attempting crisis assessment and intervention. When the patient's anxiety level is lower, he may wish to talk; the nurse tries to be available at this time. The student or new graduate functions more in the role of noting and reporting potential crisis. The new nurse can also help refer the suicidal or homicidal person to a nearby suicide prevention center or community mental health center that is equipped to handle this type of emergency.

Personal Strengths

The patient has certain personal strengths that need to be assessed. The nurse needs to be aware of what strengths can be assessed. This area of assessment may be very difficult and often cannot be completely accomplished. The assessment of personal strengths can provide valuable information, figure 8-4.

PERSONAL STRENGTHS

- Views self as a separate person.
- Sees self as others do.
- Has capacity for sustained work.
- States own wishes, desires, and hopes to others.
- Meets basic needs.
- Maintains at least one long-term, satisfying relationship.
- Speaks clearly and logically.
- States an understanding of what's happening.
- Maintains a stable life-style.
- Adapts to some changes in the environment.
- Changes the environment when it is not conducive to own welfare.

Fig. 8-4 Personal strengths to be assessed

Assessment Area	Questions to Ask
Focus on crisis	"What seems to cause this upset?" "What is upsetting you right now, today?" "What happened right before you felt upset?" "Have you any physical symptoms since feeling upset?"
Coping devices used	"Has anything like this happened before?" "What do you do to relieve tension?" "What do you do to relieve depression?" "Have you tried your usual method?" "Why not?" "What do you think would make you feel better?"
Significant other People	"Who do you live with?" "Who could you stay with tonight?" "Who can you count on to help you?"
Suicide/Homicide Potential	"Are you thinking of killing yourself?" "Are you thinking of killing someone?" "Do you have a method in mind?" "What method?" "When do you plan to carry it out?"
Perception of Crisis Significance	"Which daily activities is your crisis affecting?" "How does your wife feel about this?" "How do your friends feel?" "Are they upset?"

Fig. 8-5 Crisis assessment

Guidelines for assessment of a crisis are given in figure 8-5. The new graduate — and especially the student nurse — is not expected to be able to conduct a crisis assessment interview. It would be useful, however, to be aware of what areas are important to assess. As the nurse gains experience and confidence and finds suitable nursing supervision, crisis assessment will become an integral part of the nurse's role.

CRISIS INTERVENTION

During and after nursing assessment of crisis, the nurse selects the appropriate interventions. Major interventions include methods of communication, and prevention. In crisis intervention work, the nurse works to support the strengths of the patient.

Communication in Crisis

During crisis, the person's awareness of external surroundings may be diminished. The person in crisis is probably already overloaded with decisions, thoughts and feelings. In acute crisis when the patient's anxiety level may be high, the nurse uses short phrases to reduce sensory input. Examples of concise 3-4 word phrases include: "When did this happen?" "Describe that" "Say some more" "And then what?" "Say what you feel."

The nurse talks to the patient about what he is experiencing at the moment. She does not introduce new information, such as, "Tomorrow you'll be going to X ray," or "What would you like to know about hospital procedures?" New information is not introduced when the patient is in the early phase of crisis because it will further overwhelm him at a time when he should not have to deal with added nonrelated input. Also, new information makes focusing on the crisis more difficult. If there is any attention given, the patient may jump from the topic of the crisis to the topic introduced by the new information. Also, high anxiety levels reduce the amount of information a person hears or pays attention to so new information would probably not be heard.

Instead, by a calm tone of voice and attentive body posture, the nurse conveys "I am here" and "I am concerned." She does not interrupt a patient's fast flow of speech; the patient tells the nurse about the crisis in the best way possible at that moment. A calm, concerned person who listens to the patient can decrease the patient's anxiety.

It is not unusual for anxious people to blame others and express their anxiety by showing anger. The nurse understands that patients express their anxiety through anger. Because of this understanding, the nurse will be less likely to become angry in return.

As the patient's anxiety level is reduced, flow of speech, restlessness, and a calmer voice tone may be signs that the patient is now able to focus on solving the problems presented by the crisis. By encouraging the patient, the nurse helps him realize that he can solve the problem. She conveys that the patient must take responsibility for his own life decisions. Although the patient must make the final decision, the nurse advises that she will assist him to examine possible alternative decisions. The patient is encouraged to state the problem presented by the crisis by questions like, "What is the main problem?" or "If I hear you right, the problem is . . ." or "What problem brought you to the hospital *today*?"

Once the problem is identified, the nurse and patient work on locating resources to help with the crisis. For example, a possible resource might be a clinical specialist in psychiatric mental health nursing; another resource might be a friend who could bridge the gap between hospital stay and going home by providing companionship for the discharged patient.

To help the patient select appropriate resources, the nurse needs to be familiar with available services which include not only those in the hospital or

When patient is highly anxious	When patient is less anxious,
Use short, concise phrases.	Ask patient to restate problem.
Keep focused on crisis topic.	Explore patient's expression of feeling.
Introduce no new information.	Explore resources available to solve problem.
Convey concern and interest through calm voice and attentive posture.	Convey that patient is responsible for own life decisions.
Encourage patient's expression of feeling.	
Do not interrupt patient's flow of speech.	
Do not respond to patient's anger with anger.	

Fig. 8-6 The nurse's communication in crisis depends on the patient's level of anxiety.

clinic, but self-help groups such as Synanon, and groups such as Reach to Recovery, Cancer Care, Red Cross, Suicide Prevention Centers, Ostomy Clubs, and so on. Each nurse should become familiar with available community resources to patients. Figure 8-6 summarizes important aspects of communication during crisis.

Preventing Crises

By anticipating possible crises, the nurse practices prevention. The nurse can help to prevent some crises by anticipating where the patient may need more information, by assisting with grief work, by assessing the meaning of hospitalization, and by being aware of normal growth and development disturbances. The beginning practitioner will probably assist more experienced health personnel during crisis situations.

It is difficult to tell prior to a crisis which situations will be thought of as crises by those involved in the situations. The nurse can take steps to cut down the possibility of a crisis. For example, talking with a pregnant woman and her husband before the birth of their first child could possibly prevent a crisis. The nurse can explain what to expect and give the couple a chance to prepare themselves for the event. Husbands need to know that wives may become more irritable and have changes in their eating and sexual desires. If the couple is prepared for these changes, there is less danger of viewing these signs as crises when and if they occur.

The nurse assists the patient with grief. By allowing him to express feelings appropriate to each phase in the grief process, the nurse decreases the possibility of delayed grief reactions or later unresolved losses.

When the mother of young children is hospitalized, one of the needs assessed by the nurse is homemaker assistance. Also, the nurse determines whether it is necessary to refer a public health nurse for a home visit to help the family deal with the separation.

The nurse observes for and assesses normal growth and development disturbances. The nurse in the well or sick baby clinic or maternity ward observes the mother-infant relationship. Questions the nurse considers are: Does the mother handle her baby like an object? Does the mother handle the baby at all? Does the mother need to be taught how to relate to the baby? Does the mother need help to express her thoughts and feelings about being a mother?

All children have at least some signs of mental or interpersonal disturbance during one or more growth and development periods. When assessing disturbances of normal growth and development, the nurse realizes that these disturbances may be safety valves that allow the stressful effects of growth and development to be handled. It is the consistent inability to function — not a brief disturbance — that requires the attention and concern of the nurse in preventing crises.

The student or new graduate nurse functions more as an observer and recorder in the field of preventive crises. With supervision and added experience, the nurse can move into more active prevention. Figure 8-7, page 124, summarizes preventive nursing intervention in crisis.

BLOCKS TO CRISIS INTERVENTION

There are two major blocks to the nurse's ability to assist the patient with crises. The first block is the nurse's closeness to the patient. The second block is the structure of many hospital systems.

The Nurse's Closeness to the Patient

Because the nurse is close to the patient, the nurse is quite vulnerable to crisis situations. The nurse's vulnerability is seen when the patient's problems stimulate memories of the nurse's present or past difficulties. For example, if the nurse's father has just died and the nurse is assigned to care for a dying patient, she may be less helpful to that patient because of her own unresolved grief.

Intervention Area	Preventive Nurse Behavior
Need for information	Prepare new parents for expected changes.
	Refer clients to discussion groups centering around their role changes, e.g., preretirement group, ostomy group, multiple sclerosis group.
	Talk with mother whose child will enter school soon.
Grief Work	Accept patient's feelings of loss.
	Let patient know nurse is available to talk with about his loss.
	Talk with family of dying patient.
	Prior to surgery, talk with patient about his thoughts, feelings, and expected changes.
Meaning of Hospitalization to Family	Consult with hospitalized mother about her family's needs.
	Make referral to public health nurse or home-maker service if necessary.
Growth and Development Disturbances	Counsel parents about the effects of over-protectiveness and underprotectiveness.
	Observe for consistent (not one-time) disturbance in child and teach parents to do the same.

Fig. 8-7 Examples of nursing interventions to prevent crises

The Hospital Structure

The physician has the greater power and status in most hospitals; the hospital board is made up primarily of physicians. Nurses in leadership positions often do not give direct patient care and are responsible to the hospital board. Since doctors do not often view the nurse's talking with patients as valuable, crisis intervention (which usually involves talking) is not usually valued by doctors or nurses in leadership positions.

From a crisis view, the patient who complains or presents many interpersonal problems for the staff is the one who is experiencing the greatest situational crisis. From a hospital-focused view, the patient who complains too much may be seen as too much trouble; resolving the problem becomes a circumstance to be avoided, rather than a challenge to be attempted. Because of the hospital structure, then, crisis intervention by the nurse is not always appreciated.

The nurse who attempts to be useful to patients by using crisis intervention risks being viewed as "different" or as not part of the high status group. Hopefully, this situation can be remedied if enough nurses persist in their attempts to give comprehensive care.

SUMMARY

The nurse has special characteristics that make her especially suited for crisis work. Crisis assessment by the nurse includes evaluating the following areas: the focus on the crisis through communication and anxiety level, coping devices, significant other people, potential for suicide or homicide, perception of crisis significance, and personal strengths.

Crisis intervention work is an attempt to support the strengths of the patient. Major interventions for crisis include methods of communication and prevention. The nurse needs to be aware of her own vulnerability to patient problems and/or the hospital structure.

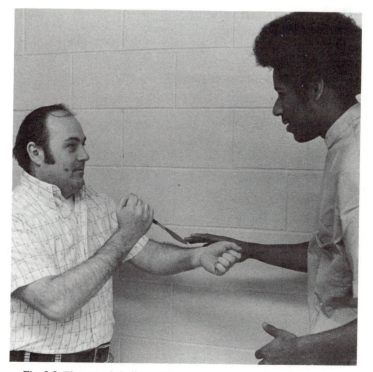

Fig. 8-8 The nurse is indispensable in crisis assessment and intervention.

ACTIVITIES AND DISCUSSION TOPICS

- Visit a community mental health center, a walk-in clinic, emergency room, or suicide prevention center. Talk with a nurse there about how he or she works with crises.

- Make a list of possible strengths a patient might have. Try to become more aware of patient strengths and health as well as patient difficulties and illness.

- Become familiar with professional and nonprofessional resources in your community. Search out at least five of the resources below and find out what services each could offer in crisis intervention. Share your findings.

  a. Suicide prevention center

  b. Self-help group

  c. Professional or nonprofessional service for patients in their home

  d. Discussion or activity group for the disabled

  e. Red Cross

  f. Voluntary ambulance squad

  g. Senior Citizen's group

  h. Police department

  i. Block association or tenant's group

  j. Liberation group such as NOW or Gay Liberation.

- Make a list of crises a patient might experience that you would be especially vulnerable to. Try to think of ways to decrease your vulnerability.

REVIEW

A. Multiple Choice. Select the best answer(s). Some questions have more than one answer.

   1. Useful ways to communicate during crisis are:

      a. Encouraging patient expression of feeling.

      b. Giving long, detailed explanations of future experiences.

      c. Exploring available resources to solve the problem.

      d. Conveying that the patient is responsible for decisions.

      e. Interrupting patient's rapid flow of speech.

      f. Asking patient to restate the problem.

2. The nurse may suspect that a crisis situation exists if the patient
   a. blows one detail of a situation out of proportion.
   b. has a restless night.
   c. jumps from one topic of conversation to another.
   d. shows no feeling in response to a stressful situation.
   e. changes the environment when it is not conducive to his own welfare.

3. Conveying an interested, nonjudgmental concern through remaining physically and emotionally present with a patient is
   a. somatization.   c. emotional support.
   b. projection.   d. role playing.

4. Suicide attempts are more likely to occur when
   a. a person is in deep depression.
   b. a depression is lifting.
   c. the person is over 44 and black.
   d. the person is under age 50 and white.

5. The nurse conveys to the patient that she is there and is concerned through
   a. calm voice tone and attentive body posture.
   b. short concise sentences.
   c. detailed descriptions of future events.
   d. siding with the patient when a disagreement occurs within his family.

B. Match the crisis assessment area in Column I with the appropriate crisis assessment question in Column II.

Column I

1. Focus on the crisis
2. Coping devices
3. Significant other people
4. Suicide or homicide potential
5. Patient perception of crisis significance

Column II

a. "What do you think would make you feel better?"

b. "What activities is your crisis affecting?"

c. "What happened right before you felt upset?"

d. "Who do you live with?"

e. "Are you thinking of killing yourself?"

C.   Briefly answer the following questions.

   1.   State three reasons the nurse is especially useful in crisis work.

   2.   Name three preventative measures for averting a crisis.

   3.   Name two blocks to the nurse's crisis intervention efforts.

chapter 9
DYNAMICS OF PAIN

STUDENT OBJECTIVES

- State two purposes of pain.
- Identify how interpersonal development is related to pain response.
- List four causes of pain.
- Identify five types of pain.
- Identify how perception influences the experience of pain.

Pain evolved as a protective device; it alerts people that danger or harm is near. Pain tells people to remove their hands from fire and not to walk on sore feet. Some people have impaired pain responses due to hereditary or acquired causes. They may create further bodily damage by walking on a broken leg or not removing their bodies from danger. Some pain, then, is useful. Pain is a symptom that alerts the patient and nurse that a need is not being met.

Although pain has a biologic or protective purpose, it may also have a communicative purpose. The patient may be trying to say something besides, "I am in pain." Perhaps the patient who complains of pain is also saying, "I need help" or "I am angry" or "Pain is the only way I allow myself to be dependent on others."

DEVELOPMENT OF PAIN RESPONSE

Response to pain has mental, physical, social and cultural components. The basic physiological response of removing a foot or arm from danger is modified at an early age by learning. Very early in life, the infant is probably unable to tell the difference between pain and anxiety. Pain arises out of a physical need; anxiety arises out of helplessness or vague discomfort. Very young infants probably can't tell whether they are anxious or need physical attention.

Since infants are helpless, they depend on significant other people such as parents to meet their needs. Pleasure and pain become associated with interactions with significant other people. If significant others pay heed to a child's hurts and complaints, there is more likelihood the child will continue to complain. If significant others do not pay attention to minor hurts of the child, the child is less likely to continue to complain of pain.

Pain and anxiety continue to be closely related in later years. For example, anxious people are apt to have a tense musculature because chronic anxiety creates ongoing stimulation to muscles. Ongoing stimulation to muscles can create pain as circulation to that area is decreased. Muscles and other body organs, then, can express feelings of anxiety. In many patients, physical pain is substituted for mental pain. This may be because physical pain is more acceptable to the patient or nurse. The patient may express mental or physical pain — both kinds are real to the patient. The nurse should never tell the patient that his pain is imaginary just because it is mental pain. Nurses who are prone to assume that mental pain is imaginary need to examine their own biases about pain.

Early in childhood, repeated exposure to pain or graded exposure to pain with emotional support from a significant other person can lead to a greater tolerance for pain. Likewise graded exposure to pain with emotional support from the nurse can help the patient to a greater tolerance for pain.

Cultural responses are varied and influence one's response to pain. In some cultural groups, children learn early that pain is to be complained about loudly. Other cultural groups are more likely to teach their children that pain should be borne in silence without complaint. The nurse is cautioned not to assume that all persons from a certain cultural group will react in the same way since the group is only one of the influences on pain response. Figure 9-1 shows factors that influence the development of pain response.

CAUSES OF PAIN

Some basic sources which are more likely to produce pain are (1) chemical, (2) mechanical, (3) thermal, and (4) psychogenic. It is important to remember that the perception of the injury may be just as important as the amount of cell or tissue destruction.

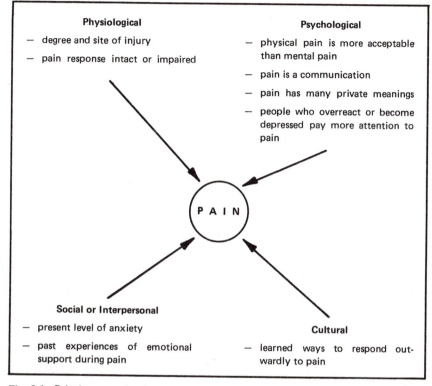

Fig. 9-1 Pain is a complex interaction of physiological, psychological, interpersonal and cultural factors.

Chemical Injury

Stimulation of free sensory nerve endings can produce pain. For example, a drop of acid or other irritating substance on the skin triggers the cells to release irritating body chemicals in reaction to the injury. These irritating substances, in turn, can also create pain.

When waste products of body metabolism accumulate in the body, pain can result. For example, running a long distance makes heavy demands on the muscles of the legs. The increase in metabolism results in increased output of lactic acid which accumulates in the leg muscles. After the run, ischemia can occur. *Ischemia* is localized tissue anemia due to the obstruction of the inflow of arterial blood. Pain can result from the ischemia as well as from the triggering of irritating chemicals from the cells. Chemical injury, then, is often twofold: pain can be caused by the chemical substance itself and by the cellular release of other chemical irritants which react to the irritant.

Mechanical Injury

Pain can be due to purely physical force. A hit in the jaw or a spanking can create pain. Pressure on nerve endings followed by the release of chemical irritants by the damaged cells causes the pain.

Mechanical pain can also result from the stretching or contracting of body tissues; this irritates nerve endings and leads to local ischemia due to some blocked blood vessels. Constriction of muscle fibers in blood vessels can also be responsible for pain. For example, in the muscle spasm of lower back pain, some pain is probably due to the constriction of small blood vessels and local ischemia.

Continued pressure on any body part such as sitting or lying in one position for long periods of time causes pressure on nerve endings and local ischemia. Well people change position frequently because of a conditioned response to the sensation of pressure. People with impaired pain perception (such as those who are paralyzed or unconscious) may not perceive this type of pain. Because this is so, nurses turn paralyzed or unconscious patients frequently to avoid ischemia and prevent pressure sores.

Thermal Injury

Extreme heat or cold damages body tissue. Minor burns create pain due to irritation and damage to nerve endings. As in the other types of injury mentioned, the pain is caused when irritating chemical substances are released from the injured cells. Because nurses frequently use heat in nursing techniques, they must be careful to protect the patient from thermal injury due to excessive heat.

Frostbite is an example of thermal injury due to extreme cold. Extreme cold cuts off the blood supply to an area by constricting or closing off the blood vessels. Nurses use applications of cold as treatment for some patients. It is important to be careful with extreme cold since pain is not always experienced by the patient until blood flow returns.

Psychogenic Influence

Once pain has been experienced in one of the ways described, the thought alone can trigger the pain. *Psychogenic pain* is a term used to describe expressions of pain where the observer can find no evidence of tissue damage. In psychogenic pain, a memory, thought, or feeling probably triggers or intensifies pain. Probably no pain is strictly physical or strictly psychogenic. It seems logical to think of all pain as an interaction where psychological, physical, interpersonal and cultural elements play a part in varying degrees.

Depression is one cause of psychogenic pain. Chronic headaches and vague complaints of pain are sometimes due to an underlying depression. This seems to occur more often in middle and older age. Some postoperative pain can also result from a depressed state. People who have developed styles of living that are characterized by an inclination to withdraw from stress, to turn anger inward, to feel helpless rather than challenged, and to dwell on body functioning are perhaps more likely to experience depression as pain.

People whose life-style is one of brief overreactions to events, of dramatic impulsiveness and helplessness may also have frequent reports of pain without organic or tissue damage. Because these people are set to overreact in general, they may also respond to organic pain in a more intense fashion. Figure 9-2 summarizes possible causes of pain.

The many aches and pains signalled by the body daily are ignored by many because attention is focused elsewhere. Soldiers in battle, firemen, and policemen may continue to fight even though they are seriously injured.

In many situations, people intensely focus on the inner body functions; they are more susceptible to body aches and pains. People with depressed living

SOURCE	EXAMPLES
Chemical injury	acid on the skin irritating materials accumulation of waste products chemicals released by cells after their damage ischemia
Mechanical injury	hitting a thumb with a hammer injection of medication spanking overeating muscle spasm sitting, lying or standing in one position too long
Thermal injury	burns frostbite
Psychogenic influence	depression overreaction to or overfocus on internal body events anxiety memories

Fig. 9-2 Pain can be triggered by a number of sources.

styles think and talk more often about their body functions. Anxiety, worry, and close attention to body functioning can result in exaggeration of body pain.

Individuals develop private meanings for pain. This is especially true of psychogenic pain. Therefore, it should not be assumed that pain in a certain body region has the same meaning for each patient. Chest pain which is unrelated to heart malfunction can elicit fears of heart attacks in some patients. Chronic headache can take on a special meaning too. A patient may interpret his headaches as a sign of a brain tumor. In general, behind the complaint of pain which has no organic basis is the patient's idea of its cause. Even when pain has an organic cause the patient may wonder why he has the pain now.

His perception of the meaning and cause for pain influences how the patient will react. Some people consider pain to be a punishment for earlier misbehavior and may bear pain silently without complaint. Others think pain is unjustified and may be angry at persons around them. Still others associate pain with inability to function at all. All of these people may become quite dependent and demanding because they feel helpless.

TYPES OF PAIN

Pain can be classified as superficial, deep, or central pain. Pain may be described in different terms, figure 9-3. The nurse may use one set of terms to describe pain, while the patient may use his own words to talk about the pain he feels.

TYPE	ARISES FROM	SOMETIMES DESCRIBED BY THE PATIENT AS:
Superficial or Cutaneous	skin or mucous membranes	pricking dull burning
Deep	bones and joints	dull aching
	muscles	sharp
	heart	viselike
	stomach and intestines	cramping gnawing burning
Central	memory or injury to sensory nerves	gnawing burning crushing nasty

Fig. 9-3 Types of pain and its descriptions

Superficial Pain

Superficial or *cutaneous pain* arises from the skin or mucous membranes of the body. Superficial pain may originate in the skin itself or in the mucous membrane which lines the canals and body cavities. Examples of mucous membrane cavities and canals are the nostrils, vagina, rectum, and mouth. The source of superficial or cutaneous pain can be located more accurately because it arises near the body surface where there are many nerve endings.

Superficial pain can be severe when the affected skin surfaces or mucous membranes are inflamed. When these surfaces are engorged with blood, they are much more sensitive to stimulation. The touch of a sheet, a quick movement of the bed, or even a loud noise can lead to increased pain. Nurses need to be aware of this sensitivity when caring for patients with superficial pain.

Superficial pain can be described as pricking, dull or burning. When caring for patients who do not complain of pain, the severe pain can be noted by the increase in blood pressure, perspiration, and muscle tension.

Deep Pain

Deep pain occurs in the inner body structures such as muscles, joints, tendons, and connective tissues (fascia). Deep pain is often due to ischemia, stretching or spasm. Patients who have had their muscles and fascia manipulated during surgery may complain of deep pain. Patients who have arthritis or rheumatism may complain of deep pain. Pain in bones is often described as dull or aching and is fairly easy to pinpoint by the patient.

Pain that is deep and severe can occur when there is a failure in homeostasis. Such failures in homeostasis can lead to nausea, vomiting, weakness, increased perspiration and a drop in blood pressure. These signs and symptoms can be observed in patients who have heart, abdominal or kidney conditions and are experiencing severe deep pain. CAUTION: Observation of sudden vomiting, drop in blood pressure and weakness should be reported immediately to a nursing instructor and/or the nurse in charge.

The source of deep pain may be difficult for the patient to identify. This difficulty occurs because (1) pain messages from the skin and inner body areas may use the same nerve pathways and (2) internal body structures have fewer nerve endings than the skin or mucous membranes. Because the brain does not receive well-defined messages, the source of pain may be identified as being elsewhere than its actual location. *Referred pain* is pain that has a source in one area but is felt or experienced in another area. For example, pain which radiates down the arm may be referred pain; the heart is the source of pain that is felt in the neck or left arm.

Pain in the stomach or intestine may be described as cramping, gnawing, or burning. Pain around the heart is often said to be viselike.

Central Pain

Central pain is pain which does not have an external stimulus. It may be due to an injury to sensory nerves or to a persistent memory that at one time a certain body area was painful. An example of central pain is phantom pain; it may be felt by a patient who has had a limb amputated. The patient has a stable body image of being whole. So enduring is this body image that patients who have had a leg amputation experience pain below the point of amputation and may continue to think of themselves as having two legs. Phantom pain is a complex interaction of psychological and physiological forces.

PATIENT'S DESCRIPTION OF PAIN

Patients may describe pain in many different ways. The way patients describe their pain may give the nurse a clue about what meaning the pain has for each patient. For example, patients who describe pain as "mean" may think they are being punished by the pain. Although patients have private meanings for their pain, it is unwise for the nurse to assume the private meaning is known by the patient. The nurse should check with the patient to see if he knows the meaning of his description of pain. For example, the patient who describes pain as "mean" might be asked, "In what way is your pain mean?" or "I wonder why you picked "mean" to describe your pain?"

The patient's description of pain should always be written in his own words and placed in quotation marks. The patient's own words will be the most useful to other nurses and health personnel. Attempting to interpret what the patient might mean often results in the introduction of the nurse's own biases and meaning for pain.

Some patients report warnings before the actual pain occurs. Increased restlessness, tremor, anxiety, and physical symptoms such as diarrhea are often reported as warnings of pain.

PERCEPTION AND THE PAIN EXPERIENCE

In order to perceive pain, the sensory nerves, sensory tracts in the spinal cord, and the thalamus as well as the cerebral cortex must all be in working order. A patient who has a spinal cord injury and is paralyzed below the waist because of injury to the sensory tracts will not feel pain below the waist.

Even if all parts of the sensory apparatus are in working order, the interpretation of pain can change the perception of pain. Pain is interpreted in the cerebral cortex of the brain; therefore, the person's individual history of pain, his present state of mind, and the response of others to his pain can alter the patient's perception of pain. Chapter 14 will consider in more depth how past and present experiences as well as expectations influence perception.

RESPONSE TO PAIN

Response to pain is a complex interaction of internal environmental processes and external environmental processes. Since pain response is such a complex process, it may be difficult for the nurse to account for the factors that are most influential. Despite this complexity, the nurse should consider all the factors when evaluating patient responses to pain, figure 9-4.

Internal Environmental Processes

Pain is a protective device signalling threat or danger. The internal environment of the person reacts to ward off the danger. Blood pressure and muscle tension are increased as blood is shunted away from the skin and digestive system and towards the muscles that move the body. Appetite decreases and diarrhea or urination may occur. These reactions are all part of the fight-flight response that occurs when a person is threatened by danger. The fight-flight

INTERNAL ENVIRONMENTAL PROCESS CONSIDERATIONS	EXTERNAL ENVIRONMENTAL PROCESS CONSIDERATIONS
Is there a change in the patient's blood pressure?	Is the patient restless?
Is the patient's pulse strong or weak?	Is the patient from a cultural group or family that teaches its members to bear pain in silence?
Has the patient's appetite changed?	
Is the patient suffering from diarrhea or frequent urination?	Is the patient from a cultural group that teaches its members to groan, cry, and tell others about their pain?
Is the patient tired or weak?	
Is the patient in a high state of anxiety or fear?	Is the nurse responding to the patient's pain with biased expectations about how patients in pain should behave?
Does the patient seem to deny, suppress, or project pain?	

Fig. 9-4 The nurse considers both internal and external environmental processes in evaluating response to pain.

response evolved early in human development. Fighting the pain or trying to escape from it are still used by people but these attempts are not always effective in reducing pain.

Patients who are experiencing severe pain may not be able to maintain balance in the internal environment. Signs such as a drop in blood pressure, a slow and weak pulse, and unconsciousness may occur.

Reactions to pain can be influenced by physical condition. Patients who are tired or weakened physically may react to minimal pain with a very strong response. Painful procedures should be scheduled for periods when the patient has rested and feels stronger.

Emotional state can also influence reaction to pain. Anxiety and fear intensify pain. The same is true conversely; that is, pain will intensify anxiety and fear. Both pain and anxiety (or fear) evoke an alarm reaction in people. If one or both of these sources of alarm are removed, homeostasis may be maintained. On the other hand, very strong fear or anxiety will sometimes block out pain, especially in life-threatening situations. As stated, the patient's interpretation of the pain can also influence the way he reacts; he may respond with anger, guilt, or helplessness. Attempts to cope with pain include defense mechanisms such as denial, suppression and projection.

External Environmental Processes

Irritability, restlessness and insomnia may be experienced by the patient in pain. Restlessness may be an attempt to restore homeostasis by maintaining freedom of movement. These covert signs or observable patient responses may be more informative about the patient's pain than overt signs such as statements by the patient. This is because people have been taught to respond to pain in different ways. Some individuals have learned to bear the pain in silence. Such behavior might be admired by others, including the nurse, since it creates less difficulty for them.

Other patients may react to pain with groans, crying, screaming or thrashing about in bed. Such behavior is often less admired by others, including the nurse, even though the response may be acceptable and useful to the patient.

SUMMARY

Pain evolved as a protective device but it also has a communicative purpose. Pain and anxiety are closely related. Different cultural groups teach their members to show different responses to pain. Pain can be set off by chemical, mechanical, thermal or psychogenic sources. Pain can be classified by the nurse

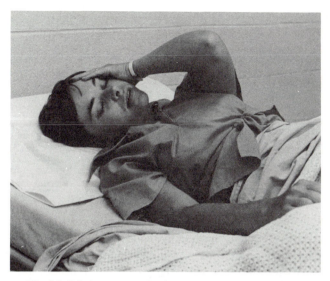

Fig. 9-5 Pain is a communicative as well as a protective device.

as superficial, deep, or central. Patients may use their own terms to describe their pain. Patients' descriptions of pain are important clues to the meaning of pain to them and should be quoted as stated by the patient without adding the nurse's interpretation or bias.

Pain perception includes both physiological and psychological factors. Response to pain is a complex interaction of internal and external environmental processes. All these factors need to be considered by the nurse. The nurse also needs to consider her own reactions to patients in pain.

ACTIVITIES AND DISCUSSION TOPICS

- Write down family or cultural patterns you have learned to follow when in pain. Examine possible biases you may have about response to pain. Be aware of the personal biases to avoid when you care for patients in pain.

- Try to discover your own private meaning for pain by remembering a painful experience and asking yourself the following questions:
  a. Did I feel I was being punished by the pain?
  b. Did I feel the pain was unjustified?
  c. Did I feel angry at unjustified pain?
  d. Did I become demanding of others and feel helpless?

- Talk with several of your classmates. Ask them to describe their pain experiences. Practice writing their descriptions, using quotation marks around their exact words.

- Make a list of patient situations that could influence pain perception.

REVIEW

A. Multiple Choice. Select the best answer(s). Some questions have more than one answer.

1. The statements that accurately state the relationship between perception and the experience of pain are:
   a. Pain is perceived in paralyzed body areas.
   b. To perceive pain, the sensory nerves, nerve tracts, thalamus and cerebral cortex must be in working order.
   c. Pain perception and how pain is experienced can be altered by past and present experiences.
   d. The cerebral cortex can override the thalamus' perception of pain.

2. Factors that influence patient response to pain are
   a. emotional state. c. learned behaviors.
   b. severity of pain. d. physical condition.

3. The statement that identifies how interpersonal development is related to pain response is:
   a. In early infancy, pain and anxiety are not differentiated.
   b. There is no relationship between pain response and interpersonal development.
   c. All people learn the same tolerance for pain.
   d. Learned, cultural responses to pain are pretty much the same in all people.

4. If a patient complains of deep pain, the pain may be in the
   a. mucous membranes. c. skin.
   b. sensory nerves. d. muscles.

5. An external environmental process the nurse can observe to suspect the patient is in pain is
   a. change in the patient's blood pressure.
   b. patient's pulse is weak.
   c. patient is restless.
   d. patient feels anxious.

B. Match the types of pain in Column II to their definition in Column I.

Column I

1. Pain felt in a limb although that limb has previously been amputated.

2. Pain experienced when joints, tendons and fáscia have been injured.

3. Pain that arises from the skin or mucous membranes of the body.

4. Pain that has a source in one area but is felt in another area.

5. A symptom that alerts people that a need is not being met.

6. Pain when the observer can find no evidence of tissue damage.

Column II

a. deep pain
b. pain
c. phantom pain
d. psychogenic pain
e. referred pain
f. superficial pain

C. Briefly answer the following questions.

1. What are the two purposes of pain?

2. Name four causes of pain.

3. What is ischemia?

4. What is the difference between pain and anxiety?

chapter 10
PAIN ASSESSMENT
AND INTERVENTION

STUDENT OBJECTIVES

- List eleven areas to assess with patients in pain.
- List five interpersonal nursing interventions in pain.
- Identify six examples of nursing interventions for pain.
- List four areas of nursing evaluation after pain intervention.

Pain is one of the most common reasons people seek help. Because pain is an experience faced by both nurse and patient, assessing and intervening in pain is a major nursing process.

PAIN ASSESSMENT

An accurate assessment of pain includes the use of observational and communication skills. The nurse watches and talks with the patient to gain information upon which to base nursing intervention. Some of the points to be covered are:

- Type and intensity of pain
- Physiological and behavioral clues
- Location of pain
- Onset and duration
- Previous experience with this type of pain
- Relationship of pain to other circumstances

- Cause and meaning of pain for the patient
- Effect on body image
- Level of anxiety
- Communicative purpose of pain
- Patient's attempt to relieve this pain

It may not be possible to gather complete information about all of the above points. However, the nurse should attempt to gather as much information about the patient's pain as is possible. This provides a broader base for assessing the needs and deciding on a nursing action or intervention.

Type and Intensity of Pain

If the patient has difficulty describing his pain, the nurse can help him by asking direct questions such as, "What does the pain feel like?" or "Use your own words to tell me what your pain is like." When describing pain, patients will most likely use terms that are familiar to them, like "splitting headache," "cutting through me" and so on.

The nurse must not ask questions like, "Is the pain sharp?" or "Does your head feel like it's being hammered on?" Such questions are called *leading questions* and may introduce ideas the patient has not thought of; this results in obtaining incorrect information from the patient. Also, leading questions tend to place the nurse in the position of second-guessing the patient. Questions that can be answered by yes or no should also be avoided. Frequently, these questions are answered more by the patient's tendency to answer most questions "yes" or most questions "no," and not whether the answer is or is not correct. For example, people who are depressed are likely to answer *no* to most questions they are asked.

Changes in intensity of pain can be significant indicators of the patient's need for assistance in maintaining homeostasis. For example, abrupt, sharp pain may indicate a recent change in the patient's internal environmental condition. Such abrupt, sharp pains should be reported to the nursing instructor or nurse in charge.

Physiological and Behavioral Clues

Some patients may give inaccurate verbal descriptions of their pain because of social or cultural experiences. Because this is so, the nurse must compare the verbal description of pain with the nonverbal clues. Nonverbal clues are less influenced by conscious will and may provide a better baseline for what is happening with the patient. At the time of pain, the nurse can take the patient's pulse, respiration and blood pressure and compare them with measurements taken prior to the pain complaint. These vital signs frequently show internal environmental changes. Excessive perspiration, complaints of nausea and vomiting, changes in skin color, restlessness, and increase in muscle tension are nonverbal clues used to assess pain.

Location of Pain

Another aspect of pain assessment is determining the location or site of the pain. Superficial pain in the skin and mucous membranes may be easily pinpointed by the patient. Deep and central pain may be more difficult for the patient to localize.

If the patient cannot describe the location of the pain, the patient can be asked to "point to where you feel the pain." The nurse can determine whether the patient's complaint is valid from his attempt to locate the pain. For example, after abdominal surgery, complaints of deep pain, which may or may not be referred to other body areas, would be expected. If a patient has had a thumb amputation, however, complaints of abdominal pain would be unexpected and would require further examination; the results of this exploration must be shared with other members of the team.

Onset and Duration

To determine the onset and duration of pain, the nurse observes when pain began and how long it lasted. When considering the time of onset it must be determined whether the pain is constant or intermittent. Pain that is not constant, but rather comes and goes is called *intermittent pain.* The *onset* is the first time the patient experiences the pain. This onset is especially important when taking a nursing history and in helping to diagnose the patient's condition. A patient with intermittent pain experiences periods of pain followed by absence of pain. The onset or periods when the pain starts must be known, as well as the length of time it persists. For example, a woman in labor may have irregular uterine contractions that become more regular and more painful. When the nurse knows the onset and duration of labor contractions, she can anticipate the approximate time of delivery.

The nurse notes nonverbal signs of the onset and duration of pain. She also uses questions to assess the onset and duration of pain. Examples of questions used include: "When did the pain begin?", "How long did the pain last?" and "Is the pain continuing while we talk?"

Previous Experience With Similar Pain

The patient may have had similar pain before this experience. Examples of questions to elicit information are: "Did you ever have pain like this before?", and "When did you have pain like this?"

While discussing any previous experience with the same type of pain, the nurse also inquires about the measures that provided relief from the pain. Examples of questions to ask about pain relief include: "What did you do to relieve the pain then?", "What helped to stop the pain?" and "What method did you use to decrease your pain?"

The patient may misinterpret the nurse's attempts to assist with pain due to past experiences with nurses or doctors when in pain. He may see the nurse in a variety of roles that may or may not reflect how the nurse really acts. The patient may see the nurse as:

- a controller who has power to deny or relieve pain.
- a communicator who tells others about his pain.
- an informant who cannot be trusted with the details of his pain.
- a judge who is more concerned about deciding if the pain is reasonable or timely than in relieving it.
- an avoider who limits his complaints of pain.
- a bargainer who gives pain relief in return for his good behavior.

The nurse should assess (1) how the patient perceives the nurse's role and (2) her own biases and stereotypes about patient pain.

Relation of Pain to Other Circumstances

Certain events and circumstances may affect the intensity of pain: the time of day, exertion, anxiety, noise, food, position in bed, and interpersonal situations. The nurse inquires about things that may have preceded the pain. Questions to elicit this type of information might include: "What was going on just before you noticed your headache?", "What time of day is your pain worse?", "Is your pain less in the morning or at night?", "How does noise affect your pain?", "What foods affect your pain?", "How does being with your family affect your pain?" and "In what position are you most comfortable?"

Cause and Meaning of Pain

Perception of the cause and meaning of pain may be assessed by examining how the patient describes it. As the nurse listens, it may become evident that:

the patient feels the pain is a punishment that is justified or unjustified; it is taken as a signal to become more dependent and demanding, or the patient thinks pain is to be borne silently.

The patient verbally communicates what the pain means to him by the words he selects to describe it; the tone of voice and facial expression also communicate his feelings. Based on knowledge and understanding of human behavior, the nurse studies the patient and his statements for unexpressed reactions. If the nurse senses that the pain has special meaning, she can develop this further; "You seem concerned about this pain. What do you think the pain means?"

Effect on Body Image

Pain can distort body image. Patients may express the distortion by statements such as "I feel unreal" or "I feel beside myself with pain."

Body image is developed from childhood, based on the child's exploration of his body, hearing the comments of others, and developing competence in the use of certain body parts. Threats to the body image can affect the amount of pain experienced; threats that affect occupational, sexual, or social roles can raise anxiety level and intensify pain. Based on knowledge of body image and its effect on pain, the nurse should be able to assess the pain of those who have had mutilating injuries or amputation with more understanding.

Level of Anxiety

Pain and anxiety are closely related from early infancy and continue to influence each other throughout the life cycle. If the anxiety level is low, the patient may appear calm, and musculature is relaxed when awake or asleep. When anxiety is increasing, the patient may show signs of restlessness, tense musculature, heavy perspiration, disconnected speech, exaggerated response to small detail, decreased eye contact, anger, and physical symptoms such as diarrhea. High levels of anxiety can intensify pain and, conversely, high levels of pain can intensify anxiety.

Communicative Purpose of Pain

The nurse tries to determine what else, besides pain, the patient may be communicating. There are other needs besides the obvious comfort and rest. The patient may be complaining of pain as a way of communicating a message like: "I need help," "I am angry," or "Pain is the only way I allow myself to be dependent on others."

If the nurse has already determined that the patient is rested and relatively comfortable, complaints of pain can be explored further. Examples of questions to ask are: "You seem rested. I wonder if there is something other than pain that is bothering you?", "I wonder if you're trying to tell me about something more besides your pain?" or "Is there something else you want to discuss?"

Patient Attempts to Relieve Pain

The nurse assesses the patient's competence in coping with his own pain. Many patients develop their own methods, and the nurse can learn new methods of intervention by carefully listening to patients' reports of how they cope with pain.

Patients may report that breathing exercises, purposeful diversion, certain body positions, or movements such as pacing, rocking, pounding, and rubbing decrease pain. A common response to pain is concentration on some factor; patients may count objects in their rooms or repeat phrases or words such as "It's almost over," "I can take this," or "Please, nurse." These words or phrases may be repeated over and over until the pain decreases. Another attempt by patients is to deliberately visualize themselves in other future situations.

Patients may try to distract themselves from their pain by talking with others, smoking, or asking others to read or do activities with them. Some people find comfort in having a roommate with whom to share pain experiences. Others may hide their real suffering from another sick person. The nurse realizes each patient is unique in his attempts to cope with pain. She tries to support and encourage constructive attempts to relieve pain. Figure 10-1, pages 148 and 149, shows areas of nursing assessment.

PAIN INTERVENTION

The nurse works together with the patient to determine what part she will play in pain relief and what part the patient will play. As in other nursing interventions, the nurse encourages the patient to assist with as much of his care as possible. Pain intervention includes both interpersonal actions and physical medications and treatments.

Interpersonal Actions

Nurses often assume that pain medication is the only way to deal with pain. There are many other nursing actions which have been shown to be effective

Area	Assessments
Type and intensity of pain	Listens to patient's words used to describe pain. Observes for abrupt, sharp pain. Asks direct questions such as: "What does the pain feel like?" or "Use your own words to tell me what your pain is like."
Physiological and behavioral clues to pain	Takes pulse, respiration, blood pressure. Compares measurements of pulse, respiration and B/P with those prior to pain. Observes for excessive perspiration, nausea and vomiting, changes in skin color, muscle tension and restlessness.
Location of pain	Asks patient to describe where pain is felt. Asks patient to point to location where pain is experienced. Determines if pain reported in area of location is to be expected.
Onset and duration of pain	Observes nonverbal behavior of patient to see when pain occurs. Asks direct questions such as "When did the pain begin?" and "How long did the pain last?" and "Are you having pain now?"
Previous experience with this type of pain	Asks direct questions such as: (1) "Did you have pain like this before?" or "When did you have pain like this?" (2) "What happened to you when you were in the pain?" (3) "What helped to relieve the pain?"
Relation of pain to other circumstances	Observes how pain changes in relation to time of day, exertion, anxiety, noise, food, position in bed and interpersonal situations. Asks questions like: (1) "What else was happening when you noticed your pain?" (2) "What time of day is your pain worst?" (3) "How does activity affect your pain?" "How does noise affect your pain? "How does being with your family affect your pain?" "In what position are you most comfortable in bed?"
Cause and meaning of pain	Listens for patient's meaning for pain (Punishment? Justified? Signal an emergency? Signal dependency? Expected to be borne in silence?) Observes if patient misinterprets attempts to assist. Asks questions like: "What do you think the pain means?"

Fig. 10-1 Nursing assessment with patient pain (continued)

Effect on body image	Listens to statements describing pain that may indicate distortion in body image. Observes for body image effects particularly in patients who have had mutilating injuries or amputations.
Level of anxiety	Observes for indications of increasing anxiety such as restlessness, tense musculature, heavy perspiration, disconnected speech, exaggeration of small detail, decreased eye contact, anger or physical symptoms.
Communicative purpose	Determines whether patient is communicating other needs besides those for comfort and rest.
Attempts to relieve pain	Listens to past efforts and successes in coping with pain.

Fig. 10-1 Nursing assessment with patient pain

for relieving the patient's pain. Pain intervention includes interpersonal actions which the nurse can take such as:

- State the intention to help relieve the pain.
- Help to decrease feelings of isolation and loneliness.
- Help to decrease fear of the unknown.
- Make joint decisions with the patient about relief measures.
- Teach relaxation exercises.
- Encourage the patient to produce pleasurable mental images.
- Show recognition of the patient's attempts to control pain.

One of the most useful interventions the nurse can make for patients in pain is to state an intention to help relieve the pain. This can be stated as, "I'm here to help relieve your pain," "You and I will work together to lessen your pain," or "I want to help you with your pain."

The patient in pain can feel very lonely because others are often unable or unwilling to understand what the patient is experiencing. To help relieve some of the feelings of isolation and loneliness, the nurse must show her interest and willingness to understand. Some ways to convey understanding are (1) listen to the patient, (2) respect the patient's preferences, (3) accept the irritable or demanding patient, and (4) be physically present or available on call.

Fear of the unknown will increase anxiety. The unknown is always more frightening when left unspoken. If the nurse has any knowledge of what the patient's pain will be like or when it will end, the nurse helps to relieve some of the fear by sharing this knowledge with the patient. Being able to speak about thoughts and feelings also decreases fear of the unknown. Some questions used to explore patient thoughts and feelings include, "What are you thinking?", "What feelings are you having now?" and "I'm here to talk with you about your pain."

The nurse directs the patient's energies to a discussion and thereby frees the energy which was bound up in the pain experience. After thoughts and feelings about pain and the unknown have been discussed, the nurse can direct a nurse-patient discussion toward analysis of the pain situation and toward joint decisions about ways to handle pain constructively.

Such discussions are initiated by the nurse not only after the patient has experienced pain, but also before anticipated pain occurs (such as surgical pain). In this way, the nurse and patient may deal with pain more constructively when it actually occurs.

Early preparation is a factor to consider when relaxation exercises are to be undertaken. The nurse can teach the patient how to deep breathe and relax before the pain experience takes place. Later, when pain occurs, the patient concentrates on the breathing and relaxation of body parts, and directs her energy toward this effort. Participants in natural childbirth classes are usually prepared in this method. A form of these relaxation exercises may be used preoperatively to decrease patient pain. They can also be used in tension-related problems such as headache.

Patients can be taught to produce mental pictures of pleasurable activities. Again, prior to the pain experience, the nurse encourages the patient to select a pleasurable experience or activity and to practice producing a mental picture of it. Then, when pain begins, it will be more likely that the patient will be able to produce the mental picture.

Another interpersonal intervention is to make verbal acknowledgment of the patient's attempt to control pain. This can be stated as, "You're making a strong effort to handle your pain," or "I see you're using activity to help with the pain." Figure 10-2 summarizes interpersonal nursing interventions with pain.

Other interpersonal interventions include behavior therapy or modification, biofeedback and hypnosis. However, these interventions require additional education and specialized experience.

Physical Care and Medications

There are four major areas where physical intervention may be directed to relieve pain: positioning and support, sensory input control, medication, and other treatments.

Positioning the patient can reduce pain. There should be no wrinkles in the bedsheets and bedclothes must not restrict movement. Patients who writhe and

Interpersonal Intervention	Verbal Examples
State intention to help with pain	"I'm here to help relieve your pain."
	"I want to help you with your pain."
Help to decrease feelings of isolation and loneliness	"What are you thinking now?"
	"I'm here to talk with you about your pain."
	"I'll sit with you and perhaps you'll feel like talking later."
	"I'll be available to be with you this morning."
Help to decrease fear of the the unknown	"You will feel a sharp pinprick."
	"After this test there is a pretty good chance you'll get a headache. You can lessen that chance by lying flat in bed for 24 hours."
Make joint decisions with patient about relief measures	"Let's work together to lessen your pain."
Teach relaxation exercises	"Take a deep breath now and when you let it out, imagine all the tension going out of your body."
Teach patient to produce pleasant mental images	"Think of a pleasant scene. Practice imagining that scene and think of it when you feel pain."
Show recognition of patient's attempts to control pain	"I see you're using activity to relieve your pain."
	"You're making a strong effort to handle your pain."

Fig. 10-2 Interpersonal nursing interventions

twist about because of their pain, may need to have their beds straightened frequently throughout the day. When turning a patient in bed, painful limbs or body areas should be supported. Telling the patient exactly what is to be done, how he can assist, and whether pain is involved will make the turn less painful. This can be stated something like, "It's time to turn on your left side. There may be some pain, but you can lessen the pain by holding your sore arm up and out to the right. When I count to three, turn."

Touch can provide emotional support in addition to the physical support given, such as in turning patients. However, touch can also be misinterpreted by some and resented by others who wish to maintain independence. The nurse listens to verbal statements and watches the patient's nonverbal communication in order to assess his attitude toward touch. The wishes of the patient should be respected and only touch necessary for physical care should be given to anyone who objects to being touched.

Control of sensory input can increase or decrease pain. Backrubs and massage are not only soothing, they also provide cutaneous stimulation, figure 10-3. Skin or cutaneous stimulation may inhibit pain transmission. A patient may discover this for himself and should not be told to stop scratching, rubbing, or massaging himself unless he is aggravating a situation.

Turning the patient frequently provides cutaneous stimulation and helps to prevent further pain by decreasing ischemia. Bathing is another nursing activity that can be soothing or stimulating to cutaneous tissue. Other aids to provide physical comfort and relief from pain are: adjusting the amount of light in a room; closing the room door to decrease noise; and providing pleasurable visual stimulation such as seating the patient at a window with a nice view, keeping his favored possessions in view, and/or encouraging the review of magazines which have appealing illustrations.

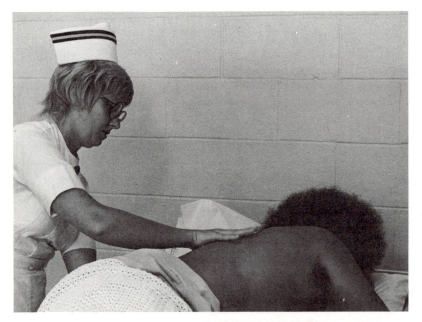

Fig. 10-3 A backrub provides cutaneous stimulation.

Social stimulation is useful for those patients who find their pain is decreased when talking with visitors or other patients. When the patient is in pain the nurse asks the patient about his preference for visitors as a way of controlling sensory input and reducing pain. Some patients prefer to be alone when in pain; they find it is draining to socialize with visitors.

Medications prescribed by the doctor can also be offered. It is important that the patient know there is a pain medication available and how often it can be given. Pain can lead to a distortion of time; patients in pain find waiting for medication a seemingly endless task. If the nurse finds pain medication does not seem to be helping, alternate measures can be discussed with the patient. Asking the head nurse to discuss the possibility of increasing the dosage or frequency of medication with the doctor may help in some cases. However, anxiety or other stress sources should also be evaluated and appropriate steps taken.

Medications often prescribed for pain include analgesics, narcotics, tranquilizers, barbiturates, and local anesthetics. The nurse's role with regard to pain medications is to:

- Know the doctor's order.

- Observe to see if the patient is in pain.

- Observe if there are any contraindications to giving the medication at that time.

- Check to determine when medication was last given to the patient.

Contraindications are conditions which forbid use of a particular treatment. For example, tranquilizers that may lower the blood pressure are contraindicated with people who have very low blood pressure already.

If pain is expected, the doctor often leaves an order for a specific medication that can be given by the nurse at stated intervals as the need arises. Such medications are referred to as *prn* medications, or medications to be given "as necessary." In deciding whether to give these medications, the nurse assesses the need of each patient as well as the drug's side effects. *Side effects* of a drug are other effects the drug may have besides the one for which the drug is prescribed.

In assessing the patient's need for medication, the nurse considers the following questions:

- Is this patient so afraid of pain that fear might be more harmful to him than the effect of the drug itself?

- Does the patient know from past experience that he has a low tolerance for pain?

- Does the patient have a negative reaction to an artificial state of well-being and so prefers some pain rather than take medication?

- Does the patient think pain indicates his condition is worsening and prefers to be under the influence of drugs most of the time?

Sometimes the doctor may order a placebo. A *placebo* is an inactive substance which is given to satisfy a demand for medication. It may be a capsule filled with sugar (glucose) or an injection of sterile water. The idea is to suggest to the patient that he is being given medication when in fact he is not. Nurses may have mixed feelings about giving any patient a placebo because they think it is not right to deceive the patient. They may feel that the patient is manipulating the staff. There is quite a bit of evidence to suggest that a large portion of the population reacts positively when a helping person tries to help a person in need. Because of this effect, it is very difficult to tell (without a controlled research study) which nursing procedures help because of the procedure itself and which help because the patient perceives he is getting aid from someone and so feels better. Since the "placebo effect" is known to occur, the nurse needs to assess and use whatever method is helpful to the patient, including the placebo.

Other treatments useful for some patients in pain are: surgical disruption of nerve impulses, electrical analgesia, acupuncture, biofeedback, and counter-irritants such as mustard plaster and liniments. None of these treatments are attempted by the nurse without special education and training. Surgical, electrical and acupuncture interventions are not nursing procedures. The nurse does use heat and cold treatments to help reduce patient pain and may use applications as prescribed by the doctor. Figure 10-4 summarizes information on physical measures nurses use to relieve pain.

PAIN EVALUATION

When working with patients in pain, the nurse not only assesses and intervenes with pain, but also evaluates how effective nursing actions have been. One form of pain evaluation is keeping a clear record of the patient's pain assessment and intervention. This record should be updated and kept current. Sometimes the Kardex is used for this record.

A second form of evaluation is the nursing conference or health team conference. When these conferences occur, information about patient pain and treatment can be shared. A third evaluation is observation of the patient. The nurse observes to see how the patient is responding to nursing actions to relieve pain. If the patient's pain is not being relieved, the nurse goes on to the fourth area of evaluation.

In the fourth area of evaluation, the nurse asks the following questions:

- Why might the patient still be in pain?

Physical Action	Examples
Positioning and Support	Straightens bedclothes. Supports painful body areas when turning patient. Asks patient to assist in turning. Evaluates patient's wish to be touched.
Sensory Input Control	Gives backrub or massage. Allows patient to massage or rub himself if not harmful. Turns patient frequently. Bathes patient or encourages patient to bathe. Shuts window blinds or curtains. Closes door to room. Provides pleasurable visual stimuli. Asks patient preference about having visitors.
Medication	Tells patient of available pain medications. Observes for early signs of pain and offers pain medication as a possible solution. Observes to see if patient's current condition contraindicates that medication. Asks patient about past experiences with medications to determine patient preferences and reactions.
Other Physical Measures	Uses heat if patient thinks it will help and there are no contraindications. Uses cold if patient thinks it will help and there are no contraindications.

Fig. 10-4 Physical nursing actions to relieve pain

- What factors in pain assessment have been missed?

- What nursing actions seem to increase patient pain?

- What nursing actions seem to decrease patient pain?

- What are realistic expectations for decreasing pain in this patient?

After completing this pain evaluation, the nurse may change the plan of care or continue on with the current plan. In some cases, it may not be possible to relieve pain; then the nurse's expectations about what can be done need to be set at a more realistic level.

SUMMARY

In pain assessment, the nurse gathers information about the patient's type and intensity of pain, physiological and behavioral clues to pain, location of pain, onset and duration of pain, previous experience with this type of pain,

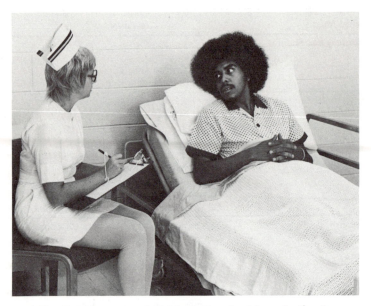

Fig. 10-5 The nurse gathers information about the patient's pain.

relationship of pain to other circumstances, cause and meaning of pain to the patient, effect on body image, level of anxiety, communicative purpose of pain and the patient's attempts to relieve his own pain.

Nursing interventions in pain can be interpersonal, physical, or a combination of the two. Interpersonal actions include: stating an intention to help with pain, decreasing isolation and loneliness, decreasing fear of the unknown, assisting the patient to make joint decisions about pain measures, teaching relaxation exercises, teaching the patient to produce pleasurable mental images, and making verbal acknowledgment of patient attempts to control pain. Physical actions include: positioning and support, sensory input control, medication, and other treatments such as application of heat and cold.

The nurse evaluates the effect of nursing action by keeping current records of patient pain, sharing information with other health workers, making sure no information on patient pain has been missed, and evaluating whether the nurse's expectations to relieve patient pain are realistic.

ACTIVITIES AND DISCUSSION TOPICS

- Find a patient or other person who is willing to talk with you about his or her pain. Use Figure 10-1, "Nursing assessment with patient pain" to make a complete assessment of the pain.

- Ask a few nurses what they think about giving placebos to patients in pain. Try to determine why they might answer as they do.
- Talk with a patient about ways he or she has found helpful in relieving their own pain. Share these observations with your fellow students.
- Attend a Lamaze or other natural childbirth class when relaxation exercises are being taught. See what you can learn to teach patients you will be working with who have pain.
- Go to the library and find out about the procedure for surgical disruption of nerve impulses, electrical analgesia, acupuncture, counterirritant therapy, or biofeedback.

REVIEW

A. Multiple Choice. Select the best answer(s). Some questions have more than one answer.

1. Leading questions should be avoided in pain assessment because they may
   a. elicit more information than the patient cares to give.
   b. result in obtaining incorrect information.
   c. introduce ideas the patient has not thought of.
   d. put the nurse in the position of second-guessing the patient.

2. Examples of physical nursing interventions that control sensory input are
   a. giving the patient a backrub or massage.
   b. observing the patient for early signs of pain.
   c. straightening the bedclothes.
   d. closing the window blinds.

3. A nursing assessment for determining the type and intensity of pain is
   a. observing for abrupt, sharp pain.
   b. asking the patient to describe where the pain is felt.
   c. observing the patient's nonverbal behavior to see when pain occurs.
   d. observing for muscle tension and restlessness.

4. A nursing intervention which is primarily an interpersonal one to relieve pain is
   a. taking measures to decrease fear of the unknown for the patient.
   b. positioning the patient in a comfortable position.
   c. asking the patient about medications taken in the past to relieve pain.
   d. telling the patient of available pain medications.

5. A capsule filled with glucose or an injection of sterile water is referred
to as
a. an analgesic.   c. a placebo.
b. a tranquilizer.   d. a narcotic.

B. Match the items in Column II to their correct definition in Column I.

Column I	Column II
1. Pain that is not constant but rather comes and goes.	a. contraindications
	b. intermittent pain
2. All the effects a drug may have besides the one positive effect for which the drug is prescribed.	c. placebo effect
	d. prn
	e. side effect
3. Positive reaction of the patient to nearly any attempt to make him feel better.	
4. Conditions which forbid use of a particular treatment.	
5. Given whenever necessary.	

C. Briefly answer the following questions.

1. Name the eleven areas in which the nurse assesses patient pain.

2. List five interpersonal nursing interventions in pain.

3. Name the four areas of nursing evaluation after pain intervention.

chapter 11
THE GRIEF PROCESS

STUDENT OBJECTIVES

- State the relationship between loss, grief and mourning.

- List three common staff reactions to death.

- Match various types of death with their definitions.

- Match patient behaviors with the appropriate stage of reaction to dying.

- Identify expected grief reactions in people who have lost a significant other person.

Relationships with other people have at least some emotional components. Relationships with family members always have a strong emotional aspect. Even brief relationships, if they have a strong symbolic meaning, can have a strong emotional impact. For example, a two-week job working with an employer who is reminiscent of one's dead mother can evoke unresolved feelings about separation from mother. Some people can become quite attached and emotionally involved with pets or cherished possessions. Whenever a relationship ends, feelings of loss, grief, and mourning are expected responses if there was an emotional involvement.

LOSS, GRIEF, AND MOURNING

One of the first things an infant must begin to learn is how to deal with loss. *Loss* refers to the lack of external or internal environmental supports that help satisfy basic needs. The mothering person who helps the infant to meet basic needs cannot always stay with the infant. When this person leaves, the infant incurs his first loss.

As the infant grows and becomes more dependent on others emotionally and less dependent physically, different losses are incurred. Throughout life, the degree (or lack) of emotional attachment to other people can result in loss. Very young infants who have been deprived of a warm, touching, caring relationship can die. Those who survive infancy and who develop emotionally involved relationships with another person are more vulnerable to the loss of that person.

Losses can be gradual with increasing separations such as in the normal developmental weaning period of infancy and childhood. Other developmental losses can be more abrupt; for example, loss of baby teeth. Losses can also be situational, such as the loss of an arm or leg due to a car accident. Developmental and situational events that result in loss were covered in chapter 7.

Life consists of a series of losses. Every time growth or change occurs, it must be traded for a loss of a comfortable environment, function, capacity or a body part.

The more the person has been emotionally involved in the relationship or situation, the greater will be the reaction to the loss. People who do not seem to respond to the loss of a significant possession or relationship may have special difficulties in resolving losses. People who denied and did not work through past separations or losses may have more trouble handling present and future losses. For example, mothers who were separated either emotionally or physically from their own parents may have more difficulty managing their own babies and may require additional support for mothering their own children.

Since emotional investment cannot be measured accurately, the nurse cannot assume that the loss of a finger is of less importance to a patient than the loss of speech or sexual ability. Emotional investment is individual and must be assessed for each patient on an individual basis. Figure 11-1 identifies some losses that could result in grief.

Grief is a series of internal emotional states in reaction to a loss. Grief is the emotional part of mourning; it allows the person to cope with an overwhelming event in a gradual way. Grief can be crucial for re-establishing homeostasis. People who are unable to grieve may appear at psychiatric clinics because they misinterpret their sadness. Those who never learned to grieve or have a series of unresolved losses may develop a life-style of depression.

The ultimate loss to be grieved is death. *Mourning* includes not only internal emotional states but also social and cultural behaviors to deal with death. Mourning is a social process. Few people can successfully grieve or mourn alone.

Loss of:	Examples
Body part	tooth extraction(s) or other loss of teeth first haircut amputation of limb or breast

Body function or capacity	change due to
	   accident
	   illness
	   aging
	loss of:
	   vision
	   memory
	   strength
	   hope
	   normal elimination route

Comfortable environment	leaving home ending a marriage loss of a favored pet changing job or home loss of friends death of loved one loss of home due to natural disaster debilitation of loved one graduation from school change in body shape and feelings during pregnancy or menopause promotion recovery of capacity organ transplant

Fig. 11-1 Losses that might result in grief.

Adaptation to a loss is assisted by religious, cultural or legal traditions and ceremonies. What is appropriate mourning behavior in Africa may not be acceptable in South America. In many religions and cultures, the funeral ceremony assists with the mourning process. Ceremonies emphasize the reality of death and serve as a focus for the expression of feeling.

Due to the increase in technology and frequent geographical moves, many Americans do not feel part of a religious or cultural group. For these reasons, people who suffer losses may be far from relatives and friends who could provide support for their mourning. Hospitalization and medical technology can also obstruct the process of mourning. Death may seem unreal and unnatural when it takes place in an intensive care unit. City life without access to cemeteries can further decrease ways to deal with mourning. Technological changes that prolong life and make the dividing line between life and death finer may also hamper mourning. Also, liberal abortion laws may increase the need for support in mourning. Some women who decide to end their pregnancies through abortion may need nursing assistance in grieving the loss of their unborn infant.

STAFF REACTIONS TO DEATH

There is strong evidence that those working with dying patients find talking about death upsetting and prefer to avoid such discussions. One of the reasons for this is that the medical culture emphasizes the preservation of life. In such a culture, death may seem like a failure.

The tendency of staff members to deny death or feel uncomfortable with it, together with the nurse's feeling of discomfort and her inexperience with talking about death, can make the dying process a lonely one for the patient. Actually, many persons, especially elderly patients, seem prepared to discuss their death and may thank the nurse who is available to share their thoughts and feelings with them. The task of dealing with the dying patient usually falls on the nursing staff. Nurses often feel ill-prepared to talk with patients about death. They feel this task belongs to the doctor so they may avoid this important aspect of patient care.

Nurses find two kinds of patient conversations in this area most disturbing. One of the most disturbing situations is when the nurse knows the patient is dying but feels she must not disclose this information to the patient. Another disturbing situation is when the patient wants to talk about dying but the nurse feels uncomfortable with the subject. In both situations, the nurse may cut off the patient's communication due to her own anxiety. Coming to grips with one's own mortality is a lifelong task that can begin with the nurse's thoughtful reflection on her personal attitudes toward death and dying, figure 11-2.

Because health personnel are constantly struggling to deal with their own feelings about death and dying, they may use specific coping devices to decrease their own anxiety. A major coping device is to emphasize tasks and procedures and ward rituals instead of relating to the dying patient on a person-to-person level. Many health personnel use withdrawal as a coping device. *Withdrawal* is a coping device where the person physically, emotionally, or socially leaves a disturbing situation. For example, the person close to death is placed in a certain room which is usually occupied by a dying patient; nursing personnel enter and leave the patient's room less and less frequently until the patient is socially isolated.

TYPES OF DEATH

Death can be defined in different ways. As the dividing line between life and death gets finer, the definition of when death occurs becomes more crucial.

Does a patient's death seem to mean I'm a failure as a nurse?

Am I uncomfortable and inexperienced in talking about death with patients?

Do I tend to deny death?

Do I resent having to deal with patients who are dying?

Do I feel "in the middle" when the doctor tells me the patient's diagnosis but won't let me tell the patient?

Do I cut off patient communication about death and dying?

Do I overemphasize tasks and procedures so I won't have to talk to a dying patient?

Do I withdraw from the dying patient either physically or emotionally?

Fig. 11-2 Questions the nurse asks about personal reactions to death and dying.

In *Deaths of Man*, Shneidman explores eight types of death. He states that *somatic death* occurs when the body's vital functions, such as heartbeat and respiration, cease. Cellular death follows. The more specialized the body organ, the more rapid the cellular death. With the advent of organ transplantation, cellular death has taken on increased importance.

Cardiac death occurs when there is an absence of electrical heart impulses. An electrocardiogram can measure this absence by making a tracing of electrical impulses from the heart. *Brain death* occurs within minutes as a result of inadequate oxygenated blood supply to the brain. *Clinical death* is the absence of audible heartbeat, but different patients may be treated as more revivable than others. The definition of clinical death always reflects the values of a society. Often it is the young patients with resources and power who are valued as revivable in our culture. The nurse must examine her values and beliefs in this area and question unequal resuscitation efforts she observes.

Subintentional death is the unconscious participation in hastening one's own death. Often death is hastened by a person's carelessness, taking of unnecessary risks, or poor judgment. People who abuse their bodies through alcohol, drugs or malnutrition may have subintentional wishes to end their lives. There are people who are so fearful of death that they scare themselves to death. This seems to be what happens in voodoo death. Death by suggestion is also probably a subintentional death; for example, some people think hospitals are places to die, and when they are brought to a hospital, they do die.

Partial death occurs whenever a phase or an aspect of life ends. Transitions between developmental periods that put a stop to expected stimuli, interpersonal relationships, or living patterns can involve grief and mourning. This grief and mourning can be as intense as the mourning caused by death. For example, a new high school graduate may experience partial death when assuming the new role of student nurse. Such a change may be intense if it involves loss of old friendships, decreased contact with family, and change in living arrangements.

Psychological death occurs when a person does not know who he is or that he exists. Health personnel are prone to think many dying geriatric patients have suffered psychological death, yet most of these patients are in intermittent or full contact with their surroundings. In our achievement-oriented society, there is a tendency to think that if the person is not behaving "sensibly" he might as well be dead; unfortunately, he may be treated as if he were dead. The nurse should avoid assuming that any patient is completely unaware at all times. Conversation and comments directed toward the patient or in his presence should always reflect consideration, kindness and courtesy.

Social death occurs when health personnel accept that death is imminent. Once this attitude is reached there is a loss of interest or concern for the dying person as a human being; the patient is treated as a body or as if he is already dead.

There are other kinds of death including anthropological or cultural death, and civil death. Death is not as clear-cut an issue as it would seem. Therefore, the nurse must examine various types of death in attempting to understand the grief process of the patient. Figure 11-3 shows different ways to define death.

THE DYING PATIENT'S REACTIONS TO DEATH

Kubler-Ross has defined five progressive stages in the grief process of dying patients. The stages are: denial, anger, bargaining, depression, and acceptance.

Type	Definition
Somatic Death	Cessation of vital body functions.
Cardiac Death	Absence of electrical heart impulses.
Brain Death	Inadequate oxygenated blood supply to the brain for a few minutes.
Clinical Death	Absence of audible heartbeat.
Subintentional Death	Unconscious participation in hastening one's own death.
Partial Death	Ending of a significant phase or aspect of life.
Psychological Death	Inability to know who one is or that one exists.
Social Death	Acceptance by significant others that death is imminent.

Fig. 11-3 Ways to define death

Denial Stage

In the *denial stage,* the dying person cannot believe he is dying. Comments the patient might make in this stage include: "No, not me. I'm getting better." or "It can't be true!" Going from doctor to doctor or acting as if one is not dying are other examples of denial. Denial seems to occur off and on throughout the dying person's progression toward death. Some patients remain in the denial stage until they die.

Anger Stage

In the *anger stage,* the patient seems to be asking, "Why me?" This stage is difficult for staff and family because the patient may direct anger toward any available target. He may complain about the doctors and nurses and about the treatment he receives. The nurse may experience a certain amount of irritation and frustration with the dying patient because whatever the nurse does, the patient is certain to complain.

In the anger stage, the person who is dying is expressing a legitimate feeling. His life is being cut off and healthy living people, like nurses, are a constant reminder that he is not healthy.

Bargaining Stage

In the *bargaining stage,* the patient attempts to postpone the inevitable death by promising good behavior in exchange for extended life. The dying person may appeal to health personnel or to a higher power such as God.

Dying patients may ask to go home once more, or promise not to complain any more if they can just live a little longer. Patients with special talents may ask to be able to perform once more; for example, sing, play the piano, or complete a work of art.

Depression Stage

In the *depression stage,* the patient comes to realize the enormity of the loss. When people have lingering deaths or are in the midst of raising a family or working at a job, the sense of guilt, anger and sadness may be great. When people die quickly or after they have completed a satisfying project, there may not be this sense of unfinished business. As loss of weight, weakness, pain or other symptoms increase, it is difficult for the patient not to begin feeling hopeless. The patient may become increasingly noncommunicative. Although what might be of most help to the patient at this time would be to express feelings of impending loss and hopelessness, he says little or nothing. If the patient does talk, he may express statements such as: "What's the use?" or "It's hopeless."

Acceptance Stage

Some patients may reach a stage in which they neither deny, become angry, or feel hopeless. In the *acceptance stage,* the patient is withdrawing from interpersonal relationships. The patient may doze frequently and be weak, but may also seem to be at peace. Interest in external surroundings may decrease too. In the stage of acceptance, a nurse's wish to prolong life contradicts the patient's wish to rest and die in peace.

Alternating Stages

Some patients may exhibit behavior characteristic of each stage, others may seem to be in one stage until they die. Still others may show brief glimpses of each stage from minute to minute, or demonstrate a combination of stages at the same moment.

Each dying patient must be seen as an individual who reacts to death depending on past and present life experiences. Often there is alternation of stages where the patient may be quite open and honest about dying, and at the next moment talk about going on a long vacation. Denial and hope seem to alternate as the dying person continues to fight to survive. Figure 11-4 summarizes stages in the grief process of the dying patient.

Stage	Examples of patient behaviors
Denial	Going to other doctors. "No, not me. I'm getting better."
Anger	"Why me? Why not you?!" "You nurses are all incompetent!"
Bargaining	"If you'll let me go home, I'll come back and die happy." "If I can live for two more months, I won't complain."
Depression	"What's the use?" "It's hopeless."
Acceptance	Peacefully dozing. Withdrawing from interpersonal relationships; no interest in external surroundings.

Fig. 11-4 Stages in the patient's grief process

THE SURVIVOR'S REACTIONS TO DEATH

The grief process may be difficult for the dying person, but it is those who are left, after the death of a significant person, who must deal with their reactions to the loss. By completing their own grief process, the survivors are able to deal with an overwhelming situation in a gradual way. In grief, the existence of the dead person is prolonged so the grievers can come to terms with the loss.

Initial reactions to a death are often shock and disbelief. Comments such as, "It didn't happen" or "I don't believe it" may be heard.

Next, the survivor may experience painful feelings of sadness and emptiness as he recalls the lost person. These painful feelings may be accompanied by crying, tightness in the throat, and sighing.

As crying subsides, the survivor is preoccupied with the image of the dead person. There is a verbal review and reliving of experiences that have been shared with the dead person. This review seems to be useful in putting the dead person to rest and in resolving the separation. Guilt about not being a good wife (mother, husband, brother, friend, or nurse) may be experienced as the survivor examines what more could have been done to prevent the death or make the dying person more comfortable. Anger often occurs when the loss and emptiness is felt. "How could you leave me alone?" or "How could you make my life so painful by dying?" are thoughts which may not be expressed but may be at the base of the angry feeling.

As the survivors bear the pain of loss, experience sadness, and review their relationship with the dead person, they can free themselves emotionally. The period of time varies for the grief process to be resolved. A year of grieving is not unusual; some people never resolve their grief and may have recurrent depressions. Also, some may overreact to future losses.

Although death is the ultimate separation and loss, the same grief process can occur when people have losses of body parts or body image, loss of a job, or even graduate from school, figure 11-5.

FIRST	Shock and disbelief.
NEXT,	Sadness, emptiness, crying, tightness in the throat, sighing.
THEN,	Preoccupation with the image of the dead person, body part, or comfortable situation accompanied by guilt and/or anger.
FINALLY,	Resolution of grief.

Fig. 11-5 Expected grief reactions for people who have lost a significant other person, body part or comfortable situation.

ANTICIPATORY GRIEF

Family members may parallel the dying patient's reactions to death by grieving prior to the actual death. Grief prior to death or loss is called *anticipatory grief*.

In anticipatory grief, there is an acceleration of feeling and reaction as the anticipated loss becomes closer to being an actual loss. This acceleration can be seen in other important losses or separations, too. For example, the anxious mother whose only child is going to kindergarten for the first time will be more upset a few days before school starts than during the preceding summer months.

Anticipatory grief is a way to begin adapting to an overwhelming loss. Family members or close friends may seek to detach themselves from the dying person and attach themselves to another object or person as a way of rehearsing for the actual loss. Such reattachments are not to be judged by the nurse but might be viewed as adaptive behaviors.

In normal growth and development, even infants may show signs that they anticipate abandonment or loss. It is not until the age of five years, however, that children begin to notice that living things can die. By observing dead animals or leaves falling from trees, children begin to notice that death occurs. About this same time, children express concern about whether their family members will die. These verbal concerns can be useful rehearsals for more serious loss and grief. There is some evidence that the anxiety and worry that often accompany observations and questions about an impending event may also be useful as rehearsals for adults. For example, preoperative patients who express moderate anxiety and concern about their surgery and subsequent loss may have a better postoperative course.

In general, family and friends who lose a person through a long, lingering death will be better prepared for the death because they have been able to do anticipatory grief work. The nurse may hear family members express anticipatory grief statements such as: "What will I do without her?" or "How will I manage the kids without him?" Although some feelings of loss can be resolved prior to the actual death, some of the grieving process remains to be done by the family after the person dies.

Anticipatory Grief and the Nurse

The emotional responses of the nurse may be the same as those of the family and friends. The nurse can feel sorrow, guilt, anger and hopelessness. Some nurses may move to help the dying patient and become so overtaxed that they cannot be of use to the dying patient or to other patients. Other nurses may try to handle their grief and anxiety by keeping distant from the patient and by being objective when giving care. Still others may be falsely optimistic, discounting the patient's fears with statements such as: "Oh, you'll live for many years yet" or "Don't be foolish, you're going to get better." Nurses need to handle their own anger and disappointment as well as the patient's and family's reactions. One way to begin to do this is for nurses to examine their own reactions and reflect on why they may be reacting so strongly.

Anticipatory Grief and the Child

Most dying children under the age of six may have no real sense of what death is about. At this time, anticipatory grief may not exist. From age six on, or even earlier, children who are dying may ask many questions about their illness and its treatment. Children in a pediatric ward may be quite observant about other children that have died, may eavesdrop on adult conversations to learn more about their condition, and may ask direct questions about the effect of medicines. Perhaps as a way to deal with their impending loss, children may learn to name their drugs and discuss the side effects, procedures, treatments and the purpose of each. In lingering conditions such as leukemia, the dying child may become aware that there are times when he feels good (remissions) and times when he feels bad (relapses) but that he is always sick. Later on in the grief process, he may have some idea of the relationship between the drugs and his relapses and remissions. Some children may enter a final stage of anticipatory grief where they realize that not only other children die but that they too will die. Figure 11-6 summarizes information on anticipatory grief and the child.

FAILURE TO GRIEVE

Patients may fail to experience normal grief if they are not in a social or cultural setting that permits and encourages grieving. For example, experiencing a loss while in another country or culture can cause difficulties. Some hospital units operate so as to deny death and discourage grieving. Patients on these units (and their families) may have unresolved losses.

Age	Expected Grief Reaction
Up to 5 years	No real sense of what death means.
5+ years	Asks questions about their condition and its treatment.
	May become aware that their condition is fatal.

Fig. 11-6 Anticipatory grief reactions and the child

```
┌─────────────────────────────────────────────────────────────┐
│           FAILURE TO GRIEVE CAN BE DUE TO:                    │
│                                                               │
│  —  Being in an inappropriate social or cultural setting.     │
│                                                               │
│  —  Being protected from information about the loss or death. │
│                                                               │
│  —  Refusing to give up the "strong" role.                    │
│                                                               │
│  —  Having mixed feelings toward the lost person or object.   │
│                                                               │
│  —  Being subjected to overwhelming or multiple losses.       │
│                                                               │
└─────────────────────────────────────────────────────────────┘
```

Fig. 11-7 Failure to grieve can be due to a number of reasons.

Unusual family attitudes or situations may interfere with grief. For example, students or employees who are not with their families when a significant family member dies may not grieve. Well-meaning family members or friends may try to protect one family member from pain by withholding the circumstances of a family death. Grieving makes the person more vulnerable and in need of support, so people who feel they must be strong may not give way to grieving. A person may fail to grieve if he has accepted the role of being the strong member in the family.

People often fail to grieve because of the *ambivalent* (mixed) feelings toward the dead person. The survivor may fail to grieve because he fears becoming aware of the intense love and hate feelings he holds toward the dead person. A natural disaster, a long series of losses, or the loss of the only significant person in one's life may be so overwhelming that the surviving person may be unable to grieve. Figure 11-7 lists some reasons why persons do not grieve.

SUMMARY

Loss, grief, and mourning are interconnected processes that concern the nurse. Some health personnel try to deny or escape the inevitability of dying and death. Because death is not as clear-cut an issue as it would seem, the nurse examines different types of death processes in order to understand the grief process as it affects the patient.

Dying patients seem to experience five stages in their grief process: denial, anger, bargaining, depression, and acceptance. Denial and hope alternate throughout the dying process. Survivors also experience a grief process that includes shock and disbelief, pain and sadness, preoccupation with the image of the dead person and review of shared experiences. Some patients, survivors, and nurses experience anticipatory grief before the death or loss actually occurs. Such grief seems to be an attempt to adapt and assist with homeostasis. The nurse must be alert to situations that might lead to failure to grieve.

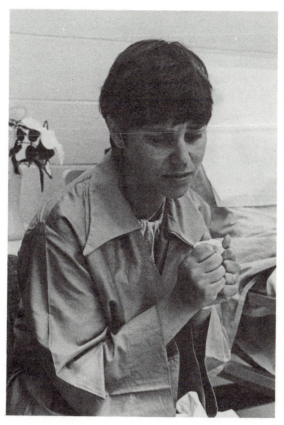

Fig. 11-8 A dying patient experiencing grief .

ACTIVITIES AND DISCUSSION TOPICS

- Spend at least 10-15 minutes with a dying person after you have conveyed an interest in whatever he or she wishes to tell you about their condition. After the discussion, write down the thoughts and feelings that occurred to you during and after the discussion. What insights have you gained into your own thoughts and feelings about death?

- Talk with one or more graduate nurses about their experiences with dying patients.

- Find out the purpose of the following:

  Euthanasia Council   the "Living Will"

  Omega   *Journal of Thanatology* (periodicals)

  Cancer Care (250 W. 57th Street, New York, New York)

REVIEW

A.   Multiple Choice. Select the best answer(s). Some questions have more than one answer.

1.   The statements that best describe how anticipatory grief affects patient and nurse are:
    a. There is no effect on either patient or nurse.
    b. The patient may grieve prior to a loss and this is referred to as anticipatory grief.
    c. The nurse may draw too close or too far away from the dying patient as an anticipatory grief response.
    d. Early childhood and adult experiences of the patient can be useful rehearsals for later losses.

2.   The grief process of survivors includes
    a. bearing the pain of loss.
    b. experiencing sadness.
    c. reviewing their relationship with the deceased.
    d. experiencing deep depression.

3.   In some cultures, the funeral ceremony assists with the mourning process by
    a. emphasizing the reality of death.
    b. serving as a focus for the expression of feeling.
    c. delaying actual separation.
    d. none of the above.

4.   Expected grief reactions in people who have lost a significant other person are
    a. disbelief, sadness, nausea and vomiting.
    b. denial, guilt, shock, anger, headache.
    c. crying and preoccupation with the image of the deceased.
    d. shock, crying, emptiness, chest pain.

5.   A coping device where the person physically, emotionally or socially leaves a disturbing situation is
    a. depression.
    b. mourning.
    c. denial.
    d. withdrawal.

B. Match the types of death in Column II to their definitions in Column I.

Column I	Column II
1. Cessation of vital body functions.	a. brain
2. Unconscious participation in hastening one's own death.	b. cardiac
c. clinical
3. Ending of phases or aspects of life.	d. partial
e. psychological
4. Absence of electrical heart impulses.	f. social
5. Inadequate oxygenated blood supply to the brain for a few minutes.	g. somatic
h. subintentional
6. Absence of audible heartbeat.
7. Acceptance that death is imminent.
8. Inability of a person to know who he is or that he exists.

C. Match the patient's behavior in Column I to the appropriate stage of reaction to dying in Column II.

Column I	Column II
1. Peaceful withdrawal from external environment.	a. acceptance
b. anger
2. Inability to believe death is occurring.	c. bargaining
3. An attempt to ask, "Why me?"	d. denial
e. depression
4. Realization of the enormity of the loss.
5. An attempt to postpone the death.

D. Briefly answer the following questions.

1. State the relationship between loss, grief, and mourning.

2. List three common staff reactions to death.

3. What is anticipatory grief?

4. Name three types of losses that could result in grief.

chapter 12
GRIEF ASSESSMENT AND INTERVENTION

STUDENT OBJECTIVES

- List three common anticipatory grief responses.
- Identify three indications of failure to grieve.
- Identify a nursing intervention for each stage in the patient's grief process.
- Identify a nursing intervention for each stage in the family's grief process.
- Identify ways nurses can handle their own grief.

Mourning is a social process in which two or more people work to resolve the loss. Because of technological and societal changes, the grief and mourning process is becoming more difficult for many persons to complete.

The nurse may be the person most available and interested in assisting with the grief process. To be of the most assistance to grieving patients, the nurse needs to be familiar with grief assessment and intervention techniques.

GRIEF ASSESSMENT

There are two main responsibilities the nurse has in assessing grief. The first responsibility is to assess the stage of grief. The second responsibility is to evaluate the patient's failure to grieve.

Stage of Grief

The nurse will be most effective if the nurse assesses both the patient's and the family's grief stage. Although these two stages may run parallel, they may be different. Frequently the patient may be ready to discuss his death while the family continues to deny the inevitable.

The Dying or Grieving Patient. It is important to assess the patient's stage of grief so the nurse will know what are useful nursing interventions at this time. In assessing the stage of grief, the nurse asks the following questions:

1. Is the person acting as if he cannot believe he is dying? If the answer is yes, the person is in the denial stage.
2. Is the person angry and irritable with frequent complaints about health personnel? If yes, the person is in the anger stage.
3. Is the person attempting to postpone death by exchanging good behavior for extended life? If yes, the person is in the bargaining stage.
4. Is the person noncommunicative, hopeless and withdrawn? If yes, the person is in the depression stage.
5. Is the person resting peacefully, with frequent naps and withdrawing interest from interpersonal relationships and the external environment? If yes, the person is in the acceptance stage.
6. Is the person constantly alternating between denial and hope? If yes, the person may be reacting in an individual manner based on his past and present experiences.

The same questions can be used to assess the grief of anyone who has had to give up a comfortable situation or suffered the loss of a body part or an alteration of body image. These patients will go through stages similar to the grief of the dying person.

The Survivors. When a person dies, the family and friends who are left are the survivors. These people must deal with the loss of a significant person. In assessing the survivor's stage of grief, the nurse asks the following questions:

1. Is the person reacting with shock and disbelief? If so, the person is in an early stage of grief.
2. Is the person experiencing sadness, emptiness and helplessness as expressed through crying? If so, the person is beginning to experience the loss.
3. Is the person preoccupied with the image of the dead person? If so, the person is moving toward resolution of the loss.

When making an assessment of survivor grief, the nurse can also determine the family's pattern of response to other losses. This should be done only if

---

THE NURSE ASKS:

— Am I spending less and less time with the dying patient?

— Do I try to evade the dying patient's family and friends?

— Do I give the patient the required physical care only?

— Do I discount the patient's fears?

— Do I listen when the patient talks about or implies fears about death?

Fig. 12-1 Questions nurses use to assess their own grief.

there is rapport with the family, and only when such questioning would be acceptable to the family. Questions the nurse can use to assess family reactions to previous losses include:

1. Who did you turn to for help at that time?
2. How did your family react to that loss?
3. How did you tell others about this loss?

Anticipatory Grief and the Nurse. Nurses can respond emotionally in the same ways as family and friends do when a person is dying. She may feel anxious, angry, sad, or hopeless. In dealing with these grief feelings, the nurse may find herself using distance, false optimism, or denial. Figure 12-1 lists some questions the nurse can use to assess her own grief responses.

Failure to Grieve

Failure to grieve can lead to later developmental problems or depressions; therefore, the nurse must observe closely for any indications that grieving has not taken place. Some indications are:

- Ongoing symptoms following the loss.
- Increased anxiety on the anniversary of the loss.
- Unresolved grief because it was not expressed at the time of the loss.
- Persistent guilt and loss of self-esteem.
- Prolonged withdrawal from family and friends.
- Increase in physical aches and pains.
- Inability to discuss the loss in a calm manner.

Most of these signs and symptoms would not indicate real problems unless they persisted more than a year after the loss was incurred. Perhaps the best clue that there has been failure to grieve is that at the time of the loss the person did not grieve. Figure 12-2 summarizes assessment questions about failure to grieve.

FAILURE TO GRIEVE CAN BE ASSESSED BY ASKING:

— Did the person grieve at the time of the loss?

— Does the person have ongoing physical or emotional symptoms more than a year after the loss?

— Does the person experience anxiety on the anniversary of the loss?

— Does the person suffer from persistent guilt?

— Does the person suffer from a decrease in self-esteem?

— Has the person withdrawn from family and friends for over a year after the loss?

— Does the person complain of an increase in physical aches and pains when there seems to be no organic basis for these complaints?

— Is the person able to discuss the loss in a calm manner?

Fig. 12-2 Questions to assess failure to grieve

GRIEF INTERVENTION

After assessing the stage of grief and determining whether there has been a failure to grieve, the nurse is ready to give more tangible assistance. She intervenes in the patient's grief, the family's grief, and her own grief.

INTERVENTION WITH THE PATIENT

The nurse intervenes in each stage of the grief process. In general, she attempts to be candid and open about death, yet tries to be consistent with the dying person's readiness for this knowledge. Those who work with a dying person can help by giving information at the rate at which the patient wants it; he will not hear or understand more than he is able to digest at that moment. In other words, the patient protects himself from hearing more than he is prepared to handle.

Should a patient ever be left to die alone? Why should there be involvement by other persons? There are a number of reasons why an interpersonal process of dying is more effective than dying without aid or support.

1. Mourning is a social process, and most people are not able to complete grief without assistance.

2. Nurses are forced to improve their care when they treat the dying person as a living person rather than as a "case."

3. The general level of morale on the ward may increase.

4. Families and friends can receive mental health benefits from such an approach.

5. The virtues of honesty, dignity and humane treatment are reaffirmed.

One of the greatest fears is that of dying alone. The presence of the nurse decreases this fear as she attempts to be physically and emotionally available to the patient. She helps the patient to talk out and express his emotions. She provides for physical and spiritual comfort and supports his right to die as he chooses.

Children also need assistance with the grief process. One of the most difficult situations for the dying child is to be unable to tell his parents that he knows he is dying. The nurse must let the child know that she will listen and talk with him. Communication is blocked if the nurse refuses to accept the fact that the dying child may know of his impending death; lying or acting as if death was not imminent can make the child feel deserted and misunderstood at a time when support is needed. After having assessed the patient's stage of grief, the nurse can proceed with the interventions appropriate for that stage.

The Denial Stage

In the denial stage, the nurse allows the patient to deny the loss, but is available to talk with him whenever he is ready. This intervention may include sitting with the patient in silence as well as telling the patient "although you

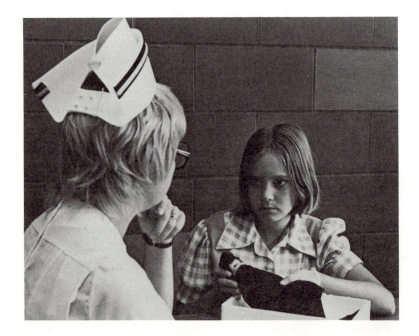

Fig. 12-3 Children can be helped to talk about grief by using dolls and other play objects.

may not feel like talking now, I am ready to talk with you any time you're ready." Then, patients may begin to share their loneliness and isolation with words or nonverbal communication.

The Anger Stage

The nurse is also available to the patient during the anger stage. She tries to understand that although the patient may seem to be angry with her, the patient is really angry about dying. A patient who is respected and understood will usually reduce the demands and begin to focus on the anger itself.

Appropriate intervention in the anger stage may be especially difficult for the nurse who believes that the patient must be kept quiet at all times. Verbalizations of patient anger may disturb the peace but are beneficial to resolving the patient's grief process.

The nurse can also help during the anger stage by allowing the patient to exert control over some aspects of his life. The dying patient should be allowed to have some control over length of visits from family and friends, times for treatments and physical care, and time chosen to talk with the nurse. This intervention is especially important now that the patient is losing much control over his death.

The Bargaining Stage

The nurse listens to the attempts of the patient to buy time and prolong life; she also lets him know that she is available for discussion or other comfort measures. Sometimes promises made by the patient during the bargaining stage may be related to quiet guilt about past behaviors. The nurse can tactfully suggest contacting a chaplain. This is one way of relieving guilt.

The Depression Stage

Encouragement and reassurance may be of little help when the patient is contemplating his own death. Expressions such as, "Don't be sad," or "Cheer up," are contraindicated and should be avoided. If the patient is allowed to express his sadness, he will move on to the acceptance stage much more easily. As a rule, the patient will be grateful to the nurse who sits with him silently and refrains from constantly telling him not to be sad. Whenever the patient says anything to convey sadness, the nurse can also use verbal statements such as "I guess words don't always help." If he shows his depression by some action, something like, "You feel sad." can provide understanding. Some patients who are in this stage may only respond to the touch of a hand or shared, silent grieving.

The Acceptance Stage

In the acceptance stage, the patient is peacefully withdrawing from environmental attachments and may wish to be left alone. This wish should be honored but the nurse should say something like, "I'll leave now, but I will check to see how you are in____minutes." In this way, the nurse shows an understanding of the patient's desire for solitude, yet also conveys a readiness for interaction should the patient wish it.

The nurse who feels unable to approach a dying patient must not approach that patient until she can deal with her own feelings. Patients generally are not as disturbed by dying itself as they are in dread of being deserted. If the nurse is able to make the patient realize that he will not be deserted, the most important intervention may have been made.

Stage of Grief	Nursing Intervention
Denial	Allows denial. Sits with patient silently until the patient is ready to talk. States intention to be available to talk with patient. Notes nonverbal communication of patient isolation and loneliness.
Anger	Available to patient physically and emotionally. Realizes patient anger directed at the nurse is really anger about dying. Allows patient to verbalize anger. Assists patient to exert control over visitors, treatments, and talking with the nurse.
Bargaining	Listens to patient's statements without promising longer life. Suggests contacting chaplain.
Depression	Does not give false reassurance or try to "cheer up" the patient. Allows patient to express sadness. Restates patient's expressions of sadness. Evaluates patient's wish to be touched or be silent and acts in accordance with wish.
Acceptance	Allows dying patient to be alone as desired. Continues to meet dying patient's needs. Evaluates and acts on patient's desires about prn medications. Encourages grieving (nondying) patient to pursue new interests and relationships.

Fig. 12-4 Nursing intervention with patient grief

In addition to providing for interpersonal needs, the nurse also tries to provide for physical and spirtual needs of the dying patient.

Physical Interventions

The nurse anticipates the patient's needs for oral hygiene, care of the skin, repositioning, care of hair and nails, intake and output, shaving, shampoos and makeup applications. In this way, the nurse conveys to the patient that he is still a person who is cared about. Pain medication may be of great help to some patients and should be given whenever necessary. A discussion with the patient may help to clarify whether he wants to remain aware of what is happening to him or whether he prefers as much medication as is ordered. These wishes of the patient should be included in team conference planning and incorporated into the nursing care plan. One of the decisions the patient and nurse may consider is whether the patient wants to stay alert in order to write final letters, draw up a will, and say farewell to friends and family.

Spiritual Interventions

Although patients may not always ask for religious consolation, the need may be there. The nurse can suggest that a chaplain come to talk with the dying patient. In this, as in other patient decisions, the patient's wish should be honored.

Other Losses

The same interventions will be useful in work with patients who have lost a body part or familiar situation. There are two differences in patient behavior. The dying patient goes through a bargaining stage, while patients who have sustained other types of losses may not. The second difference is that the acceptance stage in dying patients is evidenced through withdrawal from the environment while patients who have incurred a loss of other people, body parts, or comfortable situations will establish new relationships and interests.

INTERVENTION WITH THE FAMILY

Total care of the dying patient includes contact and intervention with the patient's family. The nurse can establish a relationship with the family during any phase of their anticipatory grief or after the loss occurs. By being available to talk with the family, the nurse can provide preventive intervention for the family. Preventive intervention includes planning for future healthy, constructive behaviors. The professional staff must decide who will be working with the family; the decision should be made well in advance of the death. Such planning increases the likelihood of effective care when the death actually occurs.

One intervention the nurse might perform for the family of the dying person is to accept their anticipatory grief responses. She must realize that family members may withdraw or form other interpersonal attachments prior to the patient's death. No attempt to judge or comment negatively on such behavior is made. Rather, the nurse understands their behavior as an attempt to regain homeostasis.

The role of the family as a unit in anticipatory grief is significant. Arrangements can be made to allow the family to be with the person at the time of death. In a busy hospital unit, family members are sometimes viewed as outsiders or persons who get in the way of the "real" treatment. It is the nurse who can insist that family members be allowed to support one another in their grief process.

The nurse is also sensitive to the switch in focus; the family moves from hope to acceptance of death. During the hope stage, the nurse will listen and help the family to discuss how they feel. The nurse is aware that the family might need to take care of unfinished business such as getting legal papers in order and saying goodbye. Therefore, when the family reaches the acceptance stage, she does not try to instill false hope or prohibit the family from completing any unfinished business.

The family may also require assistance from the nurse when the patient has reached the acceptance stage. At that time, the patient may wish peace, quiet, and no visitors. Family members who still feel guilty or angry may not understand this seeming rebuff. The nurse can help by telling them that the patient's withdrawal is an expected reaction and that the patient is more comfortable. Of course, the nurse should never make any statements unless she is sure they are valid. Figure 12-5 shows how the nurse may intervene with the family of the dying patient.

NURSES INTERVENE IN THEIR OWN GRIEF

When a nurse realizes that she is experiencing anticipatory grief or survivor grief, she is able to take certain steps to help herself. First, an attempt should be made to understand and find meaning in the death. Many persons have strong feelings about death; the nurse may be one of these. She must not be self-critical but, rather, attempt to understand the feelings she is experiencing.

Stage of Grief	Nursing Intervention
Shock and disbelief	Establishes rapport. Talks with professional staff to decide who will work with the family.
Experiencing the loss	Establishes rapport. Does not judge or prohibit other family interpersonal attachments. Defines the family role and treats the family as a unit in grief and mourning.
Preoccupation with image of the dead or dying person	Establishes rapport. Gives family information about the possible meaning of patient behavior.

Fig. 12-5 Intervention with the family of the dying patient

Another action the nurse can take is to initiate or participate in team discussions about attitudes toward death. By sharing anticipatory grief responses, health personnel can gain support from one another.

The grieving nurse may also wish to seek out a trusted nursing colleague or clinical specialist in mental health nursing who can help the nurse to talk out and work through the grief. Such intervention will be beneficial to the nurse and can affect the level of care she gives to future dying patients. Figure 12-6 suggests ways nurses assist with their own grief.

SUMMARY

The nurse may be the most available and interested person who can intervene in grief processes. In the assessment, the nurse is familiar with stages of grief and with signs of failure to grieve. Also, she is aware of her own grief responses.

NURSES INTERVENE WITH THEIR OWN GRIEF BY:

— Finding meaning in the loss.
— Trying not to dislike themselves for their strong reactions.
— Experiencing and trying to understand their feelings.
— Participating in team discussions about attitudes toward death.
— Sharing grief with a trusted colleague or mental health nursing specialist.

Fig. 12-6 Nurses intervene with their own grief.

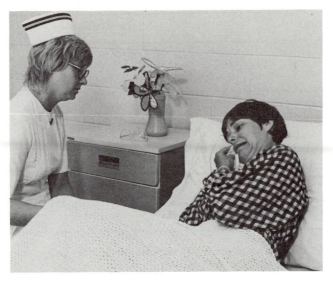

Fig. 12-7 The nurse assists with the grief process.

Nursing intervention in the care of the dying patient depends largely on an assessment of the patient's stage of grief. By being aware of behavioral differences, the nurse is able to intervene in grief which arises from losses other than death. The nurse who is assigned to work with a dying patient views the family and friends as a unit; this unit works with the patient in resolving grief and mourning. The nurse also takes steps to work through her own grief responses. By doing so, she can develop a personal understanding and provide more effective care for future dying patients.

ACTIVITIES AND DISCUSSION TOPICS

- Write one paragraph on how you conceive your own death. Include when and where you think it will occur, what would be most distasteful about death to you, and what would be most comforting. How might your conception of death be the same or different from others?

- Find another student and practice role playing the following situation: You will be the patient who keeps asking, "Am I going to die?" and the other student will play the nurse. Next, switch roles. Finally, discuss how it felt to play each role and how it might have been played differently.

- Discuss the nurse's responsibilities for the following: autopsy, donation of body parts, postmortem care, prolonging the life of a patient who requests death.

REVIEW

A.   Multiple Choice. Select the best answer(s). Some questions have more than one answer.

1.   Indications that a person has failed to grieve are
  a. crying and brief withdrawal from family and friends.
  b. anger, guilt, and preoccupation with the image of the loss.
  c. inability to discuss the loss more than a year after the loss.
  d. prolonged withdrawal from family and friends.
  e. increased anxiety on the anniversary of the loss.

2.   Nursing interventions that the nurse can use to deal with her own grief are:
  a. try to understand and find meaning in the loss.
  b. attempt to experience and understand the feelings.
  c. participate in team discussions of attitudes toward death.
  d. seek out a trusted colleague to help resolve the grief.
  e. condemn herself for reacting with strong feelings.

3.   Failure of a person to grieve over a significant loss can
  a. lead to later developmental problems.
  b. be a healthy indication of the person's stability.
  c. lead to later depression.
  d. lead to later unresolved grief.

4.   In helping the dying patient deal with the denial stage of grief, the nurse
  a. allows the patient to deny the loss.
  b. agrees with the patient's denial.
  c. gives the patient false reassurances.
  d. contacts a chaplain for the patient to talk with.

5.   The stage of grief the patient is in when he is noncommunicative, withdrawn and feels hopeless is the
  a. acceptance stage.
  b. anger stage.
  c. denial stage.
  d. depression stage.

B. Match the stage of patient grief in Column II to the appropriate nursing intervention in Column I.

Column I

1. Sits with patient silently until the patient is ready to talk.

2. Acts on patient's desires for prn medications.

3. Acts on patient's wish to be touched or to be silent.

4. Suggests contacting the chaplain.

5. Assists patient to exert control over visitors, treatments, and talking with the nurse.

Column II

a. acceptance
b. anger.
c. bargaining
d. denial
e. depression

C. Match the stage of family grief in Column II to the appropriate nursing intervention in Column I.

Column I

1. Give family information about the meaning of patient behavior.

2. Talks with professional staff to decide who will work with the family.

3. Defines the family as a unit in grief and mourning.

Column II

a. Experiencing the loss
b. Preoccupation with image of the deceased
c. Shock and disbelief

D. Briefly answer the following questions.

1. List three common anticipatory grief responses.

2. What are the two main responsibilities of the nurse in assessing grief?

3. Why is grief and mourning becoming more difficult for many people to complete?

4. Name two situations other than the loss of a significant other when people go through the grief process.

E. Associate the questions the nurse may ask, in assessing the *patient's* grief, with the grief stage in Column II.

Column I

1. Is the patient acting as if he cannot believe he is dying?

2. Is the patient attempting to postpone death by exchanging good behavior for extended life?

3. Is the patient resting peacefully, with frequent naps and withdrawing interest from interpersonal relationships and the external environment?

4. Is the patient angry and irritable with frequent complaints about health?

Column II

a. acceptance
b. anger
c. bargaining
d. denial

F. In assessing the *survivor's* grief, the nurse may ask questions. Associate each question in Column I with the grief stage in Column II.

Column I

1. Is the person experiencing sadness, emptiness and helplessness as expressed through crying?

2. Is the person preoccupied with the image of the dead person?

3. Is the person reacting with shock and disbelief?

Column II

a. early stage of grief
b. experiencing the loss
c. moving toward resolution of the loss

SECTION 3
THE OBSERVATION-PERCEPTION-COMMUNICATION PROCESS

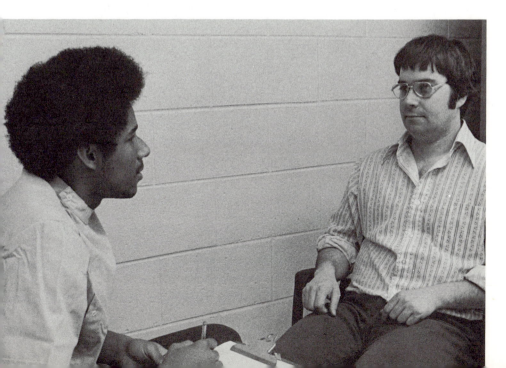

chapter 13
OBSERVATION

STUDENT OBJECTIVES

- List four methods of observation.
- Explain the difference between signs and symptoms.
- State five specific observational aspects.
- Name four types of interpersonal observation.
- Describe role playing.

The term, *observation,* has been defined as an act of recognizing or noting a fact. In nursing, observation refers to much more than the simple process of looking at what takes place. Observation is a nursing behavior that needs to be developed through practice. To become skilled in observation, the nurse must develop the ability to know what to look for. Only the major aspects of a specific situation will be obvious to the new student. With practice in the various methods of observation, the nurse can apply basic knowledge to all encounters with patients. Within a brief period of time, the nurse can learn to identify problems which require nursing intervention.

SIGNS AND SYMPTOMS

Signals to the nurse that changes are occurring in a patient are commonly called signs and symptoms. *Sign* is a term used to refer to changes that are detectable by the observer such as discoloration of skin, perspiration, increased breathing rate, or shining hair. Signs can be observed by the nurse. Some signs such as the pulse, heart rate, and respiration rate can be measured. Pulse, respiration and blood pressure are called vital signs because they give vital information about the condition of the whole body.

Symptom is the term used to refer to changes that may be less visible. Frequently the only way symptoms become evident is if the patient complains. Symptoms are experienced only by the patient. The nurse may need to question the patient in order to obtain more information about the exact symptom. Examples of symptoms are pain, itching, and sleeplessness. Look at figure 13-1 and decide whether the nurse is observing a sign or a symptom.

Even though symptoms are experienced only by the patient, the nurse can usually observe the patient and learn something about a symptom. For example, the patient in pain may moan and appear tense and irritable. However, since ways to express pain are learned, the nurse cannot assume that loud moaning means more pain than soft moaning. Figure 13-2 lists some signs and symptoms.

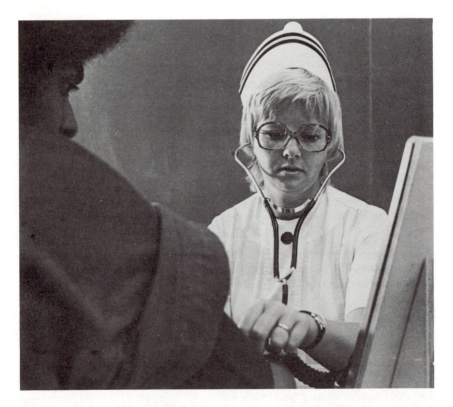

Fig. 13-1 Taking the patient's blood pressure is an example of nursing observation.

Need	Signs	Symptoms
Oxygen	Pulse Blood pressure Respiration Cyanosis	Numbness Tingling Dizziness Headache
Safety	Temperature shivering diaphoresis (perspiration) Jaundice Discolored skin Scars Prostheses (artificial appliances) Cough Swelling	Tingling Burning Pain Itching
Food and Fluid	Amount of food eaten Amount of fluid intake Decubiti Vomiting Peristalsis Weight loss Drainage from wounds Edema Warm, dry skin Obesity Sagging skin	Anorexia (lack of appetite) Nausea Pruritus Headache Weakness
Elimination of Waste	Abdominal distention Amount of urine output Type of urine Color of urine Abnormal constituents of urine, e.g. mucus, blood clots Frequency of bowel movement Type of bowel movement	Headache Discomfort Diarrhea Constipation Dysuria (difficulty urinating) Burning sensation on voiding
Interpersonal	Dilated pupils Confusion Alertness Response to commands Posture Tight body musculature Tapping fingers Pacing Withdrawal Increased or decreased speech	Headache Sadness Fatigue Fear Guilt Anger Anxiety

Fig. 13-2 Examples of signs and symptoms (continued)

Need	Signs	Symptoms
Interpersonal (Cont'd)	Maintenance of eye contact Restlessness Sighs Changing topics Talking with other patients	
Self-actualization	Knits a sweater Out of bed despite pain Practices crutch walking Learns to give own insulin injection	Anxiety Fear Fatigue Guilt Weakness
Activity/Rest	Posture rigid at sleep Naps every 2 hours Cries out in sleep Walked up and down hallway Alert Confused	Insomnia Nightmares Fatigue Pain

Fig. 13-2 Examples of signs and symptoms

METHODS OF OBSERVATION

The four basic methods of observation include use of the senses of sight, touch, smell and hearing. Nurses guide their observations by knowledge of body function and of patient reactions to the external environment. Knowledge from the fields of anatomy, physiology, biology, psychology, sociology, anthropology, and ecology is applied to nursing observations. The nurse also applies what she has learned about changes that occur as a result of disease, injury, health and stress.

Sense of Hearing

Even though pain expression is learned, nurses do use their ears to learn about changes in patient behavior. Hearing is useful in observing the patient's verbal communication. A cough, difficult breathing, and speech defects can also be observed by listening. Hearing plays an important role in techniques that require the use of a stethoscope. *Auscultation* is a term that means using the sense of hearing to interpret sounds produced within the body. Most often these body sounds are heard more clearly with a stethoscope, but direct hearing can also be used. The nurse uses auscultation to identify the sound of the heart, to measure blood pressure, and to hear the heartbeat. Hearing is also used to listen to the quality of sounds. For example, the nurse may listen to a patient who is using only the upper part of his chest to breathe. This nurse may then describe what was heard as "shallow respiration."

Nurses use auscultation to hear if peristalsis is present. *Peristalsis* is the wavelike, muscular movement of the esophagus and intestines as contents are moved through the digestive tract. The absence of peristalsis can lead to abdominal *distention* which is the accumulation of gas or fluid in the abdominal cavity. The nurse uses auscultation to observe for the presence of peristalsis in patients who are recovering from surgery.

Sense of Smell

The sense of smell enables the nurse to learn about problems of the patient or the environment. Odors may be the result of not bathing (body odor). A patient's breath can convey diabetes that is not well controlled (fruity breath). A patient's breath can also indicate a drinking problem (alcohol breath) or digestive problem (halitosis).

The odor of drainage from a wound can signal presence of infection and need for further nursing intervention. A stuffy room is a sign for the nurse to provide ventilation. The smell of smoke signals a need for nursing intervention to deal with fire.

Sense of Sight

Inspection means using the sense of sight in nursing observation. Inspection is used to compare variations in size, shape, and movement of the parts of a patient's body; deficiencies and replacements are also studied and evaluated. For example, the nurse may observe that the patient's left leg is longer and thinner than the right leg. Or, the nurse may observe that when the patient smiles, one side of the face turns up while the other side does not. Such observations may be useful in providing for the patient's needs. In the first case, the nurse watches and determines whether the patient needs assistance in walking. In the second case, the need for further assessment is clear; it will be necessary to decide if the patient had a stroke or perhaps has a brain tumor. This kind of observation can lead to further follow-up such as questioning the patient to determine whether a stroke or brain tumor could have occurred, or performing tests upon which to base a decision.

The nurse also uses the sense of sight to observe the condition of the skin. Scars and discolorations are noted, such as the yellow skin color called *jaundice.* Jaundice indicates liver malfunction. The nurse looks for *decubitus ulcers* (bedsores). This skin breakdown often develops in bed patients because of inadequate nutrition to a localized area.

Sense of Touch

Nurses use their sense of touch to determine warmth or coolness of the patient's skin. Touch is also used to determine muscle tension. For example, by walking with a patient and holding his arm, the level of general muscle tension can be noted. Nurses use touch or *palpation* to locate a patient's pulse, and to observe for unusual lumps and masses. Palpation also is used to find accumulations of fluid in the patient's body. Palpation of the lower abdomen will reveal the accumulation of fluid in the bladder. Fluid which has collected in the ankles or eyelids is palpated also. This collection of fluid in tissues near the surface of the skin is called *edema.*

Size, temperature, texture, rhythm, swelling, and hardness are observed by using palpation. Look at figure 13-3 and decide whether the nurse is using palpation or auscultation. A summary of the information on methods of observation is presented in figure 13-4.

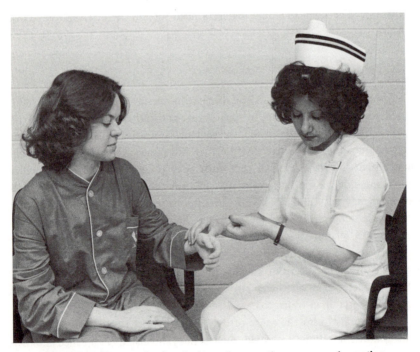

Fig. 13-3 Taking a patient's pulse is another way the nurse uses observation.

Method	Examples of Observations	Further Observation through Questioning
Hearing	Words said	"Did I hear you correctly, you said. . ."
	Difficult breathing	"You're breathing hard, when did that start?"
	Blood pressure	"Your blood pressure is hard for me to read, have others had trouble?"
	Coughing	"You've got a cough; when did you first notice it?"
Smell	Breath	"Are you having problems with your digestion?"
	Wounds	"Let me look at your wound."
	Body odor	"Do you prefer a bath or shower?"
	Room ventilation	"The room seems stuffy, shall I open the window?"
Sight	Lack of body part(s)	"I see you have dentures. Do you eat a special diet?"
	Addition to body part(s)	"You wear glasses. Are you near or farsighted?"
	Size of body part(s)	"Do you need help walking?"
	Shape of body part(s)	"The swelling in your leg is down. How does it feel to you?"
	Movement of body part(s)	"You seem to be favoring your left side. Are you in pain?"
Touch	Warmth of skin	"Your forehead is warm. Do you feel warm?"
	Muscular tension	"Your neck is tight. Do you feel tense?"
	Pulse	"Your pulse is strong. What are you feeling?"
	Distention	"Your belly is tight. How long since you urinated?"

Fig. 13-4 Several methods may be used to observe the patient.

SPECIFIC OBSERVATIONS

In observing the patient's reactions, the nurse's attention is divided and focused on the following aspects of the patient: posture, attitude and task performance, nutritional status, voice, eyes, gait, appetite and fluid balance, elimination, sleep patterns, level of orientation, bleeding, and response to hospitalization.

Posture

The nurse observes the patient's posture. The way a person holds his body is an indicator of how he feels. When a person is in pain, he may protect the painful part and seem to be bent over. When a person is depressed, he may appear dejected or sad and walk slowly with his head down. Some illness processes create changes in posture. When an abnormal posture is displayed, the nurse pursues the matter by asking further questions.

Attitude and Task Performance

The nurse observes the patient's attitude toward the illness, toward the nurse, or toward the performance of tasks such as exercises. The patient may talk about these attitudes, or convey an attitude of disgust or anxiety by his facial expression, sighs, tone of voice, and irritability. He may cry; he may become too cooperative. When these signs appear, the nurse can find out more about the patient by further questioning.

Nutritional State

The nurse observes the patient's nutritional state. Some signs of difficulty in this area include obesity, pale skin that sags, and dull, brittle hair. When these signs are observed, the nurse gathers further information by asking questions about the patient's diet and symptoms. Also, she observes the patient when he is eating; this provides valuable information about his attitude toward food and about his intake of food and fluids.

Voice

The nurse listens to the patient's voice. Hoarseness, pitch, slurring, stuttering and unfinished sentences are signs to be noted for further study. Through exploration, the nurse determines whether each sign is due to anxiety or to an illness process.

Eyes

The nurse observes the patient's eyes while talking with the patient and checks for squinting, redness, yellow discoloration of the *sclera* (white part of the eye), *pruritus* (itching), pain, tears, and unequal pupils. If any of these are noted, the nurse asks the patient if there is pain, itching, etc., and when these symptoms began.

Gait

The nurse observes the way the patient walks. This is referred to as *gait*. Gaits can be unsteady, shuffling, staggering, or limping. The patient may need support such as crutches or another person's help.

Food and Fluid Balance

The nurse observes the patient's appetite and fluid balance. Information regarding this aspect of patient care would include: Does the patient wear *dentures* (false teeth)? What are his likes and dislikes? Does the patient have any allergies or drug sensitivities? Does his skin look dry and feel warm, perhaps indicating *dehydration* (lack of fluid)? Does the patient eat all or most of the food on the meal tray? Does the patient drink fluids amounting to 8-10 glasses per day?

Elimination Habits

Changes in environment, food, activities and feelings can create drastic changes in elimination of waste materials from the body. The nurse observes the patient for diarrhea. If it is present, she makes note of frequency, amount, and the presence of blood. Color and consistency are also noted. For example, a black, tarry stool indicates the patient is bleeding or is taking an iron preparation.

Obtain information about the patient's usual habits at home. Many people do not have daily bowel movements; others have a daily habit. Bowel elimination in the hospital should be compared with the patient's usual elimination pattern. The nurse should also observe the frequency and amount of urination. *Dysuria* (pain with urination), urinary urgency, and *hematuria* (blood in the urine) are observations to be reported.

Sleep Patterns

The patient reveals verbal and nonverbal reactions to sleeping in the hospital. Facial expression and body posture are clues; relaxation or restlessness due to lack of sleep can be readily observed. Inquiries should be made about the patient's usual sleep patterns at home as some persons nap during the day.

Level of Orientation

The nurse observes the patient's level of orientation and consciousness, and observes his response. The level of consciousness and orientation is determined by watching the patient's response to light, pain, and directions. *Dilation* (increased size) and *constriction* (decreased size) of the pupils of the eye are indications of level of consciousness. Ability to respond appropriately to others' comments or behavior is also an indication of level of consciousness. Since the patient's outward behavior may belie his inner reactions, the nurse is careful to always act as if the patient is able to perceive events around him.

Bleeding

When the nurse observes blood on a patient or on his clothing, she must determine the source and amount of blood present. Bleeding can be from an external cut, fall or scrape, or from an internal body source. The nurse notes the color, amount and bleeding site.

Response to Hospitalization

The nurse continues to watch the patient and his daily progress. As time passes, changes may occur in the patient's manner. Evaluating the patient's response to hospitalization includes comparing the patient's present state with what it was on admission to the hospital. This allows the nurse to compare behavior and determine response to hospitalization. The patient's reactions to other patients, the doctor, the nurse, medications, treatments, and discharge from the hospital are also part of the total response. Figure 13-5 summarizes information on specific observations.

INTERPERSONAL OBSERVATION

In nursing, the purpose of *interpersonal observation* is to identify, clarify and verify impressions of the relationship between nurse and patient. Many intuitions about the present situation grow out of the nurse's own past experience as well as the present relationship. These so-called hunches can become the basis for further exploration with the patient.

The procedure for both physical and interpersonal observation is to note the general aspects of a situation and focus on and explore some of these aspects. This focus on only some aspects of a situation allows the nurse to be fairly sure of the meaning of what was observed. With practice, the nurse begins to develop judgment with confidence. In both physical and interpersonal observation, accuracy is achieved only when the nurse notes what is actually observable. Assumptions of biases have no place in accurate observation. Chapter 14 on perception will examine some of the sources of assumption, bias and distortion in the nurse.

Observation Aspect	Examples of Descriptive Terms
Posture	Erect. Slumped. Protecting right side.
Attitude and Task Performance	Resigned facial expression. Sighing after every sentence. Angry tone of voice. Sobbing every five minutes.
Nutritional State	Obese. Underweight. Pale skin. Dull, brittle hair.
Voice	Hoarse. Slurred speech. Stutters. Speaks in incomplete sentences.
Eyes	Squints once per minute. Sclera red. Sclera yellow. Rubbing eyes every two minutes. Right eye tears constantly. Pupils of unequal size (L $<$ R).
Gait	Unsteady. Shuffling. Staggering. Limping. Walks with cane. Asks for support of right side of body when walking.
Appetite and Fluid Balance	Wears dentures. Food likes are: mashed potatoes and chicken. Allergic to strawberries. Sensitive to penicillin. Skin dry and warm to the touch. Eats all food. Drinks no liquid.
Elimination	B.M: brown, soft formed. Voided 1000 ml clear light yellow urine, no odor.
Sleep patterns	Naps one hour in a.m. Sleeps at night with tense facial expression.
Level of Orientation and Consciousness	Responds to direct commands only. Initiates conversation with nurse. Asks questions about own care. Calls nurse, "mother."
Bleeding	Bright, red blood oozing from left nostril.
Response to Hospitalization	Initiates conversation with roommate. Has difficulty swallowing medication. Cries when dressings to left thigh are changed.

Fig. 13-5 Specific observations and how to describe them

There are at least four types of interpersonal observation: spectator, interviewer, collector, and participant.

Spectator Observation

In *spectator observation*, the patient is not aware of being observed. The nurse can watch the patient walk down the hall in order to observe his gait or watch his interactions with other persons, figure 13-6, page 202. The nurse may observe a patient while giving care to his roommate.

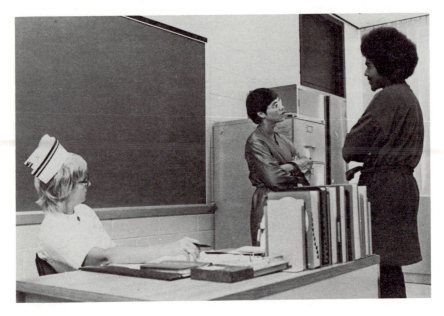

Fig. 13-6 In spectator observation, the nurse observes without interfering in patient activity.

Interviewer Observation

In *interviewer observation*, the patient is aware he is being studied to some extent. Nurses often use this type of observation when admitting patients and taking a nursing history, figure 13-7, pages 203 and 204. Note how the nursing history focuses on the basic needs which were discussed in the preceding section. Process recordings made for the purpose of studying communication patterns also reflect the results of an interviewer observation.

Collector Observation

In *collector observation*, the nurse studies records that have been made by other nurses, doctors, or other members of the health team. Partial impressions about patients can be gathered in this way. Two sources from which the nurse gathers impressions about patient behavior are the Kardex and the Nurses Notes, figures 13-9, page 205, and 13-10, page 206.

| Nursing History |

The interviewer introduces herself to the patient and proceeds:

Date: Patient Name:

Age: Sex: Allergies:

Response to Hospitalization

1. Have you been in the hospital before?
   If yes, when?
2. Have you ever been in *this* hospital before?
   If yes, when?
3. What is the reason you've come to the hospital this time?
4. What activities of the nurse were most helpful in previous hospitalizations? Most bothersome?

Expectations and Attitudes

5. What things would you like to learn about your condition?
6. What did you expect to happen in the hospital that hasn't happened?

Interpersonal Needs and Preferences

7. What restrictions would you like placed on visitors?
8. Would you rather eat alone or have company?
9. Would you like to have a nurse available to talk with you about your thoughts and feelings?

Usual Patterns of Daily Living

10. What do you usually eat for breakfast?
11. When do you usually eat breakfast?
12. When do you usually eat lunch?
13. What do you usually eat for lunch?
14. When do you have supper at home?
15. What do you have for supper?
16. Any foods you especially dislike or that disagree with you?
17. Do you like a snack?   If yes, what?
                                When?
18. What drinks do you especially like?

Fig. 13-7 This sample nursing history can be used by the nurse to gather information about the patient's needs and preferences. (continued)

19. How many hours do you usually sleep per night at home?

20. When do you usually go to sleep at night?

21. Do you like to sleep with

    an extra pillow   _____

    an extra blanket   _____

    the window open   _____

    the window closed _____

    the door open   _____

    the door closed   _____

    the curtain open   _____

    the curtain closed _____

22. What helps you to get to sleep at home?

23. How often do you bathe or shower at home?

    Which do you prefer?   _____

    When during the day?   _____

24. Do you have all your own teeth?

    If not, how many dentures or plates do you have?   _____

25. When do you usually have a bowel movement?

    How many per week?

    Any difficulties?

26. How frequently do you urinate (pass water) during the day?

    Any difficulties?

    If yes, what specifically?

Self-actualization and Barriers to Self-actualization

27. Do you have any questions to ask me about anything?

28. What special needs do you have in the following categories?

    Learning more about your condition   _____

    Hearing problems   _____

    Vision difficulties   _____

    Things that help you when you're in pain   _____

    Are you usually a very active person, or do you take things easy?   _____

    Need an interpreter?   _____

    Have trouble expressing your thoughts or feelings?   _____

    Need assistance with walking or turning?   _____

    Would you like to have the chaplain notified to visit you?   _____

        If yes, which religion?   _____

Fig. 13-7 This sample nursing history can be used by the nurse to gather information about the patient's needs and preference.

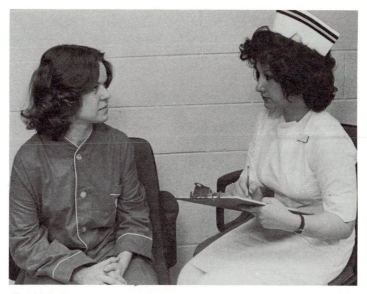

Fig. 13-8 The nurse observes the patient while completing a nursing history.

Long-range goal:	To ASSIST PATIENT TOWARD A PEACEFUL DEATH
Short-term goals and Needs	Nursing Interventions
INCREASE COMFORT	TALK c̄ PT. ABOUT HIS
	CONCERNS FOR 15 MINS. q
	4 hrs. AND p.r.n. OFFER p.r.n.
	PAIN MEDICATION TURN Pt.
	q 2 HRS. BEGINNING AT
	8 a.m.
	OFFER FAVORITE FLUIDS P.R.N.
	(7-UP. AND TEA c̄ lEMON)

Relatives or friends to contact: DREW DICKEY (SON)

Admitted on: 11/26   Religion: LUTHERAN   Age: 62

Occupation: RETIRED LAWYER   Diagnosis: CANCER OF RECTUM

Surgery: 12/6   Primary Nurse: TOM TERRY, R.N.

Room: 36 A   Patient: DICKY, JOHN   Doctor: DUMPHY.

Fig. 13-9 The Kardex is a source of information for collector observation.

Nurses Notes	
Patient's Name: JOHN SMITH	Doctor: GOODE

Date and Time	Cumulative record of nursing observations and interventions
9/21/76	
2 pm	Pt. c/o DULL, THROBBING PAIN IN OCCIPITAL REGION, OFFERED BACK RUB. Pt. AGREED
2 15 pm	Pt. STATED "I FEEL BETTER." Pt. RESTING QUIETLY
3 pm	WIFE VISITED. Pt. TURNED FACE TO WALL & REFUSED TO SPEAK c̄ WIFE. AFTER WIFE LEFT Pt. STATED "SHE ONLY COMES BECAUSE SHE FEELS GUILTY." SAT c̄ pt. FOR 15 MINUTES.
	Carolyn Clark, RN

Fig. 13-10 The patient's chart contains nurses notes, another source of information for collector observation.

Participant Observation

In *participant observation*, the nurse gives nursing care to a patient and at the same time observes the nurse-patient relationship. The patient is aware he is receiving nursing care, but may be unaware that the nurse is studying his responses, figure 13-11. The patient may be more spontaneous in his responses in a participant relationship than in an interviewer relationship. In interview situations, patients are often hesitant to make comments about their care or about their symptoms; this may be due to fear of retaliation or of being hospitalized longer if too many complaints are made.

In many ways participant observation is a more complex observation than interviewer observation. The nurse must be skilled in both physical and interpersonal nursing skills; she must be able to integrate both smoothly in order to be a competent participant observer. For this reason, physical skills and interpersonal skills are sometimes taught separately to the beginning student so that she can focus attention and develop ability in the skills under study.

As physical and interpersonal skill grows, nurses are better able to use participant observation. The most complex use of participant observation is to give physical care and carry on a patient-centered discussion at the same time. Such complex care requires practice and adequate nursing supervision in both skill areas.

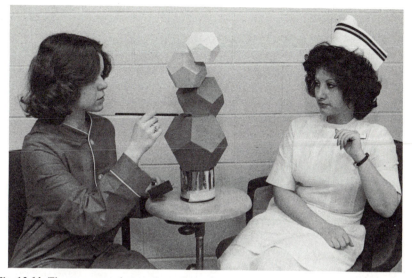

Fig. 13-11 The nurse can observe the patient when doing an activity or procedure with her.

ROLE PLAYING

Role playing is a way to improve skill in interpersonal observation. In *role playing*, two or more people are assigned to each play the part of a character or assume a role different from their own. For example, a student nurse might role play how she would teach a patient about a new procedure. Another student could role play the part of the patient. A role playing situation may be presented to the class. Members of the class can make observations of the nurse-patient interaction and then compare their observations. Often, the role players switch roles and note what it is like to be in the other role. After roles are played and switched, a general discussion follows where the audience and role players discuss what each observed. The audience can help the role players to become more aware of their communication and to suggest more effective approaches. Since role playing requires that students expose themselves to critical observation, they may experience some initital discomfort. However, anxiety created by such a situation will soon disappear. The benefits of role playing are usually worth the effort.

Role playing is a way of reliving or preplaying an experience in order to expand its meaning and sharpen observational skills. Observation of behavior is the first step in moving toward the appropriate nursing intervention. In working with patients, nurses should teach them to observe and describe their own symptoms and behavior; this is their first step toward appropriate self-intervention or nurse-intervention.

As nurses become more skilled in role playing, they may use this technique with patients. For example, the nurse may assign the role of doctor to the patient so both nurse and patient can see why the doctor may act as he does with the patient. Role playing can be used in any situation with patients, students, or families in order to understand and expand observational skills. CAUTION: Role playing skills should be developed in a supervised situation with a nursing instructor prior to being attempted in a nurse-patient interaction.

SUMMARY

Nurses develop observational skill through practice. Signs are objective observations where measurement is frequently possible. Since symptoms are subjectively experienced by the patient, the nurse may need to make additional observations by asking questions; this is done to develop sufficient information so she will know how to proceed.

Methods of observation include the use of hearing, smell, sight and touch. The nurse focuses on various aspects of patient behavior such as posture, attitude and task performance, nutritional status, voice, eyes, gait, appetite and fluid balance, elimination, sleep patterns, level of orientation, bleeding, and response to hospitalization.

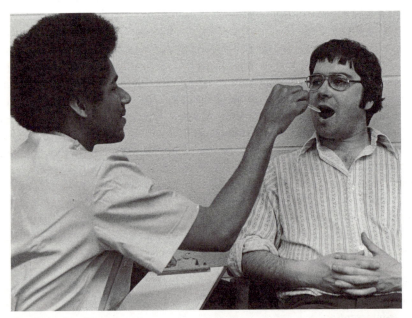

Fig. 13-12 Specific observations can be made while performing a simple nursing task.

Interpersonal observation centers on the relationship between the nurse and the patient. The nurse uses any one of the following four types of interpersonal observation: spectator, interviewer, collector and participant. Skill in interpersonal observation may be improved by role playing.

ACTIVITIES AND DISCUSSION TOPICS

- Choose a student partner and go to a moderately active clinic or ward in the hospital. Decide on an area to observe. Each partner makes her own, separate observations. If possible, take notes on whatever happens in that area for 3-5 minutes. After the observation, go to a quiet area and discuss observations. Both partners compare notes on what things each observed and what each did not observe.

- Practice types of interpersonal observation by selecting a partner and doing the following:
    a. Spend five minutes in spectator observation. Be sure your partner does not know he or she is being observed.
    b. Spend five minutes interviewing your partner. Before the interview, use figure 13-5 to develop questions to ask about each observational aspect listed. Switch roles and be interviewed. Discuss what each observed.
    c. Observe your student partner while both of you make a bed or do another activity together. Discuss what difficulties you confronted in trying to observe and participate at the same time.

- Locate a patient chart and discuss the effective and ineffective observations others have recorded. An effective observation is clear and brief, yet describes the situation so others have a sense of what took place. If you cannot find a chart, discuss the observation recorded in figure 13-10.

REVIEW

A. Multiple Choice. Select the best answer.

   1. Bed patients often develop a skin breakdown due to inadequate nutrition to a localized area called
      a. distention.
      c. jaundice.
      b. decubitus ulcer.
      d. edema.

   2. Pain, pruritus, and sleeplessness are examples of
      a. palpations.
      c. inspections.
      b. signs.
      d. symptoms.

3. A symptom that indicates the patient needs oxygen is
   a. cyanosis.
   b. shallow respiration.
   c. dizziness.
   d. anorexia.

4. A sign that an interpersonal need is not being met is
   a. insomnia.
   b. sadness.
   c. confusion.
   d. guilt.

B. Name the type of interpersonal observation described in each of the following questions.

1. The patient is not aware of being observed.

2. The nurse studies records that have been made by other members of the health team.

3. The nurse gives nursing care to a patient and at the same time observes the nurse-patient relationship.

4. The patient is aware to a certain extent that he is being observed.

C. Match the items in Column II to the correct statements in Column I.

Column I	Column II
1. Observable change that can be detected such as skin discoloration or perspiration.	a. auscultation
	b. inspection
	c. interpersonal observation
2. A distressing occurrence experienced by the patient that is usually associated with disturbed body function or illness process.	d. palpation
	e. sign
	f. symptom
3. Use of the sense of sight to determine variations in body parts.	
4. Use of touch to determine size, temperature, swelling, or hardness of various body parts.	
5. Use of hearing to interpret sounds produced within the body.	
6. Identify, clarify, and verify impressions of the relationship between nurse and patient.	

D. Briefly answer the following questions.

1. Explain the difference between signs and symptoms.

2. List four methods of observation.

3. Name five specific observations the nurse uses to observe the patient's reactions.

4. Describe role playing as follows:

   a. What is role playing?
   b. Who can participate in role playing?
   c. Where can role playing take place?
   d. What is the purpose of role playing?

chapter 14
PERCEPTION

STUDENT OBJECTIVES

- List four psychobiological factors that influence perception.

- Identify nursing interventions for sensory overload.

- Identify factors that may influence perception of time.

- Explain how group expectations influence perception and behavior.

- Identify relationships between levels of anxiety and perception.

People interact with others and organize their daily and long-term activities based on perception of themselves and the world in which they live. *Perception* is a complex process. It involves psychobiological factors: sensory organs, the central nervous system, past experiences, and future expectations. Although the process of perception is the same in everyone, no two people perceive events in exactly the same way. This is primarily because each person has different past experiences and different expectations for the future. For example, children who have the same parents and are raised in the same household can perceive their environment in completely different ways. What is perceived by each is related to what each individual's needs are at that time.

Perceptive ability is learned. Each person proceeds through stages in the ability to perceive. At first, the infant perceives a world of random lights, noises, touches and tastes which seem totally unconnected. This random state of affairs where the world is perceived as a disconnected group of events also occurs in adults experiencing high levels of anxiety.

After a number of repetitive experiences, the infant begins to realize that certain events recur regularly. For example, the infant begins to associate mother-who-gives-food-and-comfort with the pleasurable experience of feeding. This is the beginning of the infant's ability to categorize events. It is not that the infant recognizes the mother. Rather, the infant associates the two events together. In adults, moderate levels of anxiety approximate this state. In moderate anxiety, events are associated but no cause and effect relationship is noted by the person. With assistance, adults in moderate anxiety can be helped to make this cause and effect connection.

Through manipulation of objects, the infant next learns the various qualities of the objects. By this process, the child is finally able to abstract the essential qualities and learns to categorize objects by their essential qualities. The development of speech facilitates the process of categorization. Cause and effect relationships are learned by the time a child is seven or eight years old. Figure 14-1 depicts the developmental process of perception.

STABILIZING SENSORY INFORMATION

Adults screen out information that does not fit their usual perceptual categories. This screening process stabilizes perception in two ways: (1) since the number of perceptual categories is small in relation to the number of possible categories, nonclassifiable information is ignored, and (2) stability is maintained by resisting new or conflicting sensory information. This tendency to maintain stability is a protective process. Resisting information protects the person from becoming overwhelmed by excessive information from the environment. This view of perception as a protective device partially explains why some patients may be resistive to new procedures, to the nurse's attempts to teach, or even to the process of hospitalization.

Approximate Age	Developmental Events	Perceptual Ability
Newborn	Birth	Random events perceived
Up to 18 months	Feeding, toileting	Perceives association of two events, e.g., mother-who-gives-food-and-comfort is associated with pleasurable event of feeding
18 to 24 months	Speech is acquired	Manipulates objects and begins to categorize objects
7 or 8 years	Relates to more objects and people	Learns causal relationships

Fig. 14-1 The developmental process of perception

Sensory information about the surrounding environment is picked up through the eyes, ears, mouth, nose, tongue and parts of the skin and muscles. Sense organs serve to limit as well as extend the view of the world each person develops. By paying attention only to information that fits their existing perceptual categories, people limit their view of the world. When this system of limiting and extending information works well, a stable view of the environment exists. This stability can be disrupted in two ways: when there is too little or too much sensory information available, and when difficulties exist in the brain's processing or categorizing system.

Too little sensory information results in *sensory deprivation*. There is a tendency for people to produce their own information during periods of sensory deprivation, figure 14-2. Examples of such productions include hallucination, imagination, distortion, and dreaming. Hallucinations are visual (see), auditory (hear), olfactory (smell), gustatory (taste) or tactile (physical touch) sensations when there is no external stimulus.

In sensory deprivation, the goal is to stimulate available sensory organs and/or increase sensory information available to that person. For example, a person who has been alone in a private room in a nursing home and is rarely talked with may begin to suffer from sensory deprivation. Sensory deprivation can then lead to confusion. Medications can create further confusion and anxiety and decrease dream activity that is useful for emotional well-being. Study figure 14-3 to understand the assessment and intervention for sensory deprivation.

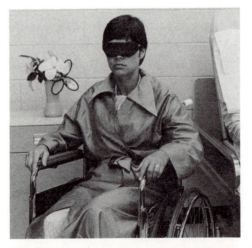

Fig. 14-2 Sensory deprivation can occur when the patient cannot use one or more modes of perception.

Assess how many of the factors below are operating and for how long	Observe for these behaviors	Determine the pattern of observed behaviors	Intervene by choosing one or more nursing intervention	Reassess pattern of observed behavior and patient response to nursing intervention
Oxygen tent Eyes patched Deafness Long periods of bedrest Physical restraints Social isolation Brain damage Medicated with hypnotics, sedatives, or tranquilizers	Hallucinations Confusion Losing track of time Decreased attention span Withdrawal Sleeplessness/ nightmares Irritability Fatigue Preoccupation with bodily functions	When do the behaviors occur? e.g., when does the patient hallucinate — morning, night, when upset? How often do the behaviors occur? e.g., does the patient report nightmares every night or after family visits? How long do the observed behaviors continue?	**ORIENT:** 1. Tell patient where things and people are in his immediate environment. 2. Explain nursing procedures to the patient step-by-step. 3. Tell hallucinating patient the nurse does not sense what the patient does. **PROVIDE REST/ACTIVITY:** 1. Provide clock, calendar, reading material, active or passive exercise, TV, or written assignments based on patient-nurse decisions. 2. Plan with patient to assume more active role in patient care. 3. Provide uninterrupted rest periods. **PROVIDE SOCIAL RELATIONSHIPS** 1. Spend additional time with patient to provide a "real" person for the patient to relate with. 2. Ask patient to describe what he is experiencing. 3. Focus on exploring patient's thoughts and feelings, not the content of the hallucination, the confusion, or the bodily function.	When do the observed behaviors occur now? How often? For how long? Should a different intervention be tried? Should there be a nursing conference to develop a consistent 24-hour approach? What does the patient verbalize about the nurse's intervention?

Fig. 14-3 Sensory deprivation: assessment and intervention

Too much, or too much of the same kind, of sensory information is called *sensory overload*. In general, the way to intervene in sensory overload is to decrease the amount of available sensory stimulation or replace it with a different kind of stimulation.

Examples of sensory overload situations are those in which the person becomes overstimulated or overexcited or is experiencing too many new or repetitive experiences. The suggested approach for sensory overload is to move to a less stimulating environment, or to decrease or change the stimulation in the present environment. Study figure 14-4 to understand the assessment and intervention for sensory overload.

NURSES STUDY PERCEPTION

Usually perception occurs automatically without conscious thought or awareness; it comes as a surprise when nurses begin to consciously study their own perceptual processes. Discomfort and anxiety may even be experienced as students focus on themselves. An important aim of nursing education is the development of self-awareness. In the study of perception, students are often asked the rationale for their behavior: for example, labelling patients as "nice," "difficult," "cooperative" and so on. Such investigations, though often uncomfortable, help nurses to widen their perceptual ability.

A perceptual device of importance to nurses is *habituation*. Habituation can occur after the nurse has become familiar with a new skill, environment or person. What at first was novel, interesting or stressful becomes boring or fails to capture attention. For example, habituation can occur after the nurse has admitted many patients or has done a procedure a number of times; the level of stress and interest in the admission and the procedure is decreased. It is important for the nurse to remind herself that although she may be familiar with the procedure, the patient is not familiar with it and may be under stress.

Since perception involves acts of categorization, there is a tendency to develop *stereotyped frames of reference* (categorizing events or people based on one or two characteristics and overlooking other qualities). If a nurse meets a patient who seems angry, it is likely that the nurse will categorize that patient as "angry." In the same manner, the nurse begins to refer to a patient as "that preop" or "that cardiac." Placing people in categories may increase efficiency but at the same time it dehumanizes the patient.

Being aware of this stereotype tendency should alert nurses to examine their own verbal and written statements for evidence of stereotyped thought. Statements which stereotype need to be altered. Nursing process requires that each patient or client be evaluated as an individual.

Assess how many of the factors below are operating and for how long	Observe for these behaviors	Determine the patterns of observed behaviors	Intervene by choosing one or more nursing intervention	Reassess pattern of observed behavior and patient response to nursing intervention
Sleep deprivation Invasion of territory or privacy Noise Extreme anxiety Crisis Social excitement Number of environmental changes Constant monitoring by machines Body catheters Number of physical exams/day Brain damage	Hallucinations Withdrawal excitement Fatigue Helplessness Disorientation Panic Sleep disturbances	When do the behaviors occur? e.g., when does the patient panic – morning, night, or when upset? How often does patient express helplessness verbally or by crying? e.g., when he is alone, with another person, when family visits?	**INTRODUCE CHANGE SLOWLY:** 1. Use short, concise statements. 2. Explain briefly and clearly the purpose of procedures. **REDUCE QUANTITY AND INTENSITY OF INPUT:** 1. Be physically present but do not force verbal interaction. 2. Arrange care to provide rest periods. 3. Decrease noise. 4. Move patient to less stimulating environment. 5. Provide for increased privacy. 6. Shelter patient from other patient's care and upsets. **PROVIDE A DIFFERENT KIND OF INPUT WHEN EXCITEMENT AND/OR WITHDRAWAL DECREASES:** 1. Assist patient to describe what he was experiencing. 2. Provide sensory stimulation to areas that were not overloaded.	When do the observed behaviors occur now? How often? For how long? Should a different intervention be tried? Does there need to be a nursing conference to develop a consistent approach over a 24-hour period? What are the patient's statements about the nursing interventions?

Fig. 14-4 Sensory overload: assessment and intervention

GROUP EXPECTATIONS, PERCEPTION AND BEHAVIOR

Group expectations can influence perception and subsequent behavior. For example, if ten people tell one person he is obnoxious, there is a great potential for that one person to begin to believe he is. Not only will he believe it, but he will often start acting obnoxious, even if he was not acting that way before.

It is obvious, therefore, that expectations which are communicated verbally or nonverbally can influence a person's behavior. Parents influence their children to behave in certain ways because of these expectations. Likewise, children influence their parents to behave in certain ways.

Group pressures on perception and behavior are active in nursing situations too. For example, if a number of nurses working in a nursing home expect a particular patient to be hopelessly confused, that patient is more likely to act confused. This probably occurs for a number of reasons. One reason is that the nurses will act on this expectation and especially notice any patient behavior that could fit the category of "confused" behavior. Another reason is that based on this assumption nurses may tend to treat that patient as if he cannot understand. They may talk about the patient rather than with him. Therefore, he will receive a decreased amount of relevant sensory information. Finally, the patient will be influenced by the nurses' expectation as well as by the decrease in sensory information. As a result of this process, the patient will probably act more confused.

Figure 14-5 depicts the self-reinforcing effect of group expectations, perception and behavior. This process does not always promote healthy behavior. It is important for nurses to recognize and break the self-reinforcing processes which do not promote healthy patient behaviors.

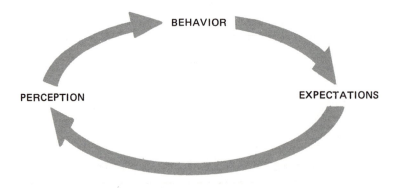

Fig. 14-5 Group expectations reinforce perception and behavior.

CULTURAL PERCEPTIONS OF THE NURSE

Patients as well as nurses have absorbed cultural stereotypes of what a nurse should be. In the United States, the traditional nurse stereotype is a white, female angel of mercy. At the same time she is pictured as a hardened person who is insensitive to suffering. Like most stereotypes, the nurse stereotype contains elements that are incongruent or do not fit together. Being an angel of mercy and a hardened person at the same time creates difficulties for both patient and nurse if the stereotype is accepted as valid.

When approaching patients, try to remember that some patients will have a stereotyped, unrealistic view of what the nurse can be. Nurses often have similar unrealistic views. Student nurses sometimes discuss their fears of being "overinvolved" with patients as well as their fears of becoming a hardened nurse. Examining such views can be a useful process for both student and graduate nurses. Stereotyped and unrealistic expectations on either the part of the nurse or the patient can lead to frustration, distorted perception, and distorted communication.

PERCEPTION OF TIME

Factors which may influence the perception of time are:

- socioeconomic and cultural orientation
- institutional orientation
- sensory orientation
- feeling orientation

These will be discussed as they influence the nurse and the patient.

Socioeconomic and Cultural Orientation

In some cultures or socioeconomic levels, people structure time based on a 24-hour cycle called *diurnal time*. To these people, time is viewed as a cycle that will recur every 24 hours. Time is approximate; there is little fuss made if people arrive one or two hours before or after the appointed hour. This is true, for example, in Greece where hardly anything has a precisely appointed time. This phenomenon also occurs in some American subcultures.

By contrast, the middle-class American believes that "time is money" and "time waits for no man." Time is measured by clock time and is divided into significance based on minutes and hours. Appointments are set for specific times.

Because of these two different views of time, patients who hold to the idea that time is an approximation may appear late for appointments, dawdle over meals, and forget to take their medications on time.

Patients adhering to the dominant middle-class view may be particularly interested in having medications and treatments right on time. These patients may judge the quality of care by how closely the nurse follows the routine time schedules.

Institutional Orientation

Institutional time is based on hours of work rather than on units of work produced. A nurse is paid for the number of hours worked, not how much was accomplished. There is also a tendency for insitutional time keepers to judge efficiency by how busy the nurse appears to be.

Thus, a nurse who is sitting and talking with a patient may be perceived to be wasting time, while a nurse who is writing at the nursing station may be perceived to be busy. These institutional perceptions and expectations encourage the nurse to be technically efficient rather than humanitarian. Figure 14-6 demonstrates how perception of institutional expectations can conflict with patient care.

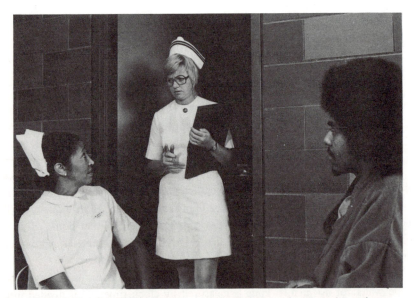

Fig. 14-6 Not all health personnel accept the usefulness of talking with patients.

Sensory Orientation and Feelings

Disturbances in sensory perception also influence how time is perceived. For example, patients in sensory deprivation or overload can experience a sense of timelessness. Patients in pain or who have sensory disturbances often over-estimate or underestimate time intervals. This perceptual disturbance can be related to demands for pain medication prior to its scheduled time.

Anxiety makes time seem to stand still since the uncomfortable experience appears unending. On the other hand, time seems to fly when pleasant or in-teresting events are being experienced.

PERCEPTION OF COLOR

The perception of color seems to be associated with emotional reactions; it is not clear whether these reactions are spontaneous or culturally learned. For example, red is associated with excitement or anger. Blue is associated with pleasurable calm. Black and grey are associated with sadness and depression.

The *Rorschach Test* is a psychological test made up of a series of inkblots presented to an individual for interpretation. The person is asked to describe what the inkblots suggest to him. Depressed people seem to perceive the ink-blots as colorless or grey. Highly emotional persons often associate the blots with blood, the sea, or sunsets.

Nurses can use color to both assess and intervene with patients. For ex-ample, the colors selected for a dress or personal belongings can clue the nurse about the patient's feelings. Likewise, room or clothing color can be used to quiet or stimulate a patient depending on the nurse's assessment of the patient's need for quiet or stimulation at the time.

PERCEPTION OF SPACE

People are able to tell where they are in space in several ways. Visual per-ception is one way. Sensations arising in the interior of the body as a response to gravity is another way. Whenever the body is tilted from an upright posi-tion, gravity presses on joints, and the muscles tense to accommodate the tilt. Another perceptual organ for space orientation is the inner ear. The inner ear registers whether the head is up, down, left or right.

In the dark, people usually lose some sense of position in space. The nurse working the late evening or night shift should be aware of the patient's in-creased need for orientation at that time. Likewise, the patient who remains in bed or a wheelchair for long periods of time can lose some sense of position in space. Passive and active exercise is important for this patient.

Patients who have lost visual, inner ear, nerve, muscle or joint action can also become confused about where their bodies are in relation to their surroundings. Because of this potential for confusion, the nurse should be especially aware of the need for orientation. Telling the patient where he is in relation to the nurse, the bed, his belongings, or his food will serve two purposes: (1) orientation decreases the potential for patient anxiety and confusion and (2) orientation will enable the patient to be more helpful and active in self-care. Figure 14-7 summarizes patient differences in perception of time, color and space. Nursing interventions are suggested for these differences.

ATTENTION AND PERCEPTION

Focused attention is a psychological-biological device. It allows a person to adapt to important changes in his environment and was probably developed to allow humans to protect themselves.

Difference	Nursing Considerations and Interventions
Socioeconomic and Sociocultural	Knows about both diurnal and clock time views.
	Allows patient to use own time view (within limits of hospital structure).
	Gives medications and treatments exactly on time to those patients who are especially concerned with time.
Institutional	Knows differences between institutional and humanitarian time.
	Is efficient, yet caring.
Sensory	Orients patient to time, e.g., "It's ten o'clock."
Color	Evaluates patient's use of color.
	Uses color to quiet or stimulate a patient.
Space	Evaluates difficulties in space perception due to loss of visual, inner ear, muscle/joint cues, or anxiety.
	Provides verbal direction in space, e.g., "the bed is one foot to your right"; "your breakfast tray includes. . ."
	Knows perception may decrease at night.
	Provides night light and/or more specific directions to patients at night.
	Assists patient with active and passive exercise.

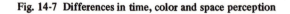

Fig. 14-7 Differences in time, color and space perception

Bright lights or loud noises can signal danger. Attention will then be focused on these events. Too much light or noise is maladaptive, however, since sensory overload is likely to occur.

Perception is how the individual views the world. It is not necessarily what the world contains. The individual focuses attention on the external environment primarily to meet his own needs and tends to perceive those things which will satisfy him.

People will often try to avoid situations that produce anxiety. They will not hear statements that evoke anxiety; this is a short-term protective device that may be detrimental in the long run. For example, a patient may sign a consent to surgery without hearing the explanation or reading what was signed; later he will deny having signed the consent. Not hearing the explanation protects the patient from anxiety during the short period of time used for consent signing but presents problems at a later date when staff and patient have to contend with the denial. Presenting the material well before the anxiety-provoking event will often allow the patient to focus attention on the material. During this time, the patient can absorb the impact of the information and will then be more able to focus attention on listening. Nurses frequently assume that patients will hear and understand the first time a statement is made. Rather, it would be wise to observe the patient and ask him to repeat what he understood the nurse to say. In this way, the nurse can assess how much the patient heard of what was said.

People perceive situations in order to meet their own needs. Their expectations about what will happen to them are based on these needs. Past experiences influence present and future experiences. Thus, patients who have had past hospitalizations that were perceived as primarily negative may tend to expect current and future hospitalizations to be negative. In other words, a number of experiences ending in the same outcome will lead to a firm expectation of future experiences.

Because of past experiences, the patient may have a *perceptual set* or preconceived idea regarding what the patient's relationship with the nurse will be like. The patient with a certain perceptual set may react negatively to an initial interaction with the nurse because of previous experience. It is important for the nurse not to automatically respond and react to this negative expectation. The nurse should pause and remember that her behavior can be influenced by the patient's expectations, just as the patient's behavior can be influenced by the way she expects him to act. Therefore, the nurse makes an objective assessment of possible distortions in the patient's perception of her. After making such an assessment, the nurse can decide on appropriate intervention. Figure 14-8, page 224, shows how anxiety and previous experience influence attention and perception.

Level of Anxiety	Past Experience	Degree of Attention and Perception
high	negative	low
low	positive	high

Fig. 14-8 Relationship between level of anxiety, past experience and perception

ANXIETY LEVEL AND PERCEPTION

During high levels of anxiety (severe anxiety) one's perceptual field is narrowed greatly. A narrowing perceptual field results in a decreased ability to be aware of what is occurring in the environment. This narrowing is probably an adaptive maneuver to shield the person from sensory information which he considers threatening. When in severe anxiety, the person may focus on one small detail of a situation, or jump from one detail to another without completely comprehending the situation. High anxiety creates a *tunnel vision effect* where perception is necessarily narrowed and distorted. Nurses working with patients who are experiencing high levels of anxiety need to be aware of this decrease in perception.

The perceptual field is also narrowed during moderate levels of anxiety. However, it is possible to help the patient focus on the topic at hand by directing his energies to it; for example, "Let's talk about your pain," or, "Before you slice your bread, finish buttering it."

In low level (mild) anxiety states, the person's perceptual ability is acute. At this time a patient is especially responsive to the nurse's direction and teaching efforts. Figure 14-9 depicts the relationship between anxiety level and perception.

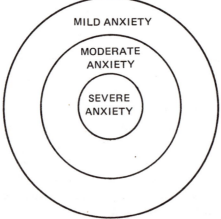

Fig. 14-9 Anxiety restricts the perceptual field.

In severe anxiety, the patient would only be able to focus on a small portion of an entire situation. In moderate anxiety, the patient perceives more of the situation, and in mild anxiety, a much greater amount of information is taken in.

BIOFEEDBACK AND PERCEPTION

A person may receive information about different parts of his or her body through biofeedback. *Biofeedback* training allows people to turn inward and even control some bodily functions. In a typical session, the subject is given feedback by hooking up to equipment that amplifies body signals. The body signals are then translated into readily observable signals such as a flashing light or a steady tone. Once a person can "see" his heartbeats or "hear" his muscle tension, he can start to control them. Biofeedback holds promise for correcting improper perception of internal states. It also provides a useful alternate to drugs. Drugs frequently have unwanted side effects while biofeedback can be used on specific problems such as high blood pressure, headache, and control of gastrointestinal disorders.

Biofeedback research supports the theory that human health depends on the integrated functioning of the entire person. The physical and psychological become parts which blend and unite to form the whole, the one system, the human person.

One way that people can enhance their perception of how mind and body interrelate is through the study of body rhythms. People develop their own individual daily rhythms for sleeping, eating, concentrating, and eliminating waste. Upsets in body rhythms can be preceded and/or followed by mood changes and symptoms of illness. By studying their own body rhythms, people can be better prepared to plan their activities to complement their body rhythms.

SUMMARY

Perception is a complex, learned process. Sensory information is restricted and categorized in order to present a stable world to the perceiver. Disturbances in sensory perception can be due to sensory deprivation or sensory overload. Nurses must study their own perceptual processes in order to decrease the effects of habituation and stereotypes on their nursing care.

Perception of time can be influenced by socioeconomic, cultural, institutional, sensory, and feeling orientation. Color perception is related to the state of feeling. Perception of space is influenced by vision, inner ear dynamics, and gravity.

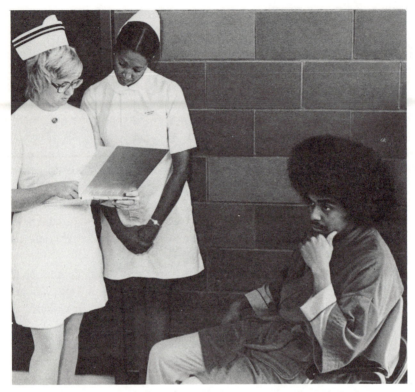

Fig. 14-10 The nurse may forget to include the patient, even though he is often aware of what is taking place.

Attention is focused on events which are important to the perceiver's needs. Anxiety and past experiences influence present perception. Biofeedback is a promising new way to improve perceptual processes.

ACTIVITIES AND DISCUSSION TOPICS

- Make a list of situations that could lead to sensory deprivation.

- Write a description of a "typical patient." Then read through the description and delete references which reflect any stereotypes.

- Keep a list of what colors you wear and your general mood every day for a week.

• Begin a body rhythm diary. (Body rhythm is related to biofeedback.) Keep records of frequency, type, and time of the following:

> sleep
> eating
> defecation
> symptoms
> activity
> moods
> concentration

Study the records and try to increase your own perception of your body rhythms.

REVIEW

A. Multiple Choice. Select the best answer(s). Some questions have more than one answer.

1. Nursing interventions useful for sensory overload are
    a. providing rest periods.
    b. encouraging patient to be more active in care planning.
    c. providing a clock, calendar, and reading material.
    d. being physically present but not forcing verbal interaction.
    e. decreasing noise and stimulating experiences.

2. Factors that may influence the perception of time include
    a. color gradient.
    b. cultural values.
    c. space dimension.
    d. institutional values.
    e. sensory disturbance.

3. A protective device that allows people to concentrate on important events in their environment is
    a. biofeedback.
    b. tunnel vision.
    c. focused attention.
    d. perception.

4. Hallucination, imagination, distortion, and dreaming may result from
    a. sensory deprivation.
    b. habituation.
    c. sensory overload.
    d. biofeedback.

5. A nursing intervention for a patient suffering from sensory deprivation is
    a. explaining nursing procedures briefly.
    b. providing increased privacy.
    c. telling the patient where things and people are in his immediate environment.
    d. moving the patient to a less stimulating environment.

B. Match the appropriate level of anxiety in Column II to the perception in Column I.

Column I

1. Perceptual ability is acute; learning takes place.

2. Perceptual ability is narrowed but patient can be helped to focus on a topic.

3. Patient able to focus on only a small portion of a situation or moves from one detail to another.

Column II

a. mild anxiety

b. moderate anxiety

c. severe anxiety

C. Briefly answer the following questions.

1. Name the four psychobiological factors that combine to influence perception.

2. How do group expectations influence perception and behavior?

3. What is the Rorschach test?

4. Explain biofeedback and its use.

chapter 15
VERBAL COMMUNICATION

STUDENT OBJECTIVES

- Define communication.
- List three functions of communication.
- Label parts of the communication process.
- Name two levels of communication.
- List five areas of assessment to determine if communication is disturbed.

People are social animals. Their behavior is defined and determined in the presence of other people. It is impossible not to communicate. Even remaining silent is a message that one does not wish to talk. *Communication* is the process of giving and getting information from others.

In order to get important information from others, people must communicate clearly. Communication helps people to find out about the world. They learn how to relate to other objects and people. Communication lets people know what to expect from one another.

People seem to want to let others know what is going on inside of them. Frustration can result when communication is prohibited. When others do not listen or respond, the person may feel isolated and lonely; thoughts, feelings, and behaviors can be distorted. Disturbed communicational patterns are thought to be the cause of some emotional or mental disorders.

Communication includes both verbal or spoken words and nonverbal messages. This unit deals only with the spoken and written word.

People are not born with the ability to communicate effectively. The infant has only a cry and a few body movements with which to convey messages.

Communication is learned in a cultural setting through interaction with other people; what may be appropriate in one cultural setting may be inappropriate in another. How people perceive themselves, the world, and their place in that world results from communication.

People from different cultures sometimes have difficulty communicating with one another. Often this is due to differences in perception. For example, in some cultures it is expected that people will be open and direct in their communication. In other cultures, it is thought to be wise to take time and present all the details to everyone. In some cultures it is expected that people will try to predict the future, while in others verbal prediction of the future may be viewed as a sign of madness.

THE FUNCTIONS OF COMMUNICATION

Communication has three functions:

- to receive messages
- to evaluate messages
- to transmit messages

In communication, the message becomes the focus of observation. A series of messages is exchanged between persons to form a communication. Communication is a dynamic process where one person affects at least one other person.

Receiving Messages

At birth, the infant perceives the world at close range only. As he matures, he learns to scan and explore the more distant environment. Memory becomes important in order to select and recall past events. Physical damage to the brain or sense organs can hamper the ability to receive messages. Emotional damage can also decrease the ability to receive messages clearly. For example, a person whose parents have warned her that the world is a dangerous place is likely to be suspicious of others' statements and to pay particular attention to remarks from others that support this suspicious idea of the world.

Emotional comfort can also influence the ability to receive messages. If the person who is to receive the message likes and feels comfortable with the sending person, the message is more apt to get through and be received.

Evaluating Messages

To evaluate a message appropriately, a person depends on (1) a combination of information from the external environment, (2) information from the person's own sense organs, and (3) past experiences or memories. Appropriate evaluation of a message requires a certain amount of openness to new information, and the necessity for taking a risk and listening closely to the other person's message.

Timing is an important element in evaluating a message. People who react too quickly or too slowly to the statements of others often make ineffective evaluations of messages.

Evaluating a message requires being able to consider different aspects of its meaning. Consideration should be given to the various meanings of a message or it will be hard to evaluate it correctly. People who expect to receive primarily one kind of message are prone to have difficulty in evaluating messages.

When strong feelings dominate the communication setting, people may not evaluate messages well. How one feels about oneself also influences the evaluation of messages received from others.

Transmitting Messages

If the person speaks so that the listener cannot understand, there will be a breakdown in communication. Talking too much or hardly at all are examples of disturbances in message transmission. The person who talks too quickly or too slowly risks not having his message received. Also, those who over-dramatize or give boring messages are apt to transmit poor messages. Slurring speech or exaggerated enunciation of words are other examples of poor message transmission.

Sending an incomplete message can also impede communication. Using unfinished sentences is one way of giving an incomplete message. Another is to use pronouns vaguely, such as "We went and so they did it." Sometimes messages are not transmitted at all, but the sender behaves as if they were. For example, the patient says, "My wife never helps me," and the nurse asks, "When did you last ask for help?" The patient replies, "She's supposed to know I need help." The nurse pursues with, "How could she know?", and the patient then says, "I guess she can't."

Effective transmission of a message requires communication that is (1) of proper length, (2) well spaced in time and tempo and (3) stated simply and clearly. How messages determine the effectiveness of communication is shown in figure 15-1, page 232.

232

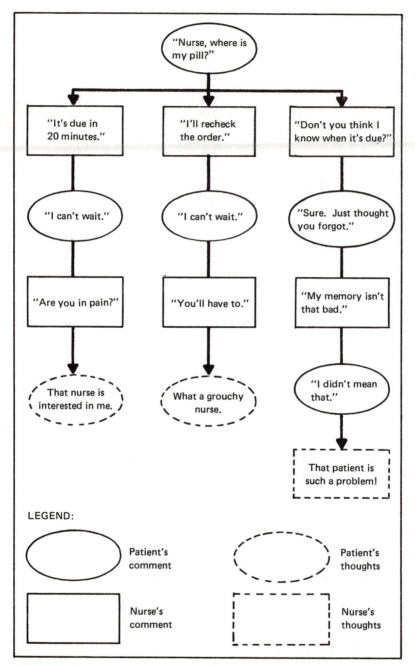

Fig. 15-1 How messages are received, evaluated and transmitted determines the effectiveness of communication.

THE COMMUNICATION PROCESS

Communication is a process. A message is not complete until it has been sent and received. When the receiver lets the sender know the message has been received and the sender recognizes this, a message has been exchanged. When one person expresses an idea in a message and the other person comments on that idea, feedback has occurred. *Feedback* is a correction device in the communication process where the sender receives correction of errors and learns about the results of his or her own statements. Learning is tied into the communication process through the feedback device. When the child says, "I go-ed to the store," and the parents say, "Not go-ed, *went*," feedback has occurred. When the patient says, "I'm thinking about going on vacation," and the nurse says, "Do you think you're strong enough for that?" feedback has also occurred. Because feedback is a powerful learning tool, the nurse is careful of when, how, and where feedback is given to the patient, figure 15-2.

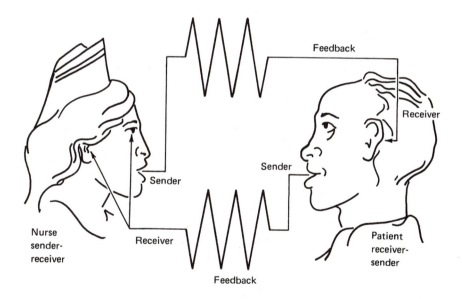

Fig. 15-2 Communication is an ongoing process where the sender is also a receiver.

It is difficult to determine whether two people ever completely understand one another. This is because people are so individual and communication is such a complex process. Words themselves can add to this problem simply because they have different meanings. For example, some meanings for the word *table* are: a piece of furniture, a list of details or numbers, a layer of bony tissue in the skull, a molding, the flat surface of a precious stone, a group of people seated at a table. Many words also have private meanings for each person. These private meanings or connotations are based on past experience. For example, a person whose mother deserted her as a child may have a different connotation of *mother* than a person whose mother was pleasant, warm, and available. Because words themselves vary in meaning, the nurse tries to clarify and qualify whatever is said. Examples of words and phrases that usually need to be qualified or clarified are:

everybody	all of them
nobody	you know
everything	all men are . . .
never	all women are . . .
always	all nurses are . . .

LEVELS OF COMMUNICATION

Verbal communication has at least two levels of meaning. One level is called the *denotative* or literal content meaning. If one person says, "It's cold in here," the person thinks the environment is cold; the communication has a literal content meaning.

The other level of communication is the metacommunication level. *Metacommunication* is the message about a message. Metacommunication tells the receiver how the sender feels about the message just sent, how the sender feels about the receiver, or how the sender feels about himself.

Whenever a person communicates, he or she asks someone for something, and expects to receive what is requested. This is the *command level of a message.* In the statement, "It's cold in here," the command level may be: "Bring me a sweater," "Close the window," "Don't pay any attention to me," or "Listen to what I say." The command aspect of a message may be clearly stated, or it may be so unclear that the receiver misses the command completely. People who miss the meaning of most messages are apt to be called psychiatric patients. They are not able to guess the thoughts and feelings of others accurately. Receivers who decide that all senders are criticizing them are likely to be called paranoid. Receivers who decide that all senders are praising them are likely to be called egocentric or self-centered.

Senders also vary in their ability to send messages. Some senders are unclear in their messages; the receiver then has to guess what is meant. Here is an example of decreasing clarity in the same message:

"Let's go to class."

"You'd like to go to class, wouldn't you?"

"If you want to go to class, we'll go."

"We might as well go to class. It's time."

"There's a class meeting about now."

"My voices are telling me to go to class."

An unclear message results when the sender refuses to take responsibility for it. Psychiatric patients are most apt to refuse to take responsibility for their messages. It is almost as if they anticipate that their messages will be refused.

Even though the sender's message is unclear, the nurse as the receiver can always ask, "Are you saying that . . .?" or "What does that mean?" in an attempt to clarify the message. Figure 15-3 shows some examples of metacommunications.

DISTURBED COMMUNICATION

The following are assessments that can be made to determine if communication is disturbed.

- identity
- relationship
- speaker's intent
- goal of action
- emotional reaction
- logic of explanations
- location of the reason for disturbance

Message	Metacommunication
"It was only a joke."	Ignore it.
"I was asking you a question."	Answer it.
"I'm telling you to pick up the paper."	Obey.
"You'll die when you hear this joke."	Laugh at it.
"Did you hear what I said?"	Pay attention.
"Boy, did that hurt."	Sympathize with me.

Fig. 15-3 Metacommunications are messages about messages.

Identity

The assessment here is who spoke to whom. If the patient refuses to call himself or be called by his own name, there is a disturbance in this area. For example, if the patient's name is Jones and he asks to be called Mr. Thompson, there is a disturbance in identity. If the sender says, "I was talking to the voice in my head" and denies that he was talking to the nurse, there is also a disturbance in identity.

The nurse who is making the assessment can do a number of things. First, she must not support the disturbance in identity. The nurse can state that she notices the patient wishes to be called Mr. Thompson even though she knows him as Mr. Jones. Secondly, the nurse must try to help the patient take responsibility for his messages. In the example above, the nurse might say, "Were you talking to me?" when the patient seems to be talking to "voices."

Relationship

The way people relate to one another can be expressed in terms of the roles they occupy in various social settings. One person may occupy the role of the nurse, mother, teacher, wife, and tennis player, depending on the social setting at the time.

When the patient reacts toward the nurse as if the nurse were a relative or old friend, there is a disturbance in the communication relationship. The nurse might then say, "I'm Ms/Mr. _____ , a nurse" and give the patient appropriate feedback to correct the disturbance about the relationship.

When the nurse reacts toward a patient who looks or acts in some way like a family member or friend, a disturbance in the communication relationship can also occur. Also, when other nurses, doctors, or health team members are hospitalized, the nurse may be confused about the role of the hospitalized person. It is best for the nurse to designate the relationship as nurse-patient, not nurse-colleague. If the nurse does not allow the ill colleague to be a patient, the nurse sets the stage for a disturbed communication relationship.

Speaker's Intent

In daily conversations, the receiver is constantly trying to guess the speaker's intent, which may be consciously or unconsciously transmitted. The receiver is probably more likely to distort the message when the intention of the speaker is not clearly demonstrated. The speaker who is aware of the conscious intent of his message, and is striving to be aware of other levels of messages he may be communicating is more apt to be a clear communicator.

Goal of Action

If the expectation of what the receiver should do is not clearly stated, the receiver will often disappoint the sender. When the speaker is unclear, the receiver is inclined to think, "What is he really after?" or "What does she want?" or "What does *that* mean?" In these instances there is likely to be a disturbance in communication.

Emotional Reaction

When the expected emotional reaction is not shown, the sender or receiver may think there is something wrong with the other person. If the sender says, "This is really sad," and the receiver says, "Let me tell you a joke," an inappropriate emotional reaction is occurring. If the nurse receives this message, it is not expected that the nurse, too, will feel sad. She is expected to allow the patient to express whatever feeling is being experienced and support him emotionally.

Logic of Explanations

When an illogical explanation is given to explain a situation, the sender-receiver may have difficulty understanding the message. For example, if the nurse asks the patient, "How did you happen to come to this hospital?" and the patient answered, "I was playing bridge this morning," the nurse will not be able to immediately grasp the connection between the question asked and the patient's answer. Such explanations are called *loose associations.* Loose associations are evident when the speaker's response does not seem to be directly connected to what was just said. The nurse not only tries to present information to the patient in a logical way, but also tries to clarify any loose associations. For example, the nurse might say, "I don't follow that" or "What does playing bridge have to do with coming to the hospital?"

Locating the Reason for the Disturbance

Communication disturbance can occur because of sensory, motor, or central nervous system abnormalities. A patient who cannot hear or see well may have trouble receiving messages. A person who cannot speak clearly due to abnormality or disease of the organs of speech will have difficulty sending a clear message. Patients with brain damage due to a tumor, blood clot, alcohol or drugs may also receive and send unclear messages.

Young children and some psychiatric patients make literal interpretations of messages that are meant to be taken abstractly. For example, a five-year-old child who is told he is "growing out of his clothes" may look in the mirror to see if the growth is visible. A psychiatric patient may be asked, "What is your view on that?", and he may reply, "Southwest." In both cases, the message was misinterpreted by the receiver and disturbed communication was the result.

Language barriers can also create disturbances in communication. If the sender speaks one language and the receiver speaks another there tends to be problems in communication.

Area of Disturbance	Questions to Ask
Identity	Who spoke to whom? Did the patient want to be called by another name than his? Did the patient deny that he was talking to the nurse?
Relationship	Did the patient act toward the nurse as if the nurse were a friend or family member? Did the nurse act toward the patient as if the patient were a friend or family member? Did the nurse treat a hospitalized colleague as a patient or colleague?
Speaker's Intent	Was the speaker clear about what he or she wanted? Did the speaker seem to be aware of conscious or unconscious intent?
Goal of Action	Was it clear what the receiver was supposed to do? Did the receiver seem puzzled about what the speaker expected from him?
Emotional Reactions	Did each person show expected emotional reactions? Did one person prevent the other from expressing thoughts or feelings?
Logic of Explanations	Did the conversation seem to flow? Were the comments related? If there were loose associations, did either party try to clarify them?
Location of the Reason for Disturbance	Were there sensory, motor, or CNS abnormalities? Did the receiver respond literally when the sender was being abstract? Were there language barriers? Was there too much noise or distraction? Was there interpersonal or intergroup disturbance?

Fig. 15-4 Assessing disturbed verbal communication

Disturbed communication can result if there is too much background noise or distraction. If the nurse hopes to communicate effectively with the patient, she must consider the amount of noise and distraction in the external environment.

Sometimes disturbed communication is located within a group; often a whole family has disturbed communication patterns. In such cases, the whole family may be treated by the family therapy method, because the disturbance is located within the group. Figure 15-4 summarizes types of disturbed verbal communication.

SUMMARY

Communication is the process of giving and getting information from others. Communication includes both verbal and nonverbal messages. The ability to receive, evaluate, and transmit messages are the three functions of communication. Feedback is a communication device that provides for learning and correction of errors. There are at least two levels of communication. One level is the denotative or literal content meaning. Another level is the metacommunication or message about the message level. In assessing disturbed communication, the nurse examines identity, relationship, speaker's intent, goal of action, emotional reaction, logic of explanations, and location of the cause for the disturbance.

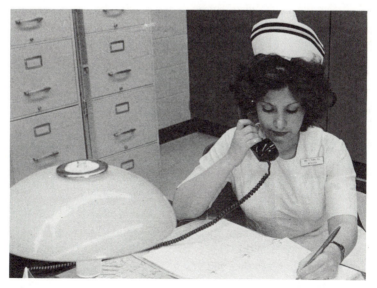

Fig. 15-5 Communication involves the ability to receive, evaluate, and transmit messages clearly.

ACTIVITIES AND DISCUSSION TOPICS

- Look up two or more meanings for the following words:

  lead   well

  table   lie

  Do you always use these words so the patient understands the meaning you have in mind?

- Listen to a conversation between two of your friends or family members. Jot down any ideas as you listen so you won't forget them. Answer the following questions after listening to the conversation?

  a. Were the messages clear?

  b. Did the receiver give the sender feedback?

  c. Did the receiver or sender use words that have more than one meaning? Did each seem to understand what was meant?

  d. What metacommunications did you hear?

  e. Were there any disturbances in identity?

  f. Were there any disturbances in relationship?

  g. Was the speaker's intent clear?

  h. Was the speaker's goal of action clear?

  i. Were the emotional reactions of the participants appropriate?

  j. Did both participants use logical explanations or were there loose associations?

  k. If there were any disturbances in communication, were they within the person, in the situation, or in the group?

REVIEW

A. Multiple Choice. Select the best answer(s). Some questions have more than one answer.

    1. The appropriate evaluation of a message depends on

        a. a combination of information from the external environment.

        b. strong feelings dominating the communication setting.

        c. information from the person's own sense organs.

        d. past experiences or memories.

    2. Effective transmission of a message requires communication that is

        a. of proper length.

        b. well spaced in time and tempo.

        c. stated very slowly.

        d. stated simply and clearly.

3. Learning is tied into the communication process through
   a. literal interpretations.   c. metacommunication.
   b. loose associations.   d. feedback.

4. In determining if a communication disturbance exists, the nurse assesses emotional reaction by questioning if
   a. the receiver seemed puzzled about what the speaker expected from him.
   b. the conversation seemed to flow naturally.
   c. one person prevented the other from expressing thoughts or feelings.
   d. the receiver responded literally when the sender was being abstract.

5. People who decide that all communication received by them is critical are
   a. egocentric.   c. paranoid.
   b. schizophrenic.   d. self-centered.

B. Match the items in Column II to the correct statements in Column I.

Column I	Column II
1. Message about a message that tells the receiver how the sender feels about the receiver, the sender, or the message.	a. command
	b. denotative
	c. feedback
	d. loose association
2. Speaker's response does not seem to follow or relate to the preceding discussion.	e. metacommunication
	f. timing

3. Level of communication with literal content meaning; usually a meaning found in the dictionary for that language.

4. Level of communication when a person asks someone for something and expects to receive what is requested.

5. A correction device in the communication process where the sender receives correction of errors and discovers the results of his own statements.

6. An important element in evaluating a message.

C. Briefly answer the following questions.

 1. Define communication.

 2. List three functions of communication.

 3. Name two levels of communication.

 4. List five areas of assessment to determine if communication is disturbed.

D. Label the parts of the communication process on the diagram below.

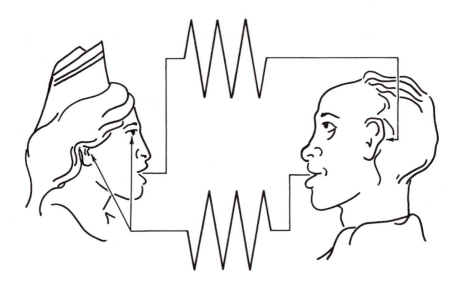

chapter 16
NONVERBAL COMMUNICATION

STUDENT OBJECTIVES

- Define nonverbal communication.
- Identify the relationship between verbal and nonverbal communication.
- List three types of nonverbal communication.
- List five aspects of nonverbal communication assessed by the nurse.

Nonverbal communication is all communication that is not spoken or written. Gestures, facial expression, posture, music and even dance are forms of nonverbal communication.

TYPES OF NONVERBAL COMMUNICATION

There are three types of nonverbal communication: sign language, action language, and object language. The nurse is challenged to use observational skills in learning to recognize these valuable indicants of health and illness.

Sign Language

Smoke signals, Morse Code, signals used by motorists, and gestures used by deaf people are types of sign language which are complicated and require some instruction. Examples of more simple sign language are the gesture of the hitchhiker, the peace sign, and the three signs shown in figures 16-1, 16-2, and 16-3, page 244. Other examples are fingerprints, footprints, cigarette butts, and worn heels on shoes.

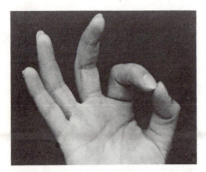

Fig. 16-1 The "o.k." or "all right" sign is a nonverbal communication.

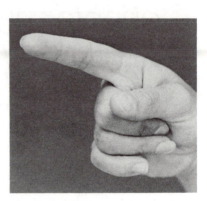

Fig. 16-2 Direction or accusation can be conveyed nonverbally.

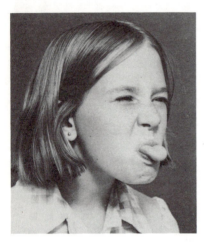

Fig. 16-3 Children often use effective nonverbal communication.

The patient conveys nonverbal information about himself through stains, calluses, discolorations in skin, and through joint changes that occur due to arthritis. The development of certain muscle groups may transmit information about that person's health and occupation. Muscle tone can convey information by nonverbal communication. For example, tense musculature may be a sign of anxiety or fear, and stooped posture can indicate depression, a lifetime of bending over books, or a physical process such as aging or arthritis.

Action Language

Action language includes all movements that are not used as signals. There are two purposes inherent in action language. For example, walking, drinking, and dancing serve two purposes. One purpose is to meet human needs. Another purpose is to suggest a message to the receiver (or observer). The message might be: "I am an active person," or "I'm in pain, but I keep moving," or even, "I have a zest for life."

Object Language

People transmit messages about themselves by displaying objects. The objects may be in the immediate environment or worn on their person. The number and kind of machines owned, art objects displayed, houses lived in, possessions owned, and clothes worn are all messages to others. People surround themselves with objects and send messages such as: "I am wealthy, admire me," or "I am orderly and attractive, hire me," or "I am poor but honest, respect me."

THE RELATIONSHIP BETWEEN NONVERBAL AND VERBAL COMMUNICATION

Nonverbal communication is not just an accompaniment to verbal communication. Nonverbal communication can be substituted for verbal communication or can complement or contradict it. For example, the very young child uses purely nonverbal communication to make his needs known. As speech and language ability develop he uses more verbal communication.

Nonverbal communication can also shape verbal communication. If one person turns away from the other, verbal communication will be shaped and affected.

Nonverbal Messages Differ From Verbal Messages

Sign, action and object languages require a certain amount of space to be effective. If arms must be swung or halls paced, there must be sufficient physical space. Written words require less space. The printed word can be vastly reduced in size through the microfilm process.

Nonverbal and verbal communication also differ in their time and order requirements. Nonverbal communication is always in the here-and-now. People get a feel for what is happening based on multiple sensory impressions that occur all at once.

Verbal and nonverbal languages do not appeal to the same senses. Spoken language is perceived by the ear. Silent language is perceived only by the eye. Action language may be perceived by the eye, ear, touch, temperature, and vibration. Action language is used to demonstrate skills when effective teaching requires more than writing or speaking. For example, a nursing student learns how to make a bed by reading and hearing about the basic principles, observing the instructor and practicing the bedmaking; action language supports the written and spoken word.

Emotions are expressed by action language. Some of these actions are nearly automatic and are more difficult to conceal than verbal messages. Slamming a fist on the table or throwing up the hands in frustration are almost universal messages. Besides signalling a feeling, action language can also shift the tension level in an interaction and make it possible to re-establish contact. The nurse who thinks tension levels are becoming too high may unconsciously begin to tap her finger or twist in her chair. Patients, too, may use action language to shift the tension level; they may pace in the hall or drum on a table top, for example.

When sign language or gestures are used with the spoken word, the relationship between nonverbal and verbal communication is clear. Gestures are often used to illustrate, emphasize, explain, or interrupt. Because of this, gestures cannot be viewed without also observing the verbal communication that is occurring.

The notion of metacommunication is the best way to understand how verbal communication is related to nonverbal communication. All messages have two parts: the statement or content part, and the command or explanation part. In order for people to understand one another, these two parts have to occur at about the same time. When a statement is made verbally, the instructions about the message (or metacommunication) tends to be nonverbal. Combinations of the verbal and nonverbal can help to clarify a message. For example, if the patient says, "I'm in pain," and then holds his abdomen and grimaces, the nurse will see more clearly that the patient is in pain.

Combinations of the verbal and the nonverbal can also confuse. For example, if a mother says to her child, "I hate you" while kissing him, the child will probably be confused. This type of message is called a *double bind*. In the double bind, two conflicting messages are given; the verbal message is not in agreement with the nonverbal message. The receiver is placed in an impossible situation because he must decide which message he should respond to. If the receiver responds to one message, the sender may wonder why there was no response to the other one. This situation is a double bind because no matter which message the receiver responds to it may be perceived by the sender as the wrong one. This type of confusion may leave the receiver with the impression that he cannot please the other person no matter what he does. Figure 16-4 shows the relationship between verbal and nonverbal communication.

Factor to Consider	Verbal Messages	Nonverbal Messages
Fit with other form of communication	Can complement or contradict nonverbal messages	Can complement or contradict verbal messages
Space	Minimal demands	Requires certain amount of space
Time	Here and now, or much later	Here and now only
Order	Serial order	Multiple impressions at once
Sense used	Hearing	Sight, hearing, touch, taste, smell
Expression of feeling	Can be disguised	Less easily disguised unless learned early in life

Fig. 16-4 The relationship of verbal to nonverbal communication

THE MEANING OF NONVERBAL COMMUNICATION

When trying to communicate with persons from different cultural groups it is important to observe and read about nonverbal behavior characteristic of that group. According to studies by Ruesch and others, nonverbal actions and gestures have meanings depending on the culture.[1] For example, both Japanese and Americans hiss; that is, they produce a sound resembling the letter *s* or *sh*. In America, the hiss is a sign of disapproval while in Japan, the hiss is a sign of courtesy to others who have more status.

The German culture is shaped by ideas of law and order. Generally, German people consider the face and spine as the most expressive areas of the body. To some Mexican-Americans, sustained direct eye contact may mean giving someone the "evil eye," so eye contact is only made if the person is also touched at the same time. (Touch is thought to ward off the "evil eye.") In Jewish societies, gesture is used to emphasize what is being said; there is physical contact through grasping, poking, and pulling. People of Scandinavian heritage may interact more freely when food is shared.

Recently there have been several attempts to predict what body movements mean. In general, it is wise not to try to understand a body movement without first observing the environment within which the movement occurs. Body movement that may be inappropriate in one setting may be quite acceptable in another.

[1] Jurgen Ruesch and Weldon Kees, *Nonverbal Communication: Notes on the Visual Perception of Human Relations* (Berkeley, Calif: University of California Press, 1956)

One factor that greatly influences the meaning of nonverbal behavior is the act of being observed. Observing someone, without saying a word, provides opportunity for feedback and influences the outcome of the situation. With practice, nurses can become good observers of nonverbal communication; as a result, they may be able to introduce less change into the observed situation.

ASSESSING AND INTERVENING IN NONVERBAL COMMUNICATION

To assess the patient's nonverbal communication, the nurse considers the following aspects: symptoms and signs, eye contact, touch, distance, posture, facial expression, appearance, movements, sounds, and correlation with verbal communication.

Symptoms and Signs

Through observing patient signs and symptoms, the nurse can gather information about the patient's physical and emotional health. Sometimes symptoms may be used by patients to signal other difficulties. For example, patients who complain of pain may actually be expressing other feelings as well as asking for nursing care. Frequently the patient who has many complaints is protesting or explaining thoughts and feelings he cannot explain more directly.

Pain complaints are often used to disguise other messages. A patient may complain "I feel as if someone were hitting me over the head." From this, the nurse might report, "The patient has a headache." But the patient's complaint could have a deeper meaning such as being figuratively hit over the head with the disapproval of his parents. By helping the patient to explore and describe symptoms, the nurse can identify more exact meanings for messages.

Eye Contact

The meaning of eyes through eye contact is an important social event. Eye contact signals a mutual openness and lack of it may hint at anxiety, distrust or fear. Even when the nurse cannot reach the patient through verbal communication, eye contact can be used to establish a relationship. It should be noted that persons who have been raised in certain cultures or families may find eye contact anxiety-provoking.

Touch

Touch is used to soothe, protest, restrain, reassure, and to gain attention. Nurses transmit a nonverbal message every time they touch patients. The nurse must, therefore, be aware of what feeling her touch may transmit to the patient during nursing procedures or other nursing intervention. Touch that may be intended to be comforting or reassuring may be interpreted differently if the nurse's hands are cold or if her personal concern cannot be conveyed.

There seem to be cultural differences in the use of touch and what part of the body can be touched. Nurses sometimes forget that to some patients the nurse's touch may be anxiety-provoking. Psychiatric patients often misunderstand its purpose. Some psychiatric patients may interpret the nurse's touch as a form of attack. The nurse must be especially careful not to touch patients who are suspicious or who are already overstimulated.

Although the nurse must use touch in some nursing procedures, it is best to tell the patient what will be done prior to the actual touch. In other situations, where words are not sufficient, the nurse may use touch to demonstrate, teach, or to soothe the patient. The backrub, hand on the arm or shoulder, and the squeeze of the hand can provide closeness between nurse and patient in many cases. Suspicious patients are less likely to become anxious if the hand or arm is touched.

Some patients may crave physical touch and may demonstrate this wish by touching the nurse or by asking the nurse to "hold my hand." Some psychiatric patients are unclear about their body boundaries and the limits of the nurse-patient relationship. These patients may test the nurse's ability to set limits regarding physical contact.

Touch can also be anxiety-provoking for the nurse. If physical contact with the patient elicits anxiety in the student or nurse, it is best to study about the meaning of touch and its therapeutic effects, and discuss the anxiety with an instructor or nursing colleague.

The use of restraints should be evaluated in light of the patient's need for freedom of movement and freedom from being touched. Geriatric or medical-surgical patients who are physically restrained often interpret restraints as an attack or attempt to limit their movement unnecessarily. Although the initial purpose of restraining a patient may be to protect the patient, patients may struggle so severely against being restrained that they may harm themselves or others in the effort.

Distance

With increased interest in nonverbal communication, a whole new study called proxemics has developed. *Proxemics* is the study of how people communicate by their use of space. When people talk, they stand or sit a certain distance away, face each other in certain ways and assume particular positions in relation to one another.

Cultural differences occur in the use of space, too. In some cultures, it is important to be close enough to smell the other person; being able to smell the other means rapport can be established. On the other hand, in the middle-class American culture, natural body smells are often replaced or suppressed as much as possible.

People who are fearful or agitated place more distance between themselves and others. The fear and agitation must be dealt with first. Trying to decrease the distance before relieving the fear or agitation worsens the discomfort. The patient may view this action as an attack by the nurse rather than the help she intended to give.

Sitting or standing too far away creates distance in a relationship and a feeling of isolation in both persons. Nursing procedures frequently require closing the distance between nurse and patient. Nurses often take this invasion of the patient's personal space for granted. It should be remembered that patients may or may not react with anxiety to the physical closeness of the nurse.

Posture

Posture can convey the inner feelings of a person. Body posture may be held by a person for a period of time as a backdrop for short, nonverbal messages such as gestures or facial expression. For example, a patient may sit rigidly at a table and commence tapping it impatiently.

Posture can express withdrawal. The nurse can often observe such changes in posture in herself and the patient if she sits with a patient for several minutes. A patient sitting alone in a slumped-over position may seem dejected. If some-one approaches him and talks with him, this same patient may sit up straight and look interested or the opposite may occur. For example, the patient may look interested until the nurse approaches, and then he may slump over. Some topics of conversation may lead to feelings that are expressed through body posture, such as dejection or interest.

Body posture also provides nonverbal clues to the nurse about pain, illness processes, occupation, and cultural history.

Facial Expression

Facial expression can indicate a wide variety of emotions which are only partly revealed by words. A smile, frown, wrinkled forehead, tight mouth, blank expression, or an angry look all announce inner feelings.

Facial expression may also belie inner feelings. In some families or cultural groups, the facial expression reports one feeling while the person really experiences another feeling.

For example, the Japanese or Spanish-American person may smile and nod "yes" only to be polite. The real feelings may be directly opposite to the smile. Some psychiatric patients may be experiencing high emotional states but show no expression on their faces. *Flat affect* is a term used to describe patients whose faces and posture are expressionless and whose tone of voice is monotonous. Patients who laugh when discussing a sad experience or cry when reporting one where laughter is expected are said to have *inappropriate affect.*

Appearance

Appearance means the way people look. Weight, height, musculature, hair, clothing, and the use of cosmetics and jewelry are all part of appearance. Appearance signals sex, age, occupational, cultural, and professional differences. Body image and self-concept are revealed; feelings can also be reflected by the colors selected for clothes, the use of flashy jewelry, the amount of makeup, hairstyle, and so on.

People learn to wear clothes that fit the setting they are in. They tell others about themselves — who they are, what they are doing, and what they intend to do — by the clothes they choose to wear.

Movements

Almost any movement that a person makes can be interpreted to be a message. Whether it is meant to be considered as a message may need further exploration. Gestures are often clear messages to the other person. Stroking the hair, tapping the foot, shifting from one foot to the other, crossing or uncrossing the legs, and smoking, are all body movements which may have one or more meanings.

Body movements can occur (1) when there is pressure on muscles or tendons, (2) when there is inner tension or anxiety, or (3) when one person wishes to signal another person. Body movements which are repetitive, seem to punctuate a conversation, or change radically from previous movements are worthwhile discussing with the patient. For example, a patient who sits quietly for a few minutes and then starts to tap his foot whenever surgery is mentioned may be conveying anxiety about the subject being discussed. When the nurse notices such an obvious body movement, she might say, "You're tapping your foot," or "What are you thinking (feeling) right now?", or "Are you anxious now?" When the nurse does comment on the patient's nonverbal behavior, she implies that the behavior may have some meaning and should be explored further.

Silence

Silences can be viewed as punctuation to conversation or as nonverbal comments about what is happening between the nurse and patient. In social situations, silences are apt to be avoided. In the nurse-patient relationship, silences provide important information for the nurse. There are different kinds of silences. The nurse needs to be able to identify these silences and intervene appropriately.

One kind of silence is the angry silence in which the patient may be trying to set up a power struggle with the nurse. The patient transmits a message such as, "I'm angry and I won't talk," or "You can't force me to talk." If the nurse responds with anxious pressure to force the patient to talk, a struggle takes place to decide who will win. A better tactic is to remain undemanding but interested. The nurse might say, "What are you feeling?" or "What's going on?" to encourage the patient to examine feelings that might be blocking more constructive discussion.

Another kind of silence is the anxious or fearful silence. This silence may occur in persons who have been criticized in the past for speaking up to others. The patient who demonstrates an anxious or fearful silence may not be able to use verbal communication because he fears relating to the nurse.

Psychiatric patients may hallucinate during silences and may remember other interpersonal situations that created anxiety. Staying physically present during anxious or fearful silences, recognizing the patient's effort to talk, accepting what he does say, and later encouraging the patient to examine the source of anxiety, are useful interventions.

The blocked silence occurs when the patient reports he "can't think of anything to say." When she finds a noncommunicative patient, the nurse can ask, "What are you feeling?" If the patient responds, "Nothing," or "I can't think of anything," the nurse might reply firmly, "You'll think of something." When the nurse communicates a positive expectation that the patient will talk during a blocked silence, the patient often does talk. As a last resort, the nurse can make an open-end suggestion on a topic that is nonthreatening such as "Tell me how you spend your day here."

The thoughtful silence occurs when the patient is thinking over what has just happened, or when he is thinking of how to word his next statement.

Factor Being Assessed	Assessment or Intervention
Eye contact	Does the patient maintain eye contact? Does the nurse maintain eye contact? Are there cultural factors that affect eye contact?
Touch	What is the meaning of touch to the patient and nurse? Could the patient perceive touch or restraint as attack? How could touch be used to soothe or reassure the patient? Does the nurse need to set limits on the patient's use of touch? Does touch elicit anxiety in the nurse or the patient? Are there cultural factors that affect use and interpretation of touch?
Distance	How does the patient use space? What distance from others does the patient seem to favor? Is the nurse's use of space helpful to the patient's need for personal space? Are there cultural factors that affect use of space?
Posture	What feelings does posture of the patient or nurse reveal? What clues about pain, illness, occupational or cultural history can the nurse observe from the patient's posture?
Facial expression	Does facial expression fit with or belie verbal communication? What emotions does the patient's facial expression indicate? Does the patient show flat or inappropriate affect?
Appearance	What does the patient's appearance show about the patient's feelings about self and others?
Movements	What repetitive, unexpected or punctuating body movements does the patient make?
Silence	What nurse-patient silences are there? Does the nurse struggle with the patient who is in an angry silence? Does the nurse stay with the patient during anxious or fearful silences? Does the nurse communicate a positive expectation to the patient during a blocked silence? Does the nurse feel uncomfortable during patient silences?
Sounds	What sounds such as cries, sighs, whistles, gasps, laughter, or voice tone, loudness and pitch are communicated?
Consistency with verbal messages	Does the metacommunication support the verbal communication? Are there double bind situations operating?

Fig. 16-5 Nursing assessments and interventions in nonverbal behavior

Thoughtful silences are best left uninterrupted. If the silence goes on for more than five minutes, the nurse might say, "What were you thinking?"

The student will need to practice sitting quietly in silence. The ability to identify types of silences will develop with experience. Students who feel too comfortable sitting in long silence should determine whether they are withdrawing from interaction with the patient; recognizing one's own feelings during silences is crucial to assisting the patient. The nurse can learn much about the reasons for silence by recalling what events occurred just before the period of silence.

Sounds

Sounds such as loudness, pitch and tone of voice, cries, sighs, whistles, gasps, and laughter are also nonverbal communications. Anxiety or comfort are often suggested by the sounds made by the patient.

Consistency with Verbal Messages

The nurse assesses whether the nonverbal message seems to be consistent with what the patient is saying. When the message does not fit the verbal statement, the nurse notes this. If this misfit occurs frequently, the nurse begins to explore this issue with the patient. Often patients are not aware of the confused messages they give others. However, they are aware of frustration, anger, and the anxious or rejecting responses of others who have been placed in a double bind by the confused message.

If the nurse is able to work with the patient over a period of time, it is possible to teach him about the confused messages. For example, the nurse might say, "You're laughing but you're talking about death," or "You're smiling but I sense you're angry." Figure 16-5, page 253, summarizes nursing assessments and interventions for nonverbal patient behavior.

SUMMARY

Nonverbal communication includes all forms of communication that are not spoken or written. Three types of nonverbal communication are sign language, action language, and object language. Although verbal and nonverbal communication differ in terms of space, time, and sensations, they can both work together to make a complete message. Nonverbal communication can complement and help to explain verbal communication or it can contradict and confuse a message.

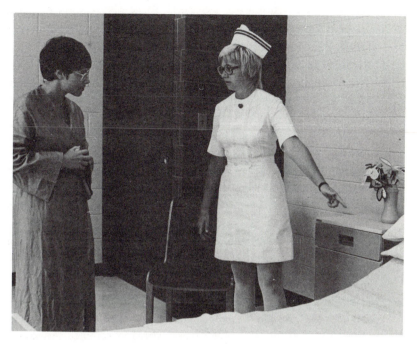

Fig. 16-6 Gestures are often used to illustrate or emphasize.

The meaning of nonverbal communication depends on the culture of the group and environment where the communication occurs. When assessing and intervening in nonverbal communication, the nurse notes the following aspects: symptoms and signs, touch, distance, posture, facial expression, appearance, movements, silence, sounds, and consistency with verbal communication.

ACTIVITIES AND DISCUSSION TOPICS

- Select one or more patients to observe. Then answer the following questions.
    - a. Describe the patient's symptoms and signs. Do any of them hint at other messages?
    - b. Describe how the patient uses touch in communicating with you.
    - c. Describe clues you have observed about the patient's wishes to be physically close or distant from you.
    - d. Describe the patient's posture when sitting, standing, walking, when apparently unobserved, and when with you. Are there changes in patient posture? When do they occur?

e. Describe the patient's facial expression when unobserved, when greeting you, when leaving you. What other facial expressions did you observe? Does the patient show flat or inappropriate affect?

f. Describe the patient's appearance. What is the patient's body build? Describe the clothing, cosmetics, jewelry, and personal hygiene habits. What does the patient's appearance tell you about his body image and self-concept?

g. Describe the patient's movements. What repetitive movements, punctuating movements, or radical change in body movement did you notice?

h. Describe the silences in your interaction with the patient. Were there angry, anxious, blocked or thoughtful silences?

i. Describe the cries, sighs, whistles, gasps, laughter, and loudness, pitch, and tone of voice.

j. Describe the consistency between verbal and nonverbal communication. Does the metacommunication support the verbal communication? Were there any double binds?

• Over a period of time (at least a week) keep a log of your own nonverbal communication. Be sure to include your eye contact with others, preference for touch (body area and when desired), preference for physical distance from others, posture(s), facial expressions, appearance, characteristic body movements, feelings during silences, and consistency of verbal with nonverbal communication. Ask a friend, classmate, or family member to help you describe all aspects of your nonverbal communication, including those of which you are not aware.

REVIEW

A. Multiple Choice. Select the best answer(s). Some questions have more than one answer.

1. The correct statements that describe the relationship between verbal and nonverbal communication are:
   a. Nonverbal communication can complement or contradict verbal communication.
   b. Nonverbal communication is never used instead of verbal communication.
   c. Nonverbal communication requires more space than verbal communication.
   d. Feelings are more accurately expressed through verbal communication.

2. Useful nursing interventions for a patient who is fearfully silent are:
   a. insisting the patient talk about his fear.
   b. being physically present during the silence.
   c. recognizing the patient's effort to talk.
   d. accepting what the patient does say.

3. Body posture can provide nonverbal clues about the patient's
   a. pain.
   b. occupation.
   c. culture.
   d. illness processes.

4. When the patient reports he can't think of anything to say, the silence is referred to as
   a. angry silence.
   b. thoughtful silence.
   c. anxious silence.
   d. blocked silence.

5. Body image and self-concept are revealed in a person's
   a. appearance.
   b. movements.
   c. facial expressions.
   d. touch.

B. Match the items in Column II to the correct statements in Column I.

Column I	Column II
1. Forms of nonverbal communication such as Morse Code and communicating with the deaf.	a. action language
	b. double bind
	c. flat affect
2. Form of nonverbal communication that includes all movements not used specifically as signals.	d. inappropriate affect
	e. object language
	f. proxemics
3. Form of nonverbal communication where people convey messages about themselves by displaying objects on or about themselves.	g. sign language
4. Two conflicting messages are given; the verbal message is not in agreement with the nonverbal message.	
5. Expressionless face, posture or tone of voice.	
6. Tone of voice, facial expression, or posture that does not fit with the situation being experienced.	
7. The study of how people communicate by their use of space.	

C. Briefly answer the following questions.

    1. Define nonverbal communication.

    2. Name three types of nonverbal communications.

    3. List five aspects of nonverbal communication the nurse assesses.

    4. Name the two parts of all messages.

chapter 17
INTERVIEWING AND COMMUNICATION SKILLS

STUDENT OBJECTIVES

- List five factors to consider in the interview situation.
- Give five purposes for the nursing interview.
- Identify what is meant by the theme of an interview.
- Match a list of communication skills with appropriate examples.
- Identify aspects of communication that will help the nurse become an effective communicator.

The *nursing interview* is conversation with a purpose. An interview may occur spontaneously or it may be planned. It may be a short-term interview or take a longer period of time to achieve its objective. Every interview reflects a major idea; this theme flows throughout the interaction. Conducting an interview with a child or by telephone requires more skill but the basic elements of a good nursing interview remain the same.

THE NURSING INTERVIEW

Several factors are considered when preparing for an interview, figure 17-1, page 260. One of the first things to consider is to establish the purpose of the interview. Sometimes an interview occurs spontaneously. A nurse may walk into a room and find the patient crying. In this case, the purpose of the inter-view would be to assist the patient to express feeling, relieve tension, and possi-'bly to help in problem solving.

Prepare for the interview depending on the purpose.

Arrange a comfortable, quiet setting.

Check with patient for consent if planning to take notes.

Assure confidentiality.

Avoid use of technical terms.

Listen actively.

Redirect the focus of conversation to the patient.

Avoid asking too many questions.

Use communication skills.

Give the patient clues close to the end of the interview that you will be leaving.

Fig. 17-1 Creating an interview climate.

At other times, the nurse may know beforehand because of an assignment to take a nursing history or to continue an ongoing process recording. In these instances, it is possible to prepare for the interview by examining previous records, reading texts and articles on the subject, and examining one's own thoughts and feelings about the upcoming experience.

Another factor to consider is the setting which should be a comfortable and quiet one. A well-ventilated room is conducive to quiet interaction; also, chairs should be provided, if necessary. If there is a choice of interview settings, the patient may be asked to choose the place which would be most comfortable for him. The nurse tells the patient about the purpose of the interview and assures him that what is discussed will be confidential; this helps to create the right climate for the interaction. If information is to be shared with others, the nurse should tell the patient just who will be given the information. Before the nurse proceeds to take any notes, the matter should be discussed and approved by the patient. If agreed upon, a small pocket notebook can be used.

The use of technical words or long explanations should be avoided. Statements should be brief and clearly made. The nurse should not ask too many questions; questions that get a "yes" or a "no" answer; or questions such as "How are you?" that get socially acceptable answers like "Fine."

Active listening requires being attentive to words and observing nonverbal communication; listening requires a lot of energy when it is done actively. As the nurse listens, asking these questions will develop the art of active listening:

"Why is he telling me *this now*?"

"Why does he choose the *words* he does?"

"What words is he *repeating* or *omitting*?"

"What *nonverbal communication* messages is he sending?"

"Is his nonverbal communication *consistent* with his verbal communication?" "Do I *understand* what he says, or should I interrupt and ask for clarification?"

If the nurse is asked a question about herself, she should redirect the focus back to the patient by saying something similar to "What about you?" or "Let's get back to you."

Questions that begin with *who, what, when* and *where* are often very effective in obtaining information about the patient. Statements such as "You should do this," or "Why don't you. . ." are to be avoided because they impose the views and values of the nurse on the patient.

When the time comes to end the interview, the nurse may terminate it smoothly by making a comment such as, "Before I leave, do you have any other questions?", or "I'll be leaving in five minutes." Such comments prepare the patient to end the discussion. It is the nurse's responsibility to end the interview but she should never end it abruptly and without warning.

Purposes of the Nursing Interview

As indicated earlier, one purpose of the nursing interview is to decrease the feeling of isolation by conveying an interest in the patient as a person. These interviews may be especially important to persons who are unable to relate to their environment because of physical or emotional factors. Some patients who might especially benefit from an interview with this purpose uppermost would be:

- Patients who are on bedrest for long periods of time.
- Patients in isolation or reverse isolation.
- Patients who find social interaction anxiety-provoking.
- Persons in homes for the aged and nursing homes.

Another purpose of the nursing interview is to establish and maintain the nurse-patient relationship. The mental health-psychiatric nurse focuses primarily on the nurse-patient relationships of those in her care. The primary nurse who works with one patient over a period of time provides for some time for nursing interviews in the overall nursing plan. This is also true of the hospital nurse who has more than one patient but she must plan her time more diligently in order to establish and maintain the relationship through nursing interviews.

The interview for the purpose of obtaining information is closely related to that of establishing and maintaining the nurse-patient relationship. The nursing history is a way to gather specific information about the patient's needs and wishes. Whenever the nurse is obtaining any information from the patient, communication occurs.

Providing for release of tension or expression of feeling is yet another purpose for the nursing interview. By talking with the nurse, the patient can channel his tension and energy into verbal and nonverbal expressions. As she assists the patient to release tension in this way, the nurse decreases the level of patient stress.

Teaching is an important purpose for the nursing interview. Providing help with diet, preparing a patient for surgery, and teaching anatomy and physiology to an expectant mother are examples of the nursing interview used to teach or give information.

The nursing interview provides the opportunity to clarify patient problems and assist with the solution of those problems. Whenever the nurse observes that the patient appears to be involved with a crisis, grief, pain, anxiety, isolation, or some other distressing situation, she may fully utilize the nursing interview.

Still another purpose of the nursing interview is referral. The nurse refers the patient to other resources as necessary; referral sources may be the doctor, the visiting nurse, the physical therapist, the family, or others who can be of assistance to the patient with the identified problem. The nurse also uses the referral technique when a patient asks her to answer for another. For example, if the patient says, "Does the doctor think I'm ready to go home?", the nurse should refer the patient to the doctor. The nurse might say, "I'm not sure. Why not ask Dr. Mason?" Figure 17-2 summarizes the purposes of the nursing interview.

The nursing interview is used to:

- Decrease isolation by conveying interest in the patient as a person.

- Establish and maintain the nurse-patient relationship.

- Obtain information.

- Provide for release of tension or expression of feeling.

- Give information or teach.

- Clarify problems and assist the patient to problem solve.

- Refer the patient to other resources.

Fig. 17-2 Purposes of the nursing interview.

Problems of the Beginning Interviewer

The beginning interviewer may have feelings of anxiety about the ability to perform adequately. There may be discomfort about the possibility of making errors and receiving criticism. Guilt feelings that the patient is being used or practiced upon may occur. The student may talk too much or too little; she may also have difficulty really listening to the patient. However, with experience based on the application of interviewing concepts, the ability to listen and observe will develop. Words, nonverbal expressions, timing, and communication will become meaningful and utilized more effectively. One step toward the goal of becoming a competent interviewer is to take notes of what was said during the interview. These notes can be expanded upon after the interaction. They should be analyzed and evaluated. The nurse can reflect on what took place and determine whether the course of action was appropriate. Regular discussions with a teacher or supervisor who is an effective communicator can also be of help toward becoming a skilled interviewer.

Short-term or Long-term Interviews

Some nursing interviews, like the nursing history, take place only once. These interviews are short-term interviews. They are done for the purpose of obtaining or giving specific information and may be completed in one or two sessions.

The long-term interview requires more frequent contact. It is used extensively during the mental health and psychiatric clinical experience. However, long-term interviewing is often carried out when the student or graduate is to develop an ongoing nurse-patient relationship such as with some medical or surgical patients or nursing home residents.

Written Reports of Interactions

Word-for-word ongoing records have become the greatest aid for the development of self-awareness and communication effectiveness. Recordings of interactions with patients and their families have proved to be of tremendous value to the patient and the nurse. A word-for-word account of the interchange is called a *process recording*; it literally records what has occurred. In addition to the verbal interaction, the process recording should include nonverbal behavior such as gestures, voice inflection, and body movement. Figure 17-3, pages 264 and 265, is an example of a three-minute process recording that was done by a student nurse.

Patient Communication	Evaluation	Nurse's Communication	Evaluation	Restatement
		① "Good morning, I'm me. Jones, a student nurse. I'd like to talk with you for ten minutes."	I've initiated the conversation.	
② "Gonna practice on me, huh!" (annoyed facial expression)	Patient is upset, but not sure why yet.	③ Silence 10 seconds.	I feel unsure and attacked.	Should have observed patient during silence but was too anxious.
④ "Just like my doctor. He doesn't tell me anything either." (tightly clutches sheet; no eye contact)	reveals anxiety.	⑤ "The doctor hasn't told you anything?"		

⑥ "Well, not about going home." (Angry voice tone; stared into space.)	Seems angry and sad.			
		⑦ "Not going home?"	I didn't know what to say, so I reflected.	I could have said, "you're concerned about going home?"
⑧ "You, what are you a parrot?"			I don't like being attacked, but I'll sit this out.	I could have said, "Are you upset?" or "Are you angry with me?"
		⑨ 1 minute silence. This one is a thoughtful silence.	Oh boy, there I go blabbering about myself. I got anxious and focused on me.	I could have said, "I'd like to understand—try me" or "tell me more so I can understand."
⑩ "But you're too young to understand. How old are you?" (Eye contact)	Patient wants to focus on me—maybe to relieve her anxiety or see if I'm interested in her.			
		⑪ "I'm 22. I'll be 23 next month. I'm a Taurus."		
⑫ Silence. Stared into space.	Withdrew when I started talking about myself.			

Fig. 17-3 A three-minute process recording with a 63-year-old female patient

Reports of interactions can be jotted down in a pocket notebook after contact with the patient. Key words and shorthand symbols for interactions (such as anxiety) can be developed. Some patients do not object to the nurse writing during the interview. However, some patients do mind, so it may be necessary to wait until after the interview is over before making notes. Some administrators may object to note-taking during patient-nurse conferences. The instructor will help students work out the best strategy to use in studying nurse-patient interactions.

Interview Themes

Every interview has a *theme* or major mood or idea that is reflected throughout the interview. Many times in short-term interviews, the planned purpose is taken over by a mood or feeling that is continually expressed. For example, a patient had been assigned to a student because it was felt the patient needed to talk about her feelings. The purpose was to provide the opportunity for this release. However, as can be concluded after reading the process recording (figure 17-3), this objective was not met. The theme that is reflected throughout the interview was the anxiety generated by both the patient and the student. They demonstrated anxiety and withdrawal.

Although many topics may be discussed, usually there are only one or two themes inherent in each interview. Most of the themes in interviews appear to be feelings. For example, patients who are taught or given information may transmit anger, depression or anxiety throughout the interview. In the process recording, figure 17-3, topics discussed included: the doctor, going home, understanding, and age.

By closely examining her notes about an interview, the nurse can begin to sense the patient's main concern; this comes through the interview theme. Note review is especially helpful when the patient does not tell the nurse directly about his problem, or when the nurse knows one exists but cannot decide what it is. If the patient and the nurse are involved in ongoing or long-term interviewing, notes should be reviewed before the next interview. They should be studied and associated with the themes of the past interviews.

Interviewing the Child

Children do not usually respond too well to the structured interview situation. There are two techniques the nurse can use to interview children. One of these techniques is role playing. Children who are frightened or angry can act out their feelings more easily if the nurse devises a role playing situation for this expression. For example, if the child is to undergo surgery, the nurse might suggest, "Let's play a game. You be the daddy who is visiting his son in the hospital. I'll play the son." As the nurse plays, she listens carefully to "daddy's" statements. If the "daddy" says, "I won't let them cut your tummy," it probably means the child fears being cut in surgery. If the "daddy" says, "You'll be fine after you wake up," it might mean the child is afraid that he will not wake up. Once the nurse has some idea of the child's thoughts and feelings, further games can be created to help the child express his feelings or give him information about what will happen during and after surgery.

Another technique is play therapy. In *play therapy* the nurse may use children's toys or play activities to help the child express feelings. For example, an angry but untalkative child may be given clay or a wooden hammer and blocks to help encourage the expression of how he feels.

To be effective in either role playing or play therapy, the student nurse will require adequate instruction and supervision.

Interview by Phone

There will be times when the nurse is unable to see the patient in person or when the patient fears person-to-person contact. The telephone may be used for interviews on occasions such as these. Suicide Prevention Centers and other crisis centers often provide purposeful conversation through use of the telephone interview. There is a special need for clarity during phone interviews or discussions as these conversations do not allow for visual nonverbal messages. Whenever the telephone is answered, the following steps are recommended for all health team members:

(1) Identify the location; for example, "Ward 3B."
(2) State name and title such as "Miss Stanley, student nurse."
(3) If unable to answer the caller's question or reach the person for whom the call is intended, take the message and write it down. Be sure it is delivered to the proper source.

COMMUNICATION SKILLS

If a nurse wishes to develop communication skills, it will be necessary to set up certain goals. By concentrating on these areas, the nurse can become an effective communicator:

- Encourage conversation.
- Help the patient to express thoughts and feelings.

- Insure a mutual understanding with the patient.
- Evaluate communication skills.

Encourage Conversation

The nurse encourages conversation by introducing herself and stating the purpose of the discussion; for example, "I'm Mary Smith, one of the student nurses from City College. I'm here to talk with you about your pain."

A major cause of anxiety or discomfort in hospitalized patients is the lack of sufficient information about their condition, treatment, or the hospital routine. When a patient is in need of information to relieve anxiety, form realistic conclusions, or make decisions, this need will often be revealed during the interaction with the nurse. By providing such information, the nurse can do much to establish and encourage communication.

By sharing information and experiences and working with the patient for his benefit, a rapport is established which encourages communication. The nurse can suggest this collaborative effort with comments such as, "Perhaps you and I can discuss what might be the reason for your anxiety" (pain, frustration, or whatever is bothering him).

The nurse may also encourage conversation by using silences effectively. When a silence occurs, it does not need to be immediately broken nor should the topic of conversation be changed by the nurse. The nurse's attention should focus on what is happening, the reason for, and meaning of the silence.

Starting the conversation with a broad opening statement or question is another way to encourage conversation. It allows the patient to set the direction of the conversation. Such questions as "Is there something you'd like to talk about?" or "I have ten minutes to spend with you. What shall we discuss?" give the patient an opportunity to begin to express himself. Upon sensing that the patient may have a need, the nurse can use a broad opening statement to initiate discussion; at the same time the patient determines what will be discussed. The nurse focuses the conversation directly on the patient and communicates to him that she is interested in him and his problems.

During the conversation, other general leads such as "Yes" or simply "Um hmm" will usually encourage the patient to continue. General leads leave the direction of the conversation to the patient. They also convey to the patient that the nurse is still listening and is interested in what he will say next. General leads can be accomplished nonverbally by nodding; facial expressions, also, demonstrate attentiveness and concern. The major purpose of general leads is to encourage the patient to continue the conversation and to speak spontaneously. In this way, the nurse can learn from him how he perceives his situation.

The nurse should be aware of a tendency to jump to conclusions regarding the nature of the patient's problem. She must resist this tendency and draw him out instead. Some additional examples of general leads which would help are: "I see," "And then. . .," "Go on," and incomplete or open-ended sentences such as "You were saying?"

By reflecting or restating all or part of the patient's statement, he is encouraged to go on. For example, if the patient says, "Everyone here ignores me" the nurse might reply, "Ignores you?" Repeating to the patient what he has just said may lead him to reconsider what he is thinking. However, reflecting can be overdone. Some patients become annoyed if their own words are continually repeated to them. Selective reflection can be used once the nurse has some idea of what the patient is trying to say. For example, if the patient says, "I feel so tired. I don't like it here." The nurse can either reflect, "Tired?" or "You don't like it here?", depending on which part of his statement she thinks is most important. Beginning interviewers often use too much reflection or restatement. This may occur because of anxiety and inability to remember or hear what the patient has said. Another reason for using too much reflection is that the student cannot think of more useful remarks because of her anxiety. With experience, and a subsequent decrease in anxiety, the student will gradually develop more skill in communications.

Referring to the self as a source of help can be used by the nurse. Statements such as, "I'll stay here with you," or "I'll sit here by you," or "I'm interested in you and will stay with you even though you don't seem to feel like talking right now" are examples of offering self.

Help the Patient to Express and Clarify Thoughts and Feelings

The nurse who wishes to further the development of communication skills must help the patient express his thoughts and feelings as clearly as possible. The following guidelines will assist her in meeting this objective:

- Encourage the description of an event.
- Explore points which need further clarification.
- Share observations with the patient.
- Verbalize implied thoughts or feelings.
- Acknowledge the patient's thoughts and feelings.
- Encourage the patient to evaluate events.
- Plan how to deal with future situations.

The patient is very much involved in this relationship and the nurse demonstrates her interest and concern while improving her communication skills.

Encourage the Description of an Event. Encouraging the patient to describe the event will help him to express himself; thoughts and feelings are clarified. Questions the nurse can ask to help the patient describe a past event more clearly are:

"Who was there?"
"When was this?"
"Where was this?"
"What was said?"   "By whom?"
"What did you think about what was said?"
"What did you feel then?"

Explore Points Which Need Further Clarification. Exploring a point more fully is an important aspect of care as well as communication development. Examples of exploring statements are: "Before you go on tell me about. . .," or "Tell me more about that," or "Describe it more fully." With practice, the student will recognize when to continue further and when to refrain from further questioning. If the patient does not wish to elaborate further, the nurse respects the patient's wishes. *Exploring* takes place when the patient introduces a topic and the nurse asks the patient to explain further. *Probing* usually occurs when the nurse introduces a topic because she is curious or anxious.

Share Observations With the Patient. The patient is often unaware of the source of his distress or may be reluctant to communicate it verbally. Tension or anxiety created by a need can be transformed into nail bitting, scratching, handclenching, or general restlessness. Frequently the nurse may be correct in her observations but incorrect in her own evaluation of what the behavior means. By sharing observations of this behavior, the nurse invites the patient to agree or disagree. Together, they attempt to find the reason for his behavior. Examples of sharing observations include: "You are trembling," or "You seem upset." Remarks should be phrased in tentative form by using words like *seem* or "I *wonder* if you are. . ." Emotionally charged words like *afraid, angry,* or *guilty* should not be used early in a relationship because they tend to evoke a patient response of denial of increased tension.

Verbalize Implied Thoughts and Feelings. When verbalizing implied thoughts or feelings, the nurse voices what the patient has expressed indirectly rather than what he has actually said. For example, if a patient says, "It's a waste of time doing these exercises!" the nurse might comment, "You feel they aren't benefiting you?" Verbalizing implied thoughts and feelings helps the nurse to verify her impressions; it also helps the patient increase his self-awareness.

Acknowledge the Patient's Thoughts and Feelings. The nurse can acknowledge any feelings that the patient may express without agreeing or disagreeing with them. A patient who feels that he is understood and accepted is more likely to express himself. If a patient were to say, "I hate it here. I wish I were at home," the nurse might reply, "It must be hard to stay in a place you hate." Such a statement places the focus on the patient, not the nurse or environment. If communication is to be successful, the nurse accepts the thoughts and feelings of the patient. If the patient feels that the nurse disapproves or disagrees with him, it is unlikely that a positive nurse-patient relationship will result.

Encourage the Patient to Evaluate Events. The nurse can help the patient learn from his experiences. Examples of evaluative statements are: "What do you think now?", or "Was your response helpful?", or "Which feeling is most difficult for you to handle?"

Plan How to Deal With Future Situations. Along with assisting the patient to evaluate events, the nurse encourages the patient to plan how to deal with future situations. Ways to do this include: "What will you do next time this happens?", "What are your plans for dealing with pain after the operation?", and "What might you do next time this happens so you'll feel more comfortable?"

Ways to Insure Mutual Understanding

Five factors which contribute to mutual understanding are: clarification, validation, summarizing, presenting reality, and voicing doubt. The nurse must develop skill in each of these in order to insure that she and the patient understand one another.

Clarification. If the nurse has not understood the meaning of the patient's statement, clarification is used. Clarifying statements include: "I'm not sure I follow what you're saying," or "Are you using this word to mean. . .?", or "What do you mean by that?" By seeking immediate clarification, the nurse can prevent miscommunication. Also, these efforts will show the patient that the nurse is interested; the patient will be more highly motivated to develop the relationship further. Meaningful communication depends upon the extent to which one person understands the other; therefore, neither should hesitate to interrupt if there is any confusion in the communication. The nurse might say, "Before you go on, I want to understand what you meant by. . ." Unclear pronouns should be clarified by asking, "Who do you mean by 'they'?", or "Who's 'him'?".

Validation. When the nurse thinks that the patient's need has been met, this impression should be confirmed with the patient. Questions to help validate are: "Do you feel more relaxed?", or "Are you feeling better now?" The nurse should not assume a patient's need has been met; validation of the outcome must be made with the patient.

Summarizing. A summary of the interview is especially important. Summarizing should be done near the end but it can also be used at crucial points during the interview. Examples of summary statements include: "As I understand it, we've been discussing your feelings today," or "Let's see if I've got this straight. . ." and "I'll try to summarize what we've agreed on so far."

Presenting Reality. The purpose of presenting reality is to indicate an alternate line of thought for the patient to consider, not to convince the patient that he is wrong. If a patient says, "There's someone else in here" (when there is not), the nurse can present reality by stating, "I don't see anyone else in the room." If a patient who hears a car backfire says, "They're trying to shoot me!", the nurse can present reality by stating, "That was a car backfiring." If the patient calls the nurse "mother," she can present reality by saying, "I'm a nurse." The nurse never tries to present reality by arguing or embarrassing the patient. Rather, she quietly and calmly expresses her own perceptions of the situation.

This technique is highly useful with patients who are confused or highly anxious. Geriatric patients in nursing homes who show signs of confusion, psychiatric patients showing high anxiety, and people who are confused due to alcohol or drugs may benefit when the nurse presents reality.

Voicing Doubt. This technique requires careful use. Only when the patient continues to express denial of a situation does the nurse consider voicing doubt. This may be done by saying something like: "Isn't that unusual?", "Really?", and "That's hard for me to believe."

Evaluate Communication Skills

In order to evaluate communication skills thoroughly, one must first consider how the communication was initiated. If it was the first interview with the patient, did the nurse or student introduce herself by name and title? Was the purpose of the interview stated? In her evaluation, the nurse also examines her ability to remain with the stated purpose and to refocus the conversation on the patient and the purpose. The evaluation includes a study of the questions that were asked and their effect. The use of open-ended questions and requests for clarification or restatement, and the way inquiries which required direct information or description were handled by the nurse are closely examined.

The nurse also evaluates the ability to listen. Listening includes being able to wait out silences and allow the patient to express a complete idea or feeling. Observation is another communication skill. The nurse notes the presence of nonverbal behavior. She evaluates her attempts to communicate with the patient, attempts which were based on the observations she had made.

Helping the patient to solve problems and learn from the experience are very important. The nurse evaluates whether the patient was helped to identify problems, explore alternatives, and form new plans of action. Figure 17-4 summarizes questions to ask when evaluating communication skills.

When the process recording method is used to describe and record encounters and interactions, it may be used as an evaluation tool. The process recording should be checked for completeness before being given to the evaluator for appraisal. It should reflect four specific points: what occurred, what was said (in quotation marks), nursing observations, and nursing evaluations; care must be taken to be sure the observations and evaluations are recognized and shown as separate nursing functions.

Did I introduce myself by name and title?

Did I clearly state the purpose of the interview?

Did I refocus the conversation to the patient and his concerns?

Did I use open-ended questions?

Did I ask for clarification or restatement when necessary?

Did I use direct questioning to obtain description of an event or to get needed information to perform nursing care?

Did I wait out silences?

Did I let the patient express a complete idea or feeling?

Did I notice the patient's and my own nonverbal behavior?

Did I notice when the patient's messages were unclear or contradictory?

Did I encourage the patient to identify and describe problems or events?

Did I encourage the patient to explore alternatives and form new plans of action?

Did I write down everything that happened as it really happened?

Did I separate my observations from my evaluations?

Fig. 17-4 Questions to ask to evaluate communication skills

SUMMARY

Nursing interviews have one or more identified purposes but may include several topics. They may be short and one-time meetings, or they can be ongoing processes. In both cases, process recordings should be done so that communication skills can be improved. Although the beginner will probably encounter some anxiety, interviewing skill will be acquired through application of principles and experience. The nurse creates the climate for a successful interview. She is aware of special skills needed for telephone interviews and interviews with children.

There are four areas which require special consideration if the nurse is to become an effective communicator. They are: encourage conversation, help the patient to express thoughts and feelings, insure mutual understanding, and evaluate the communication skills of the nurse.

ACTIVITIES AND DISCUSSION TOPICS

- Conduct a brief interview with a friend, family member, or patient. Prepare for the interview by deciding on a purpose and by setting an appropriate climate. List some of the problems you encountered.

- Do a process recording with a friend, family member or patient. Use Figure 17-4 to evaluate your communication skills. Also ask yourself the following questions:
  a. Did I set an appropriate climate?
  b. What was the theme(s) of the interview?
  c. What topics were discussed?
  d. Did I encourage conversation by giving information?
  e. Did I encourage conversation by suggesting collaboration?
  f. Did I use silence?
  g. Did I use broad opening statements?
  h. Did I use general leads?
  i. Did I reflect or restate what was said?
  j. Did I offer self?
  k. Did I encourage descriptions of events the other person mentioned?
  l. Did I explore points that seem important to me?
  m. Did I share my observations?
  n. Did I verbalize implied feelings?
  o. Did I acknowledge the other's thoughts and feelings?
  p. Did I encourage the other person to evaluate his or her own actions?
  q. Did I encourage the other person to form a new plan of action?

r. Did I use clarification?

s. Did I use validation?

t. Did I summarize?

u. Did I present reality?

v. Did I voice doubt?

After answering the above questions, explain the reason why you used or did not use each of the skills.

REVIEW

A. Match the correct communication skill in Column II to the correct example of that skill in Column I.

Column I	Column II
1. Giving information	a. "Do you feel more relaxed?"
2. Offering collaboration	b. "Who is 'they'?"
3. Giving broad openings	c. "Let's see if I have this straight."
4. Using general leads	d. "I don't hear anything."
5. Reflecting or restating	e. "Really?"
6. Offering self	f. "What might you do next time?"
7. Encouraging description	g. "What do you think now?"
8. Exploring	h. "I guess this has been difficult for you."
9. Sharing observations	i. "You seem upset."
10. Verbalizing implied thoughts or feelings	j. "Tell me more."
11. Acknowledging thoughts or feelings	k. "Go on."
12. Encouraging evaluation	l. "And then what happened?"
13. Encouraging future plans	m. "This is the syringe you will use."
14. Clarification	n. "You and I can figure it out."
15. Validation	o. "What would you like to talk about?"
16. Summarizing	p. "Tired?"
17. Presenting reality	q. "I'll sit with you for a while."
18. Voicing doubt	r. "You feel the exercises aren't benefiting you?"

B. Multiple Choice. Select the best answer(s). Some questions have more than one answer.

1. It is possible for the nurse to prepare for an interview with a patient by
    a. examining previous records.
    b. reading texts and articles on the subject.
    c. examining her own thoughts and feelings about the interview.
    d. learning effective communication skills.

2. The nurse can become an effective communicator by
    a. encouraging conversation.
    b. helping the patient to express thoughts and feelings.
    c. insuring a mutual understanding with the patient.
    d. evaluating communication skills.

3. The *theme* of an interview is the
    a. major mood or idea that is reflected throughout the interview.
    b. items discussed during the interview.
    c. actual purpose of the interview.
    d. written recording of all communications during the interview.

4. When the nurse thinks the patient's need has been met and she confirms this with the patient, it is called
    a. probing.
    b. clarification.
    c. summarizing.
    d. validation.

5. The purpose of presenting reality to the patient is to
    a. convince the patient that he is wrong.
    b. help the nurse understand the meaning of the patient's statement.
    c. indicate an alternate line of thought for the patient to consider.
    d. help the patient learn from his experiences.

C. Briefly answer the following questions.

1. List five purposes of the nursing interview.

2. State the difference between exploring and probing.

3. List five factors to consider when preparing for an interview with a patient.

4. Name two techniques the nurse can use to interview children.

5. Why is verbalizing implied thoughts and feelings useful?

chapter 18
BLOCKS TO
EFFECTIVE
COMMUNICATION

STUDENT OBJECTIVES

- Explain what is meant by communication block.
- List three ways to guard against blocks to effective communication.
- Match a list of communication blocks with appropriate examples.

Communication involves the transmission of information, thought, or feeling so that it is understood and received with satisfaction. A communication block is a barrier that hinders the transmittal of a message. When thoughts and feelings such as anxiety, conflict or stereotyped attitudes interfere with effective communication, a communication block occurs. Although the nurse cannot always change the patient's behavior, she should be aware of the importance of emotions and perception; that is, how thoughts and feelings may affect communication. In this way she can guard against communication blocks which place restrictions on the observation-perception-communication process.

Nurses may guard against communication block in the following ways:

- Utilization of process recordings.
- Discussion with an expert
- Personal reflection on the interaction

When the nurse senses an inability to talk with a certain patient or difficulty in completing nursing care effectively, a process recording will often reveal where communication was blocked. Also, nurses may talk with a third, uninvolved health team member about their interactions with patients. Psychiatric-mental health nurse specialists who are involved in ongoing one-to-one relationships with patients usually seek out ongoing supervision from an experienced therapist to make sure communication does not become blocked. Merely reflecting on an interaction with a patient will sometimes help the nurse to determine where communication was disrupted.

WHAT MAY BLOCK COMMUNICATION

Three factors which block communication are anxiety, conflict, and attitudes which are stereotyped. When the nurse-patient relationship is threatened by the presence of these factors, both parties fail to achieve the satisfaction which should be an end result of the relationship. Communication is vital to any encounter.

Anxiety

Anxiety may block communication when the patient brings up a topic of conversation or acts in a way that makes the nurse uncomfortable. For example, some nurses become anxious when patients discuss death or the possibility they may not get better. Other nurses become uncomfortable when the patient verbally attacks the doctor or nurse. Many nurses become uncomfortable with the patient who makes sexual advances or masturbates. When the nurse becomes anxious in these or other situations, perception is restricted. These high anxiety levels block communication.

Conflict

Conflict occurs when the nurse has two opposing goals to pursue. The nurse may have a strong wish or desire to help the patient talk about his fears but may wish to complete the patient's care and go to lunch. When the nurse is pulled toward both of these goals, a conflict results. Patients and nurses are not always aware that they are being pulled toward two opposing goals. However, behavior can still be influenced by goals which the nurse may not be aware of. For this reason, the nurse is always better off if she understands her goals and keeps them in proper perspective.

Conflict is present in all people at some time during their lives. In every culture, there are opposing values and attitudes about how to behave in particular situations. People learn to resolve these differences for the most part. Everyone is involved in situations which will evoke some conflict.

When a person hesitates, cannot make decisions, starts one action, stops, and then turns to another goal, conflict is taking place. Blocking is an internal action that takes place when the person cannot remember or describe a situation, wish, or goal. For example, one may stammer, stutter, or completely forget the name of a person he dislikes. In this case, the person's dislike blocks him from remembering the other's name; conflict blocks communication because of the pull between the two goals. Because the person is pulled in two directions at once, it is difficult to listen and be concerned about the other's welfare.

Stereotyped Attitudes

Stereotyped attitudes or preconceived ideas block communication. If the nurse thinks all elderly people are confused, or all men are seductive, or all women are helpless and need to be protected, communication will be blocked. Perception of the other person is restricted. Most people have some stereotyped attitudes; these attitudes or prejudices place limits on the realistic evaluation of others.

When a person stereotypes, there is a tendency to assume that all people who have one or two characteristics in common will behave in the same manner. For example, many women have prejudiced or preconceived ideas about other women. Women who hold this stereotype tend to believe that all women are fussy, complain more than men, and are more dependent. This attitude is likely to restrict the prejudiced female from noticing situations where other women are not fussy, do not complain, or exhibit independent behavior. Figure 18-1 summarizes blocks to communication.

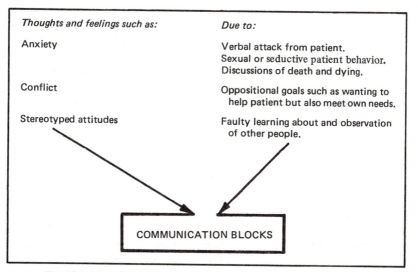

Fig. 18-1 Thoughts and feelings can lead to blocked communication.

HOW COMMUNICATION MAY BE BLOCKED

In her development and practice of communication skills, there are certain blocks to communication that the nurse must avoid. Some of these blocks to communication are:

- Maintaining social chitchat
- Using stereotyped comments
- Changing the subject
- Giving advice, approval or disapproval
- Asking for approval
- Giving false assurance
- Offering choice when none is available
- Using illogical communication
- Overgeneralizing
- Requesting impossible explanations
- Defending
- Challenging or confronting
- Breaking useful silences

Maintaining Social Chitchat

The patient may try to maintain social chitchat by talking about the weather, politics, or the nurse's social activities because he thinks this will please the nurse. Meanwhile, the patient may be worrying about himself and what will happen to him in the hospital. The nurse who gets caught up in describing herself and her social activities cannot focus on the needs of the patient.

Using Stereotyped Comments

Stereotyped comments maintain a distance between the nurse and patient because they keep conversation at a superficial level. "How are you?" or "How are you feeling?" are stereotyped comments because both people know the expected response is "Fine." By making stereotyped comments, the nurse tells the patient through metacommunication, "I do not want to hear about your problems." Other stereotyped comments such as "You'll feel better" or "It's all for the best" do not allow the patient to discuss real thoughts and feelings.

Changing the Subject

Communication is blocked when the nurse changes the subject of the conversation because it has become uncomfortable. In the example below, the nurse changed the subject when the topic of suicide began to create anxiety in her.

> Nurse: "What shall we discuss?"
> Patient: "My mother came to visit."
> Nurse: "When?"
> Patient: "I don't remember."
> Patient: "I thought about doing it last night. About ending my life."
> Nurse: "How about doing your exercises now."

Giving Advice, Approval or Disapproval

Examples of giving advice are: "What you should do is . . .", "Why don't you. . .", and "Don't ever. . .". By telling the patient what he should do, the nurse imposes her own opinions and solutions on him. It would be more helpful to explore the patient's ideas so he can arrive at his own solutions. Even when a patient clearly asks for advice, the nurse should give a cautious response which supplies only pertinent information; this information gives the patient a better basis for making his own decisions. Giving the patient advice implies that the nurse thinks she knows what is best for him and that she feels his problem can be easily solved. When advice is given and the patient does not accept it, he may resent the nurse for advising him. If the advice is accepted, the patient is then more dependent on the nurse for solutions to his problems. Instead, the nurse should help the patient to think through and attempt to resolve his problems for himself. When a patient asks for advice, the nurse can ask, "What are your feelings about that?" or "What conclusions have you reached?" She can provide pertinent information that the patient needs to solve the problems. Such pertinent information may include facts, resource people, or other services. The patient under extreme stress may be unable to solve his problems but the nurse makes every attempt to help him do so.

The nurse is careful not to agree with the patient unless there has been enough exploration of the issue. If the nurse introduces her own ideas into the conversation, the patient may hesitate to express his own ideas. If she agrees with the patient, the nurse makes it difficult for him to change his mind. Patients who are in conflict will change their minds many times as they attempt to choose the right goal for them. Sometimes patients ask the nurse to agree just to see if the nurse is really interested. The nurse who agrees or disagrees without checking to see what is behind the question may block further communication.

Giving approval can be useful when motivation or encouragement is the purpose. However, giving approval can sometimes shift the focus from the patient to the nurse. When the nurse tells the patient, "That's the right thing to do" or "That's the right attitude," the nurse implies that she can make this judgment when, in fact, it may be very difficult for the nurse to know what is right. Whenever the nurse gives approval, she takes the chance that she is approving behavior the patient really dislikes; in this case, the nurse's values and goals conflict with those of the patient. Therefore, the nurse is careful and uses approval only when it does not block communication.

Disapproving or disagreeing can also block communication. When the nurse comments; "You should stop worrying," or "You shouldn't do that," or "You're wrong," or "No you don't," a nonacceptance of the patient's behavior is indicated and communication is cut off.

Both approval and disapproval force the patient to conform to another's sense of right or wrong. The nurse must not impose standards on the patient.

Asking for Approval

When the nurse asks about her nursing care, the patient may be forced to approve. After all, the nurse controls the patient's destiny to a great extent while he is hospitalized. Since the patient is already dependent on the nurse, he may feel obligated to compliment her. Such demands use patient energy that could be better spent on dealing with stress.

Giving False Assurance

The nurse may try to convince the patient that things will turn out well. When the nurse makes such statements, even though there are no facts to bear them out, she is giving false assurance. For example, if the nurse says, "You'll be feeling better soon" or "The doctor will be right here," when she has no way of knowing what the future will bring, the nurse is giving false assurance.

Although the nurse may say, "Everything will be all right" out of a sincere wish to reduce the patient's anxiety, such encouragement is more likely to be given because the nurse is anxious. The patient who is told, "Everything will be all right" may feel the nurse is not interested in his problem if it is dismissed so easily. He may even think to himself, "That's easy for you to say." Sometimes, reassuring remarks may contradict the patient's perception of his situation. Genuine reassurance must be based on facts. A more basic reassurance is given when the nurse conveys an interested, accepting attitude.

Offering Choice When None is Available

Offering the patient a choice in his care can be a useful nursing intervention. If the nurse offers choice, but then does not let the patient choose, trust cannot be established in the relationship. When the nurse asks, "Would you like to take your bath now?" she should be prepared for "No" as well as "Yes." If there is no other time for the patient to take a bath, no choice should be offered.

Using Illogical Communication

Communication cannot be clear when it is illogical. If the nurse does not understand the patient and pretends to follow an illogical thought or conversation, a block to communication occurs; the patient will soon realize the nurse is not understanding him. Using illogical communication also occurs when the nurse changes key words used by the patient; continues conversation without clarifying unclear pronouns; asks more than one question at a time; or gives the patient two opposing messages at once (double bind).

Here is an example of the block in communication that can occur when the nurse uses illogical communication:

Nurse: "Do you want to walk or stay in your room?"
   (Two questions asked at once)
Patient: "Yes."
Nurse: "Yes what?"
Patient: "Jasari."
Nurse: "Oh" (Fails to clarify unclear word)
   SILENCE
Patient: "My parents didn't do it. But they didn't tell me that."
Nurse: "Didn't they?" (Fails to clarify the vague "they")
Patient: "No. But I fixed them. I told my cousins."
Nurse: "You did?" (Pretends to follow illogical communication)
Patient: "Yes."
   SILENCE (Communication is blocked for nurse since she
      does not understand what the patient said.)

Overgeneralizing

Freedom to express contrary ideas is restricted when there is overgeneralization. The nurse overgeneralizes by using phrases such as: "All women are. . .", "All parents are. . .", "Everybody is. . .", and "Nobody does. . .". The patient hesitates to disagree. Statements which imply that the nurse has a stereotyped idea of what people will do restrict the attempts of both patient and nurse to communicate with one another.

Requesting Impossible Explanations

"Why did you do that?", "Why are you here?" and "Why are you upset?" are examples of questions which some patients find difficult, if not impossible, to answer. Questions that call for "why" are difficult because they require people to analyze and come up with an explanation for feelings or actions. If the patient knew why he drank or why he did not follow his diet, he probably would have handled the problem himself. Patients who cannot answer "why" questions often invent answers to please the nurse. Avoid "why" except when asking simple, direct questions pertaining to patient care such as, "Why are you going to the bathroom?"

In general, the nurse is of more assistance if she helps the patient to describe his feelings and thoughts by using questions that begin with who, what, when, and where. The nurse can then help the patient begin to understand why he behaves as he does.

Defending

When the nurse feels threatened or attacked, she may try to defend her own or another's position. For example, in the statements, "Your doctor is quite capable" or "Mrs. Smith is a good nurse," the nurse seems to be defending. Whenever the patient is critical of a nurse or the care he received, the nurse may think it is important to intervene. Defending signals a nonacceptance of the patient's thoughts or feelings and sets the nurse in opposition to the patient. This may start a power struggle over who is right. Defending also shifts the focus of conversation from the patient and his concerns to the nurse and her concerns. People usually defend themselves when they feel threatened and anxious. The nurse should analyze the reason for her anxiety rather than become defensive of her actions.

Challenging or Confronting

Sometimes a nurse may feel that if she can challenge the patient he will realize he has no proof for his unrealistic ideas. She may forget that the ideas and perceptions serve a protective purpose for him; they conceal feelings and meet needs that are real. When challenged, the patient tends only to strengthen and expand any misperceptions while seeking support for his point of view.

Communication Block	Example
Maintaining social chitchat	"It's a nice day outside." "I had a great date last night."
Using stereotyped comments	"How are you?" "You'll be home in no time." "This is for your own good."
Changing the subject	"Let's talk about something less morbid." "You're feeling down? Well, let's do your exercises now."
Giving advice, approval or disapproval	"Why don't you tell her off?" "That's the right thing to do." "You shouldn't do that!"
Asking for approval	"Isn't that the best backrub you've ever had?" "Did you like your breakfast?" "I'm the best nurse you've ever had, right?"
Giving false assurance	"You'll be better." "Everything will end up O.K."
Offering choice when none is available	"Would you like to take your medicine now?" "It's bedtime. Would you like to turn out your light now?"
Using illogical communication	"It's no bother." (frowning) "I'm angry." (smiling)
Overgeneralizing	"All fathers treat their daughters that way." "All nurses give physical and emotional care."
Requesting impossible explanations	"Why are you here?" "Why are you anxious?"
Defending	"That can't be. He's a good nurse." "We know what's best for you."
Challenging or confronting	"You're acting like a child." "Can't you see your sulking isn't helping?" "If you're Jesus Christ, perform a miracle."
Breaking useful silence	Beginning to talk when the patient seems to be thinking over what was just said.

Fig. 18-2 The nurse can block communication by sending certain verbal and non-verbal messages to the patient.

Examples of challenging statements are: "Your sister couldn't be coming, she's dead," and "You are not Napoleon, you're Jimmy Jones." Rather than challenging the patient's views, the nurse might restate what she heard or ask him to "say more about that" so she can understand his viewpoint more clearly.

When the patient is confronted with his undesirable behavior or the reason for it, he is likely to withdraw or to become highly anxious. Of course, destructive behaviors need to be discussed but comments such as, "You're chewing your fingernails again" or "You're angry because you think I'm like your mother" block communication. The nurse rarely tells the patient what his behavior might mean; this information will become useful only when the patient himself comes to understand the reasons for his behavior. Confronting or challenging statements usually have the ring of a parent scolding a naughty child. This belittles the patient and places him in a dependent position.

Breaking Useful Silences

Thoughtful silences can be used by the patient to reflect on what was said or how to phrase his next words. When a thoughtful silence is broken by the nurse, the patient's stream of thought is interrupted. A patient who is interrupted during thoughtful silences may feel that the nurse does not understand; he may become more distant. Figure 18-2, page 285, summarizes how communication is blocked.

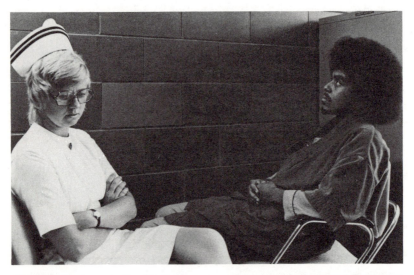

Fig. 18-3 A communication block can occur when attitudes interfere with effective communication.

SUMMARY

A communication block occurs when the nurse's or the patient's anxiety, conflict, stereotyped attitudes, or other thoughts or feelings interfere with effective communication. The nurse can block communication by maintaining social chitchat; using stereotyped comments; changing the subject; giving advice, approval or disapproval; asking for approval; giving false assurance; offering choice when none is available; using illogical communication; overgeneralizing; requesting impossible explanations; defending; challenging or confronting; or by breaking useful silences. Nurses guard against blocking communication with patients by doing process recordings, reflecting on interactions, and seeking supervision from a more experienced purposeful communicator.

ACTIVITIES AND DISCUSSION TOPICS

- Look at the picture on page 286 of this unit. Before you read on, write a brief description of what is happening in the picture. When you have finished the description, answer the following questions:
  a. Did you mention that a black and white person were in the scene?
  b. Did you describe the black person as upset or threatening?
  c. Did you describe the white person as upset, threatening, or concerned?
  d. Did you notice that communication was blocked? What led you to that conclusion?

  Do your answers tell you anything about how your attitudes might block communication?

- Pair off with a classmate. Talk for five minutes about one or more topics. Have a third person write down the blocks to communication that occurred, using the list below:
  a. Maintains social chitchat
     examples:
  b. Uses stereotyped comments
     examples:
  c. Changes the subject
     examples:
  d. Gives advice, approval or disapproval
     examples:
  e. Asks for approval
     examples:
  f. Gives false assurance
     examples:

g. Offers choice when none is available
   examples:

h. Uses illogical communication
   examples:

i. Overgeneralizes
   examples:

j. Requests impossible explanations
   examples:

k. Defends
   examples:

l. Challenges or confronts
   examples:

m. Breaks useful silence
   examples:

Are all of the previous behaviors blocks to communication in social conversations?   Which ones are not?   Use the same list to observe a nurse-patient interaction or to use in reviewing a process recording.

REVIEW

A.   Multiple Choice.   Select the best answer(s).   Some questions have more than one answer.

1.   "Why" questions should be used sparingly when communicating with a patient because the patient
     a. is required to analyze and explain his feelings or actions.
     b. may not want to give the nurse this information.
     c. may invent answers to please the nurse.
     d. probably does not know the answer.

2.   The nurse should not interrupt a patient's thoughtful silence because the patient may be
     a. hoping the nurse will leave him alone.
     b. thinking how to phrase his next words.
     c. reflecting on what was said.
     d. angry with the nurse.

3.   An internal action that takes place when a person cannot remember or describe a situation, wish or goal is called
     a. challenging.   c. illogical communication.
     b. blocking.   d. anxiety.

4. When the patient brings up a topic of conversation that makes the nurse uncomfortable, communication may be blocked because of
   a. conflict. c. anxiety.
   b. stereotyping. d. blocking.

5. Conflict blocks communication because the person in conflict
   a. is pulled in two directions at once.
   b. feels threatened and becomes defensive.
   c. uses illogical communications.
   d. always remains silent.

B. Match the communication block in Column II to the appropriate example in Column I.

Column I	Column II
1. "I was only trying to help."	a. Asks for approval
2. "Do you want to take your medicine now?"	b. Challenges or confronts
	c. Changes the subject
3. "Do you like the way I arranged your flowers?"	d. Defends
	e. Gives advice, approval or disapproval
4. "Don't worry. Everything will turn out all right."	f. Gives false assurance
	g. Maintains social chitchat
5. "Yes, I went to school in South Dakota."	h. Offers choice when none is available
6. "You really should get a divorce."	i. Overgeneralizes
	j. Requests impossible explanations
7. "Why did you try to kill yourself?"	k. Uses illogical communication
8. "Don't do that!" (smiling)	l. Uses stereotyped comments
9. "Oh, all mothers are like that."	
10. "How can you be Jesus Christ. He's dead."	
11. "That's too morbid. Let's talk about your going home instead."	
12. "You'll feel better soon."	

C. Briefly answer the following questions.

    1. What is a communication block?

    2. When does a communication block occur?

    3. Name three ways the nurse may guard against communication blocks.

    4. How is overgeneralizing a block to communication?

chapter 19
NURSING PROCESS

STUDENT OBJECTIVES

- Identify how communication is related to the nursing process.
- Define nursing diagnosis.
- List four steps in the nursing process.
- Identify a patient-centered goal and objective.
- Identify an effectively stated nursing order.

In nursing, a *process* is a series of actions that meet a goal or need. The nursing process is a way of thinking and acting in a purposeful way when giving nursing care. Every nursing activity is preceded by (1) assessment of patient needs, problems and strengths, and (2) deciding on goals, priorities or actions. Intervention is the actual carrying out of the proposed nursing action. Every nursing action or intervention is followed by evaluation and, if necessary, revision of the goal or the nursing action. Using the nursing process makes nursing care systematic. This is because all of the nurses follow the same series of steps in providing care. When care is systematic, it is more scientific and nursing practices can be studied to determine whether they are useful or whether other actions might be more useful. As research in nursing proceeds, nurses test out nursing actions and develop new nursing theories. Briefly, the nursing process is a series of actions:

- Assessment
- Deciding on goals, priorities, and nursing actions.
- Intervention
- Evaluation and/or revision

Nursing Assessment

When the nurse assesses the needs of the patient, she uses observation, perception and communication. In observation she gathers information through use of the senses of sight, touch, and hearing. Tools such as the thermometer and stethoscope also help the nurse to assess the patient's needs. The nurse's perception is influenced by past and present experiences. Communication is used in nursing assessment to receive written, spoken, or nonverbal information and to help the patient express thoughts and feelings and clarify needs and problems.

Knowledge from previous experience and courses of study is used in nursing assessment. Knowledge of physiology and anatomy, growth and development, the behavioral sciences and the humanities help the nurse to predict patient behavior. Textbooks and other sources of information are often kept on the hospital unit for nurses to use.

The patient's chart includes information for patient assessment such as nurses' notes, medical history and progress notes, medication and treatments ordered for the patient, findings from various laboratory tests given to the patient, as well as information written by the social worker, physical therapist, and occupational therapist. In some hospitals, all patient assessment information appears in the form of the Problem-Oriented Record (POR). In this system, the nurse, doctor, and other health team members do not keep separate records. All health personnel use the same recording sheets. Information on the POR is organized by patient problems rather than written entries by the health professional. In the POR system, a problem could be a diagnosis (such as multiple sclerosis), a symptom (confusion), a sign (elevated temperature), an abnormal finding in a laboratory or psychological test (elevated white blood count), a risk factor (smoking and high cholesterol in a patient with hypertension), or an operation (such as prefrontal lobotomy or appendectomy). In psychiatric hospitals where the POR system is used, patient strengths or assets are also included in an assessment. It is thought that including the patient's strengths and resources gives health personnel a better chance of re-establishing patient equilibrium. Assets could include special skills, resources, abilities or motivations, family ties or supportive friends, or community agencies available to give care. Figures 19-1 and 19-2 (page 294) show differences between the recording method where each professional records in a different place, and the POR record where recording is organized around patient problems or strengths. Each problem or strength has a subjective statement, objective observation, assessment and plan (S-O-A-P). Date, time and signature are included, figure 19-2. Some Problem-Oriented Record systems also include intervention (I)

Nurses Notes

Patient's Name: John Lenard

Doctor: Wentworth

Date and Time	Cumulative record of nursing observations and interventions
9/21	
12 n.	Completed nursing history. Pt. 2+ - 3+ anxiety. Repeating the same question, perspiring profusely, unable to concentrate on nurses' questions.
	Carolyn Clark, R.N.

Date and Time

9/21

Doctors Progress Notes
Cumulative record of Patient's progress

Preparing patient for Blalock
Will ask anesthesiologist
to talk with patient
B. Blake, M.D.

Fig. 19-1 In some systems, each health professional records on a different form.

Progress Sheet	
Date	Notes

#1 ANXIETY ABOUT SURGERY

9/21
Nson

S: "THIS IS HAPPENING SO FAST - I ONLY WENT FOR MY ANNUAL PHYSICAL LAST WEEK."
O: INABILITY TO CONCENTRATE ON TASK. ASKED SAME QUESTION REPEATEDLY PERSPIRING PROFUSELY.
A: 2+ - 3+ ANXIETY
P: STAY WITH PATIENT; BE AVAILABLE TO HELP PATIENT VERBALIZE.
　　　　Carolyn Clark, R.N.

9/21
7pm

#2 Preparation for Surgery

S:
O: + Hgb = 12g.
A: Anemia associated with bleeding from lower bowel
P: Type and crossmatch blood. Ask anesthesiologist to see patient. Explain procedures to patient.
　　　　D. Reade, M.D.

9/21
2pm

#3 Bloody Stool

S: Patient stated he had "blood in the bedpan"
O: Large, amount bright red blood in stool
A: Bleeding
P: Report to charge nurse tell patient the nurse will be notified
　　　　Clifford Brown, Aide

Fig. 19-2 In the Problem-Oriented Record system, all health personnel make consecutive entires on the same form. The letters represent: S = Subjective (patient statement), O = Objective (observation by the health team member), A = Assessment, P = Plan.

Progress Sheet	
Date	Notes
9/16 3 a.m.	#1 Anxiety about surgery S: "This is happening so fast – I only went for my annual physical examination last week." O: Inability to concentrate on task. Asked same questions repeatedly. Perspiring profusely. A: 2+ – 3+ Anxiety P: Stay with patient; be available to help patient verbalize. I: Spent 15 minutes with patient encouraging verbalization. E: Patient's posture became more relaxed. Patient stated, "I think I can sleep now."

Fig. 19-3 Some Problem-Oriented Record systems also include intervention (I) and Evaluation (E).

and evaluation (E), figure 19-3. Nursing interventions (I) could include such actions as notifying the doctor or changing a plan after talking with the patient. Nursing evaluations (E) are used to explain the effectiveness of the nursing action; patient behaviors that indicate the nursing action was effective or ineffective are recorded.

Assessment Tools. There are three tools nurses use most often to assess patient needs, strengths, and problems. The first tool is the nursing history. The *nursing history* describes the patient's response to hospitalization, expectations and attitudes regarding hospitalization, interpersonal needs and preferences, usual patterns of daily living, and self-actualization needs. The nursing history differs from the medical history because the nurse focuses on the meaning of illness and health to the patient and family. The nurse obtains most of the information for the nursing history by talking with the patient. Figure 19-4, pages 296 and 297, shows a nursing history that the nurse has completed.

Nursing History

(The interviewer introduces herself to the patient and proceeds)

Date: *9/21*   Patient Name: *Mr. J.L.*

Age: *48*   Sex: *Male*   Allergies: *None*

Response to Hospitalization

1. Have you been in the hospital before? *No*
   If yes, when?

2. Have you ever been in *this* hospital before? *No*
   If yes, when?

3. What is the reason you've come to the hospital this time?
   For a Colostomy

4. What activities of the nurse were most helpful in previous hospitalizations? —
   Most bothersome? —

Expectations and Attitudes

5. What things would you like to learn about your condition?
   What is it? How will I handle it?

6. What did you expect to happen in the hospital that hasn't happened?
   Everything is done so quickly I didn't expect surgery so soon.

Interpersonal Needs and Preferences

7. What restrictions would you like placed on visitors? *No visitors*

8. Would you rather eat alone or have company? *alone*

9. Would you like to have a nurse available to talk with you about your thoughts
   and feelings? *I don't know*

Usual Patterns of Daily Living

10. What do you usually eat for breakfast? *eggs and muffins ē Sanka*

11. When do you usually eat? *9 a.m.*

12. When do you usually eat lunch? *1 p.m.*

13. What do you usually eat for lunch? *raw vegetables, fruit, nuts, cheese*

14. When do you eat supper? *6:30 p.m.*

15. What do you eat for supper? *Lean meat, fish, potatoes or rice; bread. salad, chocolate dessert or ice cream*

16. Any food you especially dislike or that disagrees with you?
    Coffee, soy sauce, spinach

17. Do you like a snack? *Yes*   If yes, when? *8 p.m.*
    what? *dried fruit or ice cream*

18. What drinks do you especially like? *Sanka, 7up, grapefruit juice*

19. How many hours do you usually sleep per night at home? *9*

20. When do you usually go to sleep at night? *9 - 11 p.m.*

21. Do you like to sleep with an extra pillow *no*
    an extra blanket *yes*
    the window closed _____
    the door closed _____
    the curtain closed _____
    the window open *yes*
    the door open _____
    the curtain open *yes*

22. What helps you to get to sleep at home? *reading, exercises*

23. How often do you bathe or shower at home? *every day*
    Which do you prefer? *shower*
    When during the day? *morning*

24. Do you have all your own teeth? *no.*
    If not, how many dentures or plates do you have? *upper and lower dentures*

25. When do you usually have a bowel movement? *morning*
    How many per week? *4-7* Any difficulties? *bleeding and had to force it last 2 weeks*

26. How frequently do you urinate (pass water) during the day? *4-5*
    Any difficulties? *dull pain in morning*
    If yes, what specifically?

Self-Actualization and Barriers to Self-Actualization

27. What questions do you have to ask me? *What will I be like?*

28. What special needs do you have in the following categories?

    Need to learn *all about colostomy*
    Hearing problem *deaf in left ear*
    Vision difficulties *glasses to read*
    Things that help you when you're in pain *backrub, heating pad, quiet*
    Are you usually a very active person, or do you take things easy? *active*
    Need an interpreter? *no*
    Have trouble expressing your thoughts or feelings? *sometimes*
    Need assistance walking or turning? *no*
    Would you like to have the chaplain notified to visit you? *yes*
    If yes, what religion? *Lutheran*

    Signature of Interviewer *Carolyn Clark, R.N.*

Fig. 19-4 A nursing history is one assessment tool.

The second tool the nurse uses to assess patient needs is nursing diagnosis. *Nursing diagnosis* consists of identifying patient needs and problems. To assess patient needs, the nurse considers all of the following: interpersonal needs, self-actualization needs, need for oxygen, need for activity and rest, need for safety, need for food and fluid, and need to eliminate waste. A *patient problem* occurs when the person is unable to meet a need. Patient problems lead to a disturbance in homeostasis.

Patient problems can be due to a lack of function such as movement or to a lack of a need such as food or companionship. Problems can also occur when there is too much input (sensory overload) or when excessive psychological or physiological demands are placed on a person. Generally speaking, patient problems can arise when there is economic, psychological, social, physiological, or spiritual danger that poses a real or perceived threat.

When a nursing diagnosis is made, a decision to focus on certain aspects of patient behavior is also made. A nursing diagnosis differs from a medical diagnosis in that the nursing diagnosis is concerned with human responses to health problems. Physicians are concerned primarily with the health problem, its causes and treatment. Some nursing diagnoses are anxiety, lack of understanding, impaired mobility, reactions to pain, ineffective sleep/rest pattern, disturbed communication, deprivation, sensory overload, irregular bowel function, decubitus ulcer, and noncompliance. *Noncompliance* is a nursing diagnosis used to describe behavior where the patient refuses to go along with the nurse's goals for care.

The third tool nurses use is a systematic assessment guide. The *systematic assessment* focuses on areas that change depending on the patient's degree of health or illness. The assessment guide often differs from the nursing history as the nursing history focuses on information that changes very little from admission to discharge. The patient's ability to maintain homeostasis may change several times during a hospital stay. The student nurse may not use a systematic assessment guide since it may be impossible to follow a patient from admission through discharge. However, some nursing history forms include systematic assessment features.

There are several systematic assessment guides that have been developed to assess primary areas of the patient's physiological and psychosocial needs. Areas which are important to assess on an ongoing basis are:

- General condition

- Social, economic and cultural factors

- Mental, perceptual, interpersonal and developmental state

- Self-actualization state

- Respiratory state

- Circulatory state

- Body temperature state

- Motor ability

- Sleep/rest/comfort state

- Food and fluid state

- State of skin

- Elimination state

- Sexual and reproductive state

- Ability to avoid injury and repair damage

Figure 19-5, pages 300-302, shows a completed sample systematic assessment.

Through the use of the three tools of nursing assessment, the nurse is able to decide what areas of assessment require attention. Now the nurse is ready for the next step in the nursing process.

Deciding on Goals, Priorities, and Nursing Actions

At this point, the nurse is armed with a great mass of information. Sorting out priorities may be difficult. In situations of crises, the area which demands attention could be oxygen supply, suicide attempt, fluid balance, or other pressing area. In less critical situations, the student may have difficulty setting goals and priorities. *Nursing goals* or *objectives* are statements that describe the desired result or change in patient behavior that will restore homeostasis.

The nurse must first separate nursing goals (or objectives) into long-term and short-term goals. Long-term goals are things like "return to work," "help to accept disability," or "assist to peaceful death." Short-term goals might be to "establish the nurse-patient relationship," "increase oxygen supply," "assist family during a crisis," and "prevent skin breakdown." Both long-term and short-term goals should be as specific as possible so there is no misunderstanding about the nurse's intent. After deciding on the goals, the next step is to separate and classify them as either nurse-centered or patient-centered objectives.

Nurse-centered objectives or goals tell what the nurse hopes to accomplish. Nurse-centered objectives begin with action verbs such as maintain, increase, provide, establish, prevent, end, teach, modify, identify, compare, remove, develop, allow, and accept. The nurse strives to write objectives that are specific,

---

Systematic Assessment of Patient Needs

Date begun: 9/21   Patient: Mr. J.L.   Medical diagnosis: Cancer of rectum and anus

1. *General Condition*

    9/21   Preoperative for colostomy

    9/22   Surgery; colostomy performed

    9/26   Convalescent

2. *Social, Economic, and Cultural Factors*

    9/21   Age: 48
    Has taught 8th grade shop for past 10 yrs.
    Divorced last year.
    Lives alone with dog; parents on West coast; brother lives ten minutes away.
    Lutheran religious affiliation.
    German-American cultural group.
    Has Major Medical group coverage for hospitalization.

3. *Mental, Perceptual, Interpersonal and Developmental State*

    9/21   Aware of time, place and person.
    Shows anxiety by his inability to concentrate on task, repeatedly asking the same question, and profuse perspiration.
    Said several times, "This is happening so fast — I only went for my annual physical last week."
    Wears glasses to read. Eyes clear; conjunctiva pink.
    Unable to hear from left ear since birth.

    9/22   Helps to guide the next generation by being a teacher.

    9/24   Verbalizing fears of having "more cancer" and of "soiling."
    Sad facial expression; seems to be still grieving separation from wife.
    Said, "I thought I was over her, but this illness makes me lonely for her."

    9/26   Asked to have brother called to visit.

4. *Self-actualization State*

    9/21   Seemed disorganized by anxiety, but did request more information on colostomy.
    Requested glasses be kept nearby in bedstand drawer.
    Asked to be spoken to into right ear.

    9/26   Asked for literature on colostomy care.

Fig. 19-5 The systematic assessment focuses on changes that occur during a patient's hospitalization. (continued)

5. *Respiratory State*

   9/21   Rate = 24; shallow and irregular.

   9/26   Rate = 16; regular.

   Has morning cough which patient attributes to "smoking too much."

6. *Circulatory State*

   9/21   Pulse = 126; regular and strong.

   B/P = 140/90
   No evidence of edema or dehydration.

   9/26   Pulse = 96; regular and strong.

   B/P = 130/80
   No evidence of edema or dehydration.

7. *Body Temperature State*

   9/21   Temperature 99.0 at 3 p.m.

   9/26   Temperature 98.6 at 9 a.m.

8. *Motor Ability*

   9/21   Up and active.
   Full range of motion in all joints. Erect posture when seated and standing.
   No muscle or nerve atrophy. Well developed, muscular male.

   9/22   Confined to bed. IV infusing in left arm.

   9/23   Out of bed. Sat in chair for one hour in morning and afternoon.

   9/26   Up walking in hall by himself twice today.

9. *Sleep/Rest/Comfort State*

   9/21   Stated he "slept 12 hours last night," but still felt "tired."
   At home rises at 7 a.m. and goes to bed between 9 and 11 p.m.
   Plays tennis and jogs 3-4 times per week.
   c/o "tendonitis" in left lower leg.

   9/22   Drowsy. Awake at hourly intervals. Moving restlessly in bed. c/o "pain" in peritoneal area. Preferred not to take pain medication. Asked for backrub.

   9/26   Refused sleep medication, despite being awake every three hours tonight.

Fig. 19-5 The systematic assessment focuses on changes that occur during a patient's hospitalization. (continued on page 302)

10. *Food and Fluid State*

    9/21   Patient described his garden and stated a preference for raw, uncooked vegetables and fruits. Likes chocolate desserts and dried fruit.
                c/o decreased appetite and loss of energy for past month.
                Ht: 5' 10"   Wt: 144 pounds.
                Dislikes coffee, soy sauce and spinach.
                Has upper and lower dentures.
                NPO after 6 p.m.

    9/22   IV infusing into left arm. 1000 cc dextrose in water absorbed between 2 p.m. and midnight.
                c/o thirst, was given ice chips to suck.

    9/23   Clear liquid diet. c/o slight nausea. Drank 400 cc gingerale, 300 cc water, 250 cc jello

    9/24   Full liquid diet. Ate bowl gruel, 2 custards, 200 cc eggnog, 200 cc milk, 800 cc water.

    9/25   Low residue diet. Ate whole tray.

11. *State of Skin*

    9/21   Clear skin. Medium complexion with pale face and perspiration on forehead and chest.
                No breaks, ulcers, bruises, rashes, or pigmentation noted.
                Small scar behind left ear.
                Forehead wrinkled, circles under eyes. Appears tense.
                Balding with clean, dull hair on side and back of head.
                Long, horny nails on feet and hands.

    9/26   Skin clear with pink color in cheeks.

12. *Elimination State*

    9/21   Had some "diarrhea" prior to hospitalization with bright, red blood in feces.
                c/o "dull pain" at times when voiding.

    9/22   Colostomy dressings in place. Many liquid stools.

    9/24   Patient observed nurse irrigating colostomy. Stool less liquid. Off I and O

    9/26   Patient refused to look at colostomy or help with irrigation.

13. *Sexual and Reproductive State*

    9/21   No children.

    9/26   Reports being impotent since divorce.

14. *Ability to Avoid Injury and Repair Damage*

    9/21   Reports undigested food and blood in stool for past month.
                Biopsy shows presence of cancerous cells.
                Hemoglobin = 12 g.

    9/22   Thrashing in bed; injured left wrist.

Fig. 19-5 The systematic assessment focuses on changes that occur during a patient's hospitalization.

measurable, and realistic. In certain areas, such as the nurse-patient relationship, it may be difficult to be specific. In such cases, the nurse can ask, "How will I know when it has happened?", or "What patient behaviors will tell me I've reached my goal?"   These questions will help the nurse to be more specific in stating the objective. For example, if the goal is to establish the nurse-patient relationship, patient behaviors which may indicate this goal has been met may be "patient talks freely with nurse," "patient maintains eye contact," and "patient waits for nurse to return." In other need areas, objectives can be stated more specifically from the start. For example, the nurse will know the objective "teach the patient to administer his own insulin" has been met when the patient shows the nurse he can give himself the injection.

Patient-centered objectives or goals are also stated in action terms. *Patient-centered objectives* indicate what the patient will do. These objectives are stated in a positive manner because the expectation of the nurse is that the patient will accomplish the objective. Patient-centered objectives include the exact time of the behavior, how long the behavior will continue, and what will be accomplished during the time period. Examples of patient-centered objectives are:

Patient will sit in chair by bed for one hour at 10 a.m. and 4 p.m.

Patient will drink 100 ml water q hour

Patient will attend occupational therapy at 10 a.m. and 4 p.m.

Patient will sit with nurse for 5 minutes at 11 a.m. and 5 p.m.

It is useful to try to keep a balance of two objectives for each patient problem or priority. One of these objectives is usually patient centered. The other objective is usually nurse centered.

After objectives or goals have been specified, the nurse decides on the nursing action. The *nursing action* tells the reader what is to be achieved for or with the patient. Nursing actions are stated using action verbs such as turn, feed, walk, rub, irrigate, and give. Nursing actions also include when and how the action should occur. The nurse who prescribes the action initials the order. Statements of nursing actions, then, may be called *nursing orders.* The following are examples of nursing actions or orders:

Change dressing to left lower arm using sterile 2x2s at 8 a.m.

C.E.

Walk patient to physical therapy at 10 a.m. holding patient's left arm firmly   R.F.

Feed patient slowly, telling patient what each food is, at 8 a.m., 12n, 4 p.m. and 8 p.m.   T.C.

Intervention

The third step in the nursing process is intervention. *Intervention* includes action with a purpose; each action has a scientific rationale or reason. Scientific rationale is based on knowledge and theory from nursing, and the behavioral and physical sciences. Without a rationale for action, the nurse's treatment of the patient becomes mechanical, meaningless, and often ineffective.

When the nurse has a sound knowledge base for action, it becomes possible to examine whether the action is effective. For example, the necessity of giving a patient a daily bath can be examined. The nurse decides whether the patient is bathed daily because he always has been, or is bathed daily in order to increase circulation, maintain musculoskeletal function, or establish communication. Other nursing actions can be examined and tested in the same way to see how patient's needs are best met.

Nursing interventions are based on sound nursing judgment. They help the patient meet basic needs and function at the highest level of wellness. Intervention includes actions taken to promote the patient's comfort, hygiene, safety, learning, rest, activity, and any steps taken to restore homeostasis. Counseling, listening, making appropriate referrals and rehabilitation efforts, and carrying out medical orders are also nursing interventions.

Evaluation

Although the nursing process includes steps, it is really a circular process. Closing the circle of the nursing process is evaluation. The nursing process is a continual circle where reassessments, reordering of priorities, restating of objectives, and re-evaluation of nursing interventions occurs. In the *evaluation* step, the nurse reconsiders her objectives and determines whether they have been met satisfactorily. Questions such as, "Were my objectives met?", "How do I know my objectives were met?" and "What evidence do I have that the patient's needs were met?" are asked.

In the evaluation step, the nurse also considers the patient's response to the nurse's interventions. Some questions the nurse might use to evaluate patient response are:

Did the patient re-establish homeostasis?

Did he say he felt better or worse?

Did he appear calmer, stronger, in less pain, less pale, less anxious, more confident?

Did he seem to understand more fully?

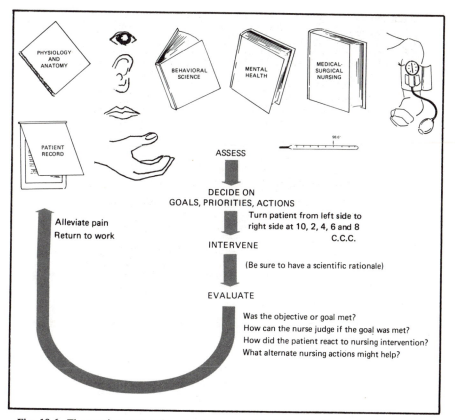

Fig. 19-6 The nursing process is a circular one that includes thinking and acting in a purposeful way.

Did his vital signs or laboratory tests show a move toward the normal range?

What alternative actions can I perform to achieve the objective?

Figure 19-6 shows the nursing process as a circular event.

SUMMARY

The nursing process is a way of thinking and acting in a purposeful way to meet a patient goal or need. Every nursing action is preceded by an assessment of patient needs, problems and strengths, and a decision on goals, priorities or actions. Every nursing action or intervention is followed by evaluation, and, if necessary, revision of the goal or nursing action. Nursing process makes nursing intervention systematic, testable, and potentially more effective.

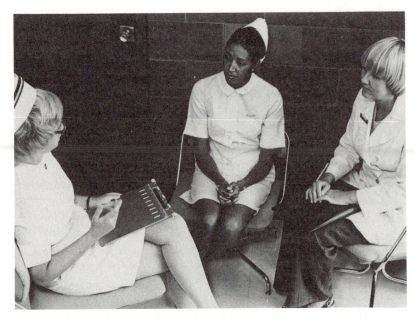

Fig. 19-7 Deciding on goals priorities, and nursing actions based on systematic assessment of the patient's needs.

The primary tools of nursing assessment are the nursing history, nursing diagnosis, and the systematic assessment guide.

In the second step of the nursing process, the nurse defines goals or objectives in specific terms using action verbs. Short-term, long-term, nursing-centered, and patient-centered goals and objectives are identified.

During the intervention step of the nursing process, the nurse acts in a purposeful way based on scientific rationales. In the evaluation step, the nurse considers whether objectives were met, and, if necessary, identifies alternate actions which will meet the objectives.

ACTIVITIES AND DISCUSSION TOPICS

- Read about or visit a hospital where problem-oriented records are used. Find out the pros and cons of this method. Practice recording patient information using the POR method.

- Talk with several graduate nurses about nursing diagnosis. Do they seem to understand what a nursing diagnosis is? If not, does there seem to be a confusion over nursing diagnosis and medical diagnosis? What are the differences?

- Practice writing nursing goals and objectives.
  a. Write two long-term and two short-term goals.
  b. Write four nurse-centered and four patient-centered objectives.
  If possible, write these goals and objectives for actual patients.
- After working with several patients, write some nursing orders that could assist other health personnel in caring for these patients.

REVIEW

A.   Multiple Choice. Select the best answer.

1. The statement that best describes the relationship between communication and nursing process is:
   a. Communication is related to observation and perception, but is not part of the nursing process.
   b. Communication is used most frequently in the evaluation step of the nursing process.
   c. Communication is not used in the assessment step of the nursing process.
   d. Communication is used throughout the nursing process.

2. An effectively stated patient-centered goal and objective is:
   a. Help the patient understand his condition.
   b. Teach patient to irrigate her colostomy by 10/30. C.T.
   c. Patient will walk from his room to the solarium with walker at 10 a.m., 2 p.m. and 6 p.m.
   d. Increase oxygen supply.

3. An effectively stated short-term nursing goal is:
   a. Patient will stand on left leg for five minutes every hour.
   b. Patient will drink 200 ml water q 2 hours. R.R.
   c. Patient will straighten own bed q day before noon.
   d. Turn patient from right to left side q even hour (12, 2, 4, 6, 8, 10) C.C.
   e. Renew Demerol order.

4. The systematic assessment focuses on
   a. areas that change depending on the patient's degree of health or illness.
   b. the patient's response to hospitalization, interpersonal needs, and patterns of daily living.
   c. identifying patient needs and problems.
   d. the desired result or change in patient behavior that will restore homeostasis.

5. In the Problem-Oriented Record (POR) system
   a. all health team members keep separate records.
   b. all health team members use the same recording sheet.
   c. only problems dealing with treatment are recorded.
   d. only the patient's symptoms are recorded.

B. Match the items in Column II to the correct statements in Column I.

Column I	Column II
1. A series of actions that meet a goal or need.	a. noncompliance
	b. nursing action
2. Nursing diagnosis used to describe behavior where the patient refuses to go along with the nurse's goals for care.	c. nursing goals
	d. patient problem
	e. process
3. The end product of a person being unable to meet a need which results in disturbed homeostasis.	
4. Statements that describe the desired result or change in patient behavior that will restore homeostasis.	
5. Statement of what is to be achieved for or with the patient, including when and how the action should occur.	

C. Briefly answer the following questions.
   1. List four steps in the nursing process.
   2. Define nursing diagnosis.
   3. How does a nursing diagnosis differ from a medical diagnosis?
   4. What are the three tools nurses use most often to assess patient needs, strengths, and problems?
   5. What is the purpose of nursing interventions?
   6. In the Problem-Oriented Record (POR) system, what do the letters S.O.A.P. stand for?

chapter 20
NURSING
CARE PLANS

STUDENT OBJECTIVES

- Define nursing care plan.
- List four purposes of the nursing care plan.
- Write a nursing care plan using the Kardex system.
- Write a nursing care plan using the student nursing care plan guide.
- List four suggestions for writing effective nursing care plans.
- State the usefulness of the Kardex in nursing rounds.

Nursing care plans are records that summarize information necessary to provide nursing care for patients and families. Nursing care plans are revised as necessary; they reflect patient problems from the time of admission through discharge. In developing nursing care plans, the nursing process is used. The individual plan is based on assessment of the patient's needs and includes the nursing diagnosis, goals, and interventions. The student's nursing care plans should also include rationales or scientific reasons for choosing an objective or intervention. An evaluation of the objectives and interventions is also necessary.

In the past few years, nursing care plans have become more comprehensive and more scientifically based. It takes time and effort to develop a comprehensive nursing care plan. Because of the time and work pressures, nursing care plans in some hospitals are not comprehensive. The student may experience mixed feelings about what is taught in nursing class about nursing care plans and those nursing care plans which are actually in effect on the hospital units.

As a student, one may not be able to change the status quo, but as a graduate nurse it is possible to add to the body of nursing knowledge by creating in-depth nursing care plans and testing out their effectiveness.

PURPOSES OF THE NURSING CARE PLAN

One purpose of the nursing care plan is to individualize patient care. Since each patient is different, it is important to plan care that takes into account the special needs, preferences and goals of each patient.

Another purpose of the nursing care plan is to set priorities for care. It is impossible for the nurse to meet all the needs of the patient; sometimes the patient does not reveal them or will not allow the nurse to help him meet them. Therefore, the nurse makes a list of patient needs and problems based on a systematic assessment and then selects problems that have priority for nursing intervention.

A third purpose of the nursing care plan is to communicate. Since there are three shifts of nursing personnel and constant change takes place, it is necessary to maintain a written record about the care of each patient. By writing the goals and interventions, nurses are required to clarify their thinking so they may work together to meet the needs of each patient.

Another purpose of the nursing care plan is to provide continuity and coordination of care. Having a written record makes it possible to plan an even flow of nursing care through the various stages of the illness. The nursing care plan also assists in the planning of various diagnostic tests, therapies, and nursing activities with the minimum of stress. From this written record, health personnel in departments throughout the hospital receive the information needed to assist the patient.

Nursing care plans also assist in the evaluation of care and can indicate when goals or objectives are being met. They also point out the need for changes in interventions or objectives. Nursing care plans can add to the body of knowledge used to help future patients. The collection of a number of care plans makes it possible for the nurse to test approaches for use with patients whose problems and characteristics are similar.

Developing nursing care plans can increase skill in observation, perception, and communication. With practice, nurses begin to see where there are gaps in assessment, goals, interventions, or evaluation. By working with other members of the nursing staff, effective and challenging nursing care plans can be developed.

FORMS FOR THE NURSING CARE PLAN

A number of forms and systems are available for use to record nursing care plans. One system is the Kardex. A *Kardex* is a special holder that contains a card for each patient. The Kardex card usually has space for objectives, special needs and preferences, patient problems and nursing interventions, figure 20-1. The flip side of nursing order section of the Kardex often shows the medical orders or plan for the patient which includes medications and treatments ordered by the doctor. Figure 20-2, page 312, shows that portion of a Kardex card used to record medical orders.

Long-Term Goal: Assist to reach and maintain highest level of wellness	
Problems	Action/Intervention
6/21 Confusion	Identify self by name and title when entering room Orient patient to person, place + time prn Sit c̄ patient at 10 a.m. + 2 pm encouraging her to share thoughts and feelings C.F.
6/22 Decreased Motor function	Walk c̄ patient to end of hall at 10 a.m., 2 p.m. + 7 p.m. R.T.
6/24 Unsteadiness on feet	Hold pt's arm firmly when walking. Assist pt. in + out of bathtub. Side rails prn L.S.
6/26 Dehydration	Give pt. 100 ml water or fruit juice q hr. G.R.

Admitted: 6/18   Discharged   Allergies: *none*

Medical diagnoses: *organic brain Syndrome; arthritis of hip*   Safety measures: *low bed side rails up prn*   Activity: *Walking c̄ assistance*

Surgery: *Total hip replacement 3/3*   Hygiene: *Prefers tub bath*

Age: *75*   Diet: *regular; force fluids*

Name: *Whitaker, Sybil*   Bowel/bladder measures: *none*

Fig. 20-1 The Kardex is one system used in many hospitals to record nursing care plans. What could you add or change in this plan?

MEDICATIONS				
Date	Medication	Time	Route	Instructions to patient or family
12/2	Elavil 25 mgm	8-4-8	oral	Teach pt. purpose of medication and precautions
	Coumadin 5 mgm	8 a.m.	IM	
	Edecrin 50 mgm	8 a.m.	Rectal (suppository)	

TREATMENTS				
Date	Treatment	Time	Other Comments	Instructions to patient or family
12/2	Fasting blood Sugar	8 am.		Do not eat after midnight on preceeding day.
	Blood pressure	8-12-4-8		Teach pt to take + monitor own blood pressure

Patient: Charles, Don   Doctor: Blythe

Fig. 20-2 Some Kardex cards have a section to record medical orders.

Another system for using nursing care plans is the loose-leaf notebook form which allows for more space to record patient information. One or more separate pages are used for recording the plan of care for each patient.

There are other kinds of nursing care plans. In some settings, the patient's plan of care is left at the bedside or in the home. This method is used when the patient or family takes an especially active part in care. Nursing care plans that focus on teaching or learning may be developed on a separate checklist or outline form. Some nursing care plans may include routine orders. In some settings, routine postoperative or rehabilitation orders are stamped on the order sheet or are mimeographed and added to the patient's chart. Standard care plans have developed based on the care of groups of patients with similar problems and nursing procedures. For example, some hospitals now have a standard care routine for the patient who is preoperative, postoperative, or about to be discharged. Although these orders are fixed, there is space provided to add special objectives or problems. This method has the advantage of combining the commonalities of a group of patients with individualized care.

The student may see any of these methods of planned patient care in practice. Assignments to write nursing care plans will involve detailed nursing care plans. These will require statements of (1) the basic need, (2) the patient problem arising from an inability to meet the need, (3) objectives, (4) interventions, (5) rationale for action, and (6) an evaluation of whether patient problems were solved or whether the plan requires revision.

By putting all of this information in one place, the student is more likely to understand how needs, problems, objectives, interventions, and rationales fit together. In order to develop skills in nursing assessment, it is essential that the student learn to correlate theory with the scientific reasons for nursing actions.

It may be easier for the student to collect the necessary information for a nursing care plan if three words are remembered: what, how, and why. The *what* of a nursing care plan is, "What is the patient's need?", "What interfered with meeting the need that created a patient problem?", and "What does the nurse want to achieve?" The *how* of a nursing care plan is, "How does the nurse intervene to restore homeostasis?" The *why* of a nursing care plan is, "Why the intervention? What is the reason or rationale that gives it a scientific base?" Figure 20-3, pages 314 and 315, shows a nursing care plan commonly used by student nurses.

DEVELOPING AN EFFECTIVE NURSING CARE PLAN

With experience, the student will become more skilled in developing nursing care plans. In the meantime, the following questions should be considered when preparing a nursing care plan:

- Did I fill in all the information requested on the nursing care plan guide?

- Did I look up terms or words I did not understand?

- Is the plan realistic?

- Is the plan specific for this patient?

- Did I relate theory to nursing intervention?

- Did I include the patient and/or family in the plan?

- Did I include teaching in the plan?

- Are both physiological and psychosocial needs considered?

- Did I write what I meant to convey in a clear and simple manner?

Patient's Initials	Sex	Age	Occupation	Cultural Group	Marital Status	Diet	Admitted	Discharged	Diagnoses
R.T.	F	59	Teacher	Lithuanian	Married	Low Residual	9/21		Carcinoma of rectum and anus

NEED (What?)	PROBLEM (What interfered with homeostasis?)	OBJECTIVE (What to do to restore homeostasis?)	INTERVENTION (How to do it)	RATIONALE (Why is it a good idea?)	EVALUATION (Did it work?)
Interpersonal	Anxiety	Provide clear, open communication.	Introduce self. Explain procedures. Answer patient questions. Offer to stay with patient.	Offering self and explaining the unknown decrease anxiety.	Patient still anxious; will need continued communication efforts.
	Changed body image due to stoma	Assist patient to incorporate change into body image.	Allow patient to view stoma and discuss reactions. Show nonverbal acceptance of stoma.	Others' acceptance will help the patient to accept body change.	Patient talking about stoma, described feeling.
Oxygen	Dyspnea	Increase oxygen supply.	Elevate head of bed 45°. Ask patient to deep breathe with supervision.	Gravity assists with breathing and lungs are expanded, allowing more oxygen in arterioles of lung.	Patient breathing more easily. Respirations decreased from 24 to 18 and were deeper.
Eliminate waste	Unfamiliar route of eliminating feces.	Keep colostomy patent and draining.	Give fluids. Check drainage from colostomy every hr. Change dressings as needed.	Forcing fluids helps eliminate waste; checking drainage frequently will decrease possibility of nonpatency.	Colostomy is open and draining.

Food and Fluid	None				
Avoid injury Repair damage	Unsteadiness on feet.	Assist patient when walking.	Hold onto patient's arm firmly. Walk slowly.	Firm assistance may prevent patient from a fall.	Patient did not fall.
Activity/Rest/Comfort	Unable to Sleep at night.	Assist patient to sleep.	Ask patient what she does at home to sleep. Encourage patient to be active during day. Reposition. Suggest patient ask for a backrub.	Patients often know what will help. Inactivity interferes with sleep pattern. Circulation and comfort is increased when body is positioned correctly.	Sleeplessness decreased.
Self-actualization	Enforced dependency.	Allow patient to be as independent as possible.	Encourage patient to assist with own care. Develop teaching plan for colostomy care with patient. Ask patient to talk with nurse and family about colostomy care at home.	Total dependency leads to feelings of low self-esteem. Independency and mastery of the environment leads to increased self-esteem.	Patient agreed to become more independent and seemed pleased to start learning more about colostomy.

Fig. 20-3 Student nurses use detailed nursing care plans to learn how theory relates to clinical practice.

USING THE NURSING CARE PLAN

The student who is assigned to a clinical area will usually receive a report from the instructor or nurse in charge. The report covers the condition of the assigned patients, their progress, and their specific needs and preferences. It should also include pertinent information about the care given by nurses on the previous shift of duty. The student then gives the patient care and follows through on required procedures and observations. When reporting off duty, it is important to be clear, specific and thorough; any unusual occurrences such as the patient's refusal to take medication or a change in vital signs must be reported. Before giving a report to the nurse in charge (or the team leader), it may be useful to mentally check through the systematic assessment guide categories discussed earlier. Although all information about patient care may be important to the patient, the nurse in charge may focus on new or unusual information. This difference in attitude sometimes leads students to think that the nurse in charge is not interested in what the student has to report. However, the student should continue to give a thorough report and the nurse will assume the responsibility of determining what to pass on to others.

The nursing staff gathers to convey information to one another at each change of shift. Discussion at this time is focused on the Kardex and the nursing care plan. Important additions or changes in the patient's plan of care are entered on the record.

Sometimes the nurse who is in charge of coordinating the work of several health team members will take the Kardex along when visiting and evaluating the patients under the care of these staff members. These evaluation visits are called *nursing rounds*. The nurse in charge of coordinating the care given by several health team members is called a *team leader*. The team leader may call for a *team report*; all members of the team share information about each of the patients in their care. The Kardex is used to check and change care plans at this time.

Nurses are often called upon to plan nursing care for patients who are transferred to other services or units within the hospital or to other care facilities. The written nursing care plan may be sent with these transferred patients. In addition, nurses who are interested in continuity of care may include a note on the patient's progress and a request to be called to share further information about patient problems and approaches.

SUMMARY

Nursing care plans are records that summarize information necessary to provide nursing care for patients and families. Nursing care plans individualize

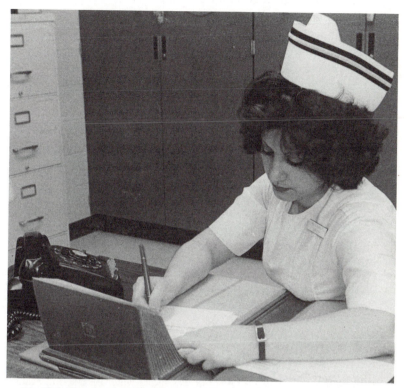

Fig. 20-4 The nurse records patient problems and care on the nursing care plan.

care, help to set priorities, improve communication, provide continuity and coordination of care, assist in the evaluation of care, and develop the nurse's skill in observation, perception, and communication. In developing effective nursing care plans, the nurse asks, "What is the patient's need?", "What interfered with the patient's ability to meet the need?", "What does the nurse want to achieve?", "How can the nurse assist the patient to re-establish homeostasis?", and "What is the scientific rationale for the nursing action?"

ACTIVITIES AND DISCUSSION TOPICS

- Look through the Kardex in the clinical area where you are assigned. Ask yourself the following questions as you examine the entries:
  a. Are there attempts to individualize care for each patient?
  b. What are the priorities for (1) general care on this unit and, (2) specific care for each patient?

c. Is sufficient material recorded to communicate essential information among the three nursing shifts?

d. Is continuity of care provided for? What gaps or inconsistencies do you notice?

e. Look at the Kardex cards of two or three patients who have similar patient problems. What new knowledge about effective nursing care could you add or learn?

f. What strengths and weaknesses in observation, perception, and communication are there?

- Listen to the report given at a change of shifts.
  a. What did you learn about nursing care plans for these patients?
  b. What was not discussed that might have been helpful?
  c. Was medical care and orders mixed in with nursing care and orders? Was the report primarily focused on medical care?
  d. Did you feel free to ask questions about patient care?

- Next time a patient you have worked with is transferred, speak or write a note to the receiving nurse about patient problems and approaches. Ask for feedback from the nurse about future patient care and responses.

REVIEW

A. Briefly answer the following questions.

1. Define nursing care plan.

2. List four purposes of the nursing care plan.

3. List four suggestions for writing effective nursing care plans.

4. State the usefulness of the Kardex in nursing rounds.

5. What three words are helpful in collecting necessary information for a nursing care plan?

6. What is a team report?

B. Read the following patient information, look up any unfamiliar words, and then fill in the sample Kardex card appropriately.

Mr. S., age 68, has diabetes. He had difficulty voiding for two weeks before coming to the hospital. Two days ago, on April 22, Mr. S. had surgery to correct a benign prostatic hypertrophy. He now complains of bladder spasms and some

pain at intervals. He also seems confused about where he is at times. His wife's voice and presence seems to orient him to the present situation. You are assigned to provide the following care for the patient: partial bath and backcare, blood pressure at 10 a.m., Foley catheter to straight drainage, Foley hygiene care, intake and output, out of bed (OOB) in chair after bath, check urine for sugar and acetone (S and A), check dressing and reinforce as necessary with sterile 2 x 2s, encourage patient to verbalize thoughts and feelings. Do a process recording.

SAMPLE KARDEX CARD

Long-term goal:	
Problem/Objectives	**Action/Intervention**
5/24 Body image change	1.
	2.
	3.
5/24 Confusion	1.
	2.
	3.
5/24 Bladder pain and spasms	1.
	2.

Admitted: Discharged:	Allergies: none
Medical diagnoses:	Safety measures:
Surgery: Transurethral resection	Activity:
	Hygiene:
Age:	Diet: 1500 calorie diabetic
Name	Bowel/bladder measures:

C. After completing the Kardex card, use the same patient information to
develop a nursing care plan using the form provided below.

				Sample Nursing Care Plan Form			Student:		
Patient's Initials	Sex	Age	Occupa- tion	Cultural Group	Marital Status	Diet	Admission Date	Dis- charge Date	Diag- noses

Need	Problem	Objective	Intervention	Rationale	Evaluation
Interpersonal					
Oxygen					
Elimination of waste					
Food and fluid					
Safety					
Activity/ Rest/ Comfort					
Self- actualization					

D.   Fill in the missing information (dosage time, route, instructions to patient or family) for the medications and treatments listed below.

MEDICATIONS				
Date	Medication	Time	Route	Instructions to patient or family
10/4	Nitrofurantoin Glutethimide Digitalis			

TREATMENTS				
Date	Treatment	Time	Other Comments	Instructions to patient or family
10/6	Hot packs to left leg oxygen tent			

SECTION 4
COPING
WITH
ILLNESS

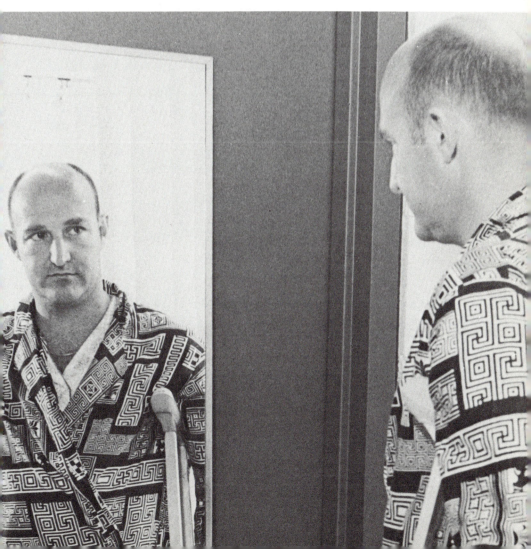

chapter 21
THE HOSPITAL
AND THE INSTITUTION

STUDENT OBJECTIVES

- Identify factors that contribute to the operation and atmosphere of the hospital unit.

- List two ways the communication structure can influence patient ability to cope with illness.

- Identify effects of illness and hospitalization.

- List three ways the nurse can recognize the overcooperative patient.

- List four characteristics of total institutions.

To a great extent, the health personnel assigned to a unit determines how the hospital unit will operate. Many factors contribute to the operation and atmosphere of the unit. One of these factors is the educational preparation obtained in nursing and medical institutions. Cultural background also affects the behavior of the health personnel. Lastly, individual personalities play an important part in providing a favorable clinical setting.

THE HOSPITAL SOCIAL SYSTEM

Although one may think of a social system on a wider scale, it may apply to institutional environments as well as the outside community. When health personnel continually interact and develop shared expectations, norms, and values, the whole operation can be called a *social system*. Social systems have both formal and informal rules for behavior; formal rules are written or spoken while the informal rules are those which are understood or tolerated. The former are based on the statements of philosophy made by the institution or health-related facility; what actually happens in practice (the informal rules) is sometime another story.

Within the social system, a culture develops. *Culture* includes such things as language, proper ways to communicate, proper ways to act, appropriate punishment for those who do not act as expected (*negative sanctions*) and appropriate reward for those who do act as expected (*positive sanctions*).

The people in a social system not only work toward common goals, they also try to get along with one another. Health personnel who work together develop a mutual idea of what to expect. These expectations are composed of ideas and behaviors which are built on values and norms, respectively. Social systems are constantly changing; therefore, at times, more energy may be directed on establishing cooperation and staff conformity than on patient care. When change in patient and staff occurs frequently because of frequent turnover, disjointed communication and weak leadership may result.

Each hospital unit has an atmosphere which may differ from others; some are noisy, others are chaotic with constant crises, others convey anxiety, hopelessness, or apathy, and others are quiet, yet cheerful. Much depends on the way staff members handle crises. Again, this may differ with each unit. Reactions vary when a crisis occurs regardless of whether it is a patient crisis, such as death, or a staff crisis, such as the loss of a head nurse or chief doctor. Staff members may react by: (1) banding together and supporting each other, (2) pulling apart and going separate ways, (3) ignoring the crisis and continuing with the usual activities and routines, or (4) trying to change the situation so that homeostasis can be restored.

Communication Structures

Any social system has a power structure. The appointed leaders of the unit, such as the head nurse or the chief doctor, are the formal leaders. The informal leaders are often those persons who stay on the job for many years and exert power by sticking together. On some units, the nursing aides may be the informal leaders. The new student or graduate nurse may not be aware of the power structure of a unit at first. It is useful to examine this structure so the nurse will not become caught in the middle of power struggles or reinforce destructive power.

One way to assess the power structure is to examine the communication channels on the unit. In a *horizontal* or *free flowing structure*, every staff member has access to all other staff members. The flow of communication is fluid and diverse. Each person on the staff is considered to have some expertise and voice in patient care. In a *hierarchical communication structure*, the flow of communication is primarily one way, from the top to the bottom. The aides probably never talk to the doctor except through the nurse. In a very strict hierarchical structure each person may be able to talk to co-workers but must contact only the immediate supervisor to share or get information pertaining to the care of the patient.

No matter what the structure, however, some formal and informal channels of communication do exist. Formal channels of communication include nurses' and doctors' notes, staff meetings, and nursing reports. Informal communication can take place during coffee breaks, lunch, and/or brief verbal interactions with other staff members. Informal notes are also used for communicating with others.

The communication structure not only influences the nurse but the patient, too, is affected. A strict hierarchical communication structure will make it much more difficult for the patient to communicate his wants and needs. Such a structure also decreases the possibility of the patient receiving assistance with his communicated wants and needs. Figure 21-1, page 328, depicts a hierarchical communication structure. Figure 21-2, page 329, depicts a horizontal or free flowing communication structure.

Another way the patient is influenced by the communication flow is through mixed or conflicting messages. If the nurse disagrees with the doctor's order, the patient may receive a confused picture of what is expected. For example, the nurse may repeat the doctor's words but nonverbally communicate disagreement with the doctor. Mixed or conflicting messages often occur when there is a power struggle between nurse and doctor about who knows what is best for the patient. In general, the patient receives less attention when the nurse and doctor are using their energies to struggles with one another.

The student or graduate nurse can be helpful to the patient in coping with his illness if she assesses the social system of the unit. Factors the nurse can consider when a unit social system is assessed are:

- Informal and formal rules for behavior (norms)

- Leadership patterns

- Stability of staff and patient population

- Unit atmosphere

- Channels for communication

- Intervention in crises

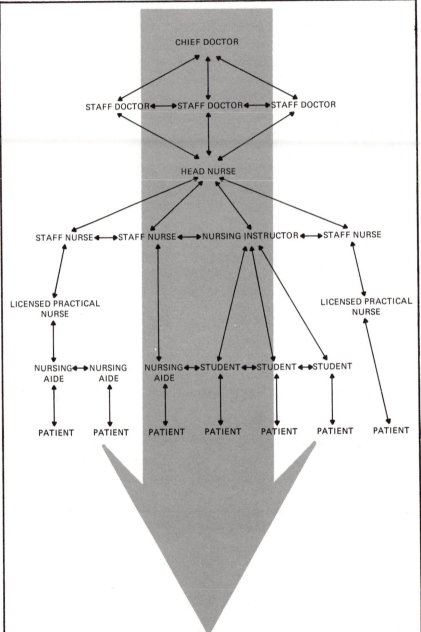

Fig. 21-1 In a hierarchical structure, communication flows mainly downward. Any upward communication is only to the next highest level, while communication between the staff remains at the same levels.

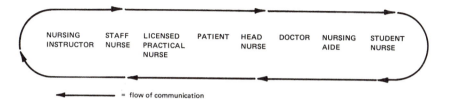

| NURSING INSTRUCTOR | STAFF NURSE | LICENSED PRACTICAL NURSE | PATIENT | HEAD NURSE | DOCTOR | NURSING AIDE | STUDENT NURSE |

───────── = flow of communication

Fig. 21-2 In a horizontal or free flowing communication structure, no one staff member is above another. The communication flows freely, with each staff member able to communicate to the patient and all other staff members.

Figure 21-3 presents some questions the nurse can use to assess a unit social system.

The Patient's View

To the patient who arrives at a hospital for the first time, the hospital environment may seem quite strange. For example, the degree of privacy is not the same; most persons are used to more privacy than hospitalization offers. Unfamiliar machines and equipment and unusual sights, sounds, and smells are encountered. Doctors and nurses use new terms and phrases which they seem to expect the patient to understand. There are strict routines for eating, treatment, rising and bathing. All of these changes and differences are likely to create anxiety in the patient.

1. What are the formal expectations for staff and patient behavior?
2. What actually occurs between patient and staff?
3. Who are the formal leaders?
4. Who are the informal leaders?
5. How often does the staff population change?
6. How often does the patient population change?
7. What kind of atmosphere exists?
8. What formal channels are there for communication?
9. What are the informal channels for communication?
10. What does the staff do during a crisis?

Fig. 21-3 Questions to ask when assessing the social system of a hospital or institutional unit.

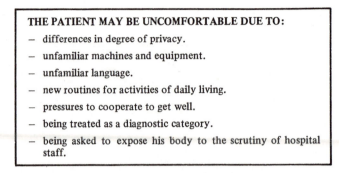

Fig. 21-4 Reasons which contribute to an unfavorable concept of the hospital.

The patient soon learns that cooperation with the hospital staff is a rule to be followed in order to get well. The patient is expected to follow the directions of the staff. Patients who do not do as the staff says may receive negative sanctions such as a frown, an angry glance, or inattention to requests for comfort measures.

Many of the practices which nurses and doctors take for granted can be viewed by the patient as dehumanizing. For example, when nurses or doctors discuss the patient as if he were not present, the patient may feel less human. Being referred to as a diagnostic category such as "the hernia case" is also dehumanizing and should not be used either within the patient's hearing or away from it. Exposing one's body to the scrutiny of the nurse or doctor and not being asked about or even told about future treatment plans can cause distress and takes away the patient's dignity. Figure 21-4 summarizes hospital factors that may create discomfort in the newly admitted patient.

EFFECTS OF ILLNESS

One of the major effects of illness the nurse will observe is a tendency for the patient to *regress*; there is a tendency to go back to a previous state or condition. This regression can be viewed as one of the patient's attempts to cope with illness. Regression includes four aspects:

1. An increased need to control the external environment as a result of feeling less in control of what is happening to him.

   This may take the form of telling the nurse how to perform nursing care.

2. A narrowing of interest from the external environment and a focus on basic needs such as food, rest, and physical comfort.

   The student may find it curious that some patients should be so concerned about their blood pressure, pulse, urine, or feces. If the nurse realizes that this concern is part of the attempt to cope with illness, she can be more understanding with anxious or irritable patients who ask many questions about their body functions.

3. A resentment or anger that the illness has occurred. Many times this anger or resentment is not verbalized for fear of being punished or sanctioned.

4. An increased dependency.

   This need to be dependent on others for care creates *ambivalent feelings.* When a person has ambivalent feelings he feels two ways about a situation. A patient may feel grateful to the person helping him yet dislike the loss of power and control that dependency demands.

Pain and its ability to create isolation is another common effect of illness. Patients who suffer pain are really isolated as others cannot share the pain experience. Assessment and intervention in the pain experience was discussed in more detail in chapters 9 and 10.

Anxiety and fear are also common effects of illness. Patients can experience anxiety because of an unawareness of the importance of treatments and lack of familiarity with the hospital and procedures. Being kept waiting for long periods of time for a diagnosis or treatment add to these anxious feelings. Fear of the unknown, of cancer, of dying, being abandoned, and suffering without relief are common fears. Generally, fear of the unknown, that is not knowing what will happen next, is a predominant, frequently experienced cause for anxiety which is a common effect of illness. Nurses can diminish this effect by keeping the patient informed and explaining the purpose and technique of ordered treatments. Figure 21-5 summarizes possible effects of illness.

EFFECTS OF ILLNESS INCLUDE:

- increased need to control the external environment including the nurse.

- focus of interest in basic needs for food, rest and physical comfort.

- resentment or anger.

- increased dependency.

- ambivalent feelings about being dependent.

- isolation due to pain.

- anxiety.

- fear.

Fig. 21-5 Possible effects of illness

EFFECTS OF HOSPITALIZATION

The effects of hospitalization depend on the patient's perception of the immediate environment. However, the nurse should be familiar with common effects of hospitalization: depersonalization, loneliness, invasion of privacy, anxiety about physical contacts, and forced passive acceptance.

Depersonalization. *Depersonalization* means not treating the patient as a person. The patient is depersonalized when he is given a patient number, referred to by diagnosis or room number, given hospital clothing and forced into a dependent role, and is kept waiting for long periods of time for unknown people to do unfamiliar procedures.

Loneliness. Another effect of hospitalization is loneliness. Even though a patient may share a room with another person, both are ill and may feel apart from one another because each is focusing on himself and his body processes. Time may seem to drag. Minutes may seem like hours. The last time the patient saw the nurse may seem like days. Since the usual household, business, or social activity is no longer being done, there is little to occupy one's time and patients become isolated and lonely.

Loss of Privacy. An effect of hospitalization that nurses often overlook is the loss of privacy. Giving a bedbath or taking a rectal temperature may become so routine that the nurse may overlook the fact that they are invasions of privacy. Some loss of the patient's privacy will occur no matter how many precautions the nurse takes as many procedures require some invasion of the patient's privacy. The nurse can provide adequate draping and shielding of the patient from the view of others, explain and prepare the patient for any procedure, and make allowance for the patient to make some decisions about his privacy; for example, asking whether his room door is to be left open or closed.

Physical Contact with Patients. Related to lack of privacy is the anxiety which may be felt about close physical contact with strangers. It will be necessary that the nurse, doctor, lab technician, and others make contact with parts of the patient's body; such contact is considered to be socially or culturally unacceptable outside of the hospital.

Assuming a Passive Role. When a person is hospitalized, it becomes necessary to assume a passive patient role; this contributes to a loss of dignity and worth. When a person is active and in control of the environment, feelings of self-worth

```
COMMON EFFECTS OF HOSPITALIZATION:
 –  depersonalization.
 –  loneliness.
 –  loss of privacy.
 –  anxiety about close physical contact with strangers.
 –  forced assumption of passive role.
```

Fig. 21-6 Effects of hospitalization

are strong. The passive patient role decreases the potential for action and mastery of the environment and thereby the possibility for ways to feel good about oneself.

Dealing With the Effects of Hospitalization

The patient can deal with the effects of hospitalization in a number of ways. One way is to turn anxiety into hostility and resentment. The patient who uses this coping method orders the nurse around, refuses to comply with the nurse's requests, and makes constant requests for attention. If the nurse realizes the patient is using anger to cope with the effects of hospitalization, it may be easier to understand the patient's behavior and not take it as a personal attack.

Another method patients use to deal with their anxiety about hospitalization is to withdraw from relating with others. A common reaction to being hospitalized is to adopt the "good" or "overcooperative" patient rule. Figure 21-7 summarizes some ways patients deal with the effects of hospitalization.

The Overcooperative Patient Role. The good patient is usually overly cooperative; he is careful not to be demanding or overdependent. He is more concerned about pleasing the nurse than he is about decreasing his own conflict and tension. The patient might very well benefit from being demanding but he refuses to make his needs known for fear of displeasing the nurse. Since the patient appears all right, nurses may easily overlook the real needs of this patient.

```
THE PATIENT CAN DEAL WITH THE EFFECTS OF
HOSPITALIZATION BY:
 –  becoming hostile and resentful.
 –  withdrawing from relationships with others.
 –  adopting the "good" or "overcooperative" patient
    role.
```

Fig. 21-7 There are a number of ways patients deal with the effects of hospitalization.

The overcooperative patient probably feels the usual hospital pressures to get well. These pressures are intensified by observing doctors and nurses who seem to be overworked and rushed. The patient may compare his illness with that of his roommate. Thinking that most other patients must be sicker than he, this patient may feel guilty about asking for help. It is the overcooperative patient who is often not able to state exactly what the rights of patients are. If the nurse asks this patient how care could be improved, he is likely to be vague or noncommittal in an effort to please the nurse.

Patients may share societal biases that physical complaints are legitimate but requests for emotional or supportive care are not. The overcooperative patient is even less likely to receive emotional or supportive care because he neither asks for it nor appears to need it.

The nurse has several clues that a patient has assumed the role of an over-cooperative patient. For example, patients may say everything is all right but may grimace or convey through tone of voice that they are in distress. Getting up to give their own care even though they are on bedrest or watching the nurse's every move to see what will please her are other clues that the patient is assuming the role of the good patient.

Many persons wish to appear cooperative but also want to receive emotional and supportive care. This often leads to unrealistic expectations that the nurse

PATIENT ASSESSMENT	NURSING INTERVENTION
Patient:	Nurse states:
— does not demand care.	"People think I'm too busy, so they don't ask for what they want. I do have time, and I'd like to help you."
— is overly cooperative with nurse.	
— verbally denies need for assistance, but gives nonverbal clues implying need for help.	OR
— is vague or noncommittal when asked how patient care could be improved.	"I can only help you if you tell me what you want and need."
— states others are sicker and more in need of care than he is.	
— gets up to do own care although on bedrest.	
— watches nurse's every move to discover what will please the nurse.	

Fig. 21-8 The overcooperative patient: assessment and intervention

will somehow know that help is needed. This behavior — where people expect things to occur merely because they wish it — is called *magical thinking*. In early childhood, magical thinking occurs as a part of growth and development. For example, young children think they can reach up and touch a rainbow because they wish to be able to do so. In adults, magical thinking creates frustration in both parties of an interaction. The magical thinker assumes others know exactly what he wants and sees no reason why he should verbally state his needs. The other party in the interaction will also feel frustrated since she has no way of knowing what the other wants unless he tells her.

Nurses can decrease patient frustration due to magical thinking by making comments such as, "People think I'm too busy so they don't ask for what they want. I do have time, and I'd like to help you." Later, if the nurse has established a good relationship with the overcooperative patient, she might comment, "I can't read your mind. I only can help you if you tell me what you want and need." In this way, the patient may give up magical thinking and learn new ways of relating with others. Figure 21-8 shows nursing assessments and interventions for the good or overcooperative patient.

OTHER INSTITUTIONS

Institutions are established to care for people who are unable to look after themselves or who are considered to be a threat to the community. The occupants are confined or restricted to some degree, and the institution is considered their residence. Examples of these institutions are mental hospitals, and prisons.

In *Asylums*, Goffman has explored the characteristics of these institutions.[1] He refers to them as "total institutions." The nurse may be employed in a total institution; it is important that its cultural elements be understood. One of the characteristics of a total institution is the breakdown of barriers which in ordinary life separate places where people sleep, play, and work. Unfortunately, there is a tendency to treat people by bureaucratic organization; human needs are not given individual attention. The chief activity of the staff may be surveillance where looking for those who break the rules becomes more important than giving care. Lines of communication are distant and restricted. For the most part a hierarchical communication structure exists. This leads to staff perception of patients or inmates as untrustworthy, and patient perception of staff as mean and uncaring. Past ties to family or employer are broken. These breaks are reinforced when it is difficult or impossible for the resident to have visitors or to go home for a visit.

[1] Erving Goffman, *Asylums* (Garden City: Anchor, 1961)

Admission to institutions can be very dehumanizing; the new arrival is often stripped, bathed, and coded with an identification number and/or tag. There may be a lack of locker space. Periodic searches of private possessions by the staff reinforce feelings of low self-esteem and dehumanization. Actions which were taken for granted at home may now require special permission. In some institutions it is necessary for residents to beg or humbly ask for matches, a drink of water, or permission to use the telephone.

Those persons who must reside in total institutions lose their privacy when (1) they are forced to tell facts about themselves they would rather withhold, (2) they are humiliated in front of others, (3) their waste products are scrutinized for evidence of hidden objects, (4) they are called by their first name without prior permission, and (5) their sexual behavior is discussed.

Because staying out of trouble is a primary goal for residents of total institutions, they often forego socializing with others in order to avoid staff confrontation. Talking with staff members is often minimal since the staff may disregard their statements.

Total institutions tend to reinforce or increase the already problematic feelings of the residents: isolation, low self-esteem, confusion, and inability to control their impulses to act. As a coping device, people who spend long periods of time in total institutions often adopt an apathetic, hopeless approach to their living environment.

Students who have clinical experiences in total institutions often feel frustrated, angry, and hopeless. They are apt to blame the staff for the residents' condition without considering that the standardized culture of total institutions tends to decrease potential for individualized care. In such a culture, both staff members and residents may be caught in a self-reinforcing social system. Figure 21-9 lists characteristics frequently found in total institutions. However,

---

- A breakdown in the barriers which usually separate sleeping, playing, and working areas.
- Bureaucratic organization is more important than personalized care.
- Surveillance is more important than resident care.
- Lines of communication are distant and restricted.
- Staff and resident groups perceive each other in a stereotyped way.
- A stripping process occurs at the time of admission.
- Patients must ask permission to act in ways they took for granted at home.
- There is a nearly complete lack of privacy.
- Staying out of trouble is a primary resident goal.
- A self-reinforcing cycle of apathy and hopelessness is produced in staff, residents, and students.

Fig. 21-9 Common characteristics of total institutions

some progress (although slow) is being made toward improving the situations found in many of these residences.

SUMMARY

Each hospital develops its own culture including values, norms, sanctions, leadership, communication patterns, and atmosphere. Communication structure and the patient's view of the hospital social system are major factors to consider in establishing an environment conducive to effective nurse-patient relationships.

Common effects of illness include regression, isolation, fear, and anxiety. In addition to these effects, the patient must also deal with the effects of hospitalization: depersonalization, loneliness, lack of privacy, anxiety related to close physical contact, and pressures to assume the passive patient role. The patient tries to deal with the effects of hospitalization by becoming angry, withdrawn, or overly cooperative. The needs of the overcooperative patient may be overlooked by the nurse because he appears to be all right.

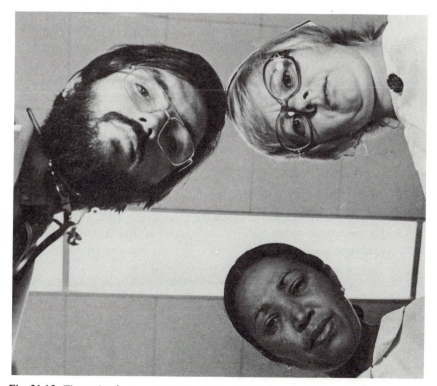

Fig. 21-10 The patient's view of the hospital social system should be considered in establishing a therapeutic environment.

In contrast to hospitals, institutions are places where people live for a longer period of time. Total institutions have the following characteristics: the barriers which usually separate sleeping, playing, and working areas are broken down; bureaucratic organization is more important than personalized care; surveillance is more important than resident care; lines of communication are distant, restricted and stereotyped; admission is a stripping process; permission must be asked for actions that were taken for granted at home; there is a nearly complete lack of privacy; staying out of trouble is a primary resident goal; and a self-reinforcing cycle of apathy and hopelessness is likely to occur in staff, residents and student nurses.

ACTIVITIES AND DISCUSSION TOPICS

- Select a hospital or total institution. Evaluate the social system used on one of their units. Use figure 21-3 as a guide.
- Evaluate how three different patients seem to deal with the effects of hospitalization. To do this evaluation, ask yourself, "Does this patient become hostile, withdraw from others, or adopt the overcooperative patient role?"
- Visit a total institution such as a state or county mental hospital, state or county home for the mentally retarded, prison, or home for the blind. Write down your reactions to the visit. Which characteristics of total institutions did you find to be operating?

REVIEW

A. Multiple Choice. Select the best answer(s). Some questions have more than one answer.
1. Some common effects of illness are
    a. regression.
    b. depersonalization.
    c. isolation due to pain.
    d. anxiety and fear.
2. Some common effects of hospitalization are
    a. loneliness.
    b. loss of privacy.
    c. depersonalization.
    d. anxiety.
3. Factors that contribute to the operation and atmosphere of the hospital unit are
    a. individual personalities of the staff.
    b. communication structures.
    c. educational preparation of the staff.
    d. cultural background of the staff.

4. When a patient is more concerned about pleasing the nurse than he is about decreasing his own conflict and tension, he is being
   a. passive.
   c. supportive.
   b. overcooperative.
   d. depersonalized.

5. A group of people who continually interact and develop shared expectations, norms and values can be referred to as a
   a. hierarchical structure.
   c. culture.
   b. horizontal structure.
   d. social system.

B. Match the items in Column II to the appropriate statement in Column I.

Column I	Column II
1. The flow of communication primarily from the top down.	a. ambivalent feelings
	b. culture.
2. Assuming others know what is wanted without stating the need.	c. hierarchical structure
	d. horizontal structure
3. When a person feels two ways about a situation.	e. magical thinking
	f. negative sanction
	g. positive sanction
4. The language, beliefs, communication, and behavior of a group of people.	h. regression
5. Appropriate punishment for those who do not act as expected.	
6. Every staff member has access to all other staff members; free flow of information.	
7. To go back to a previous state or condition.	
8. Appropriate reward for those who act as expected.	

C. Briefly answer the following questions.
   1. Name two ways the communication structure can influence the patient's ability to cope with illness.
   2. List three ways the nurse can recognize the overcooperative patient.
   3. State two ways the nurse can intervene with the overcooperative patient.
   4. List four characteristics of total institutions.
   5. Name the four aspects of regression.

chapter 22
THE
THERAPEUTIC
ENVIRONMENT

STUDENT OBJECTIVES

- Name six elements of the physical environment to be assessed for therapeutic effectiveness.
- Identify ways the staff members can provide a more therapeutic interpersonal environment.
- Explain the purpose of a therapeutic environment.
- List four ways the nurse can enhance the therapeutic environment during patient admission.
- List four ways the nurse can enhance the therapeutic environment during patient discharge.

A *therapeutic environment* enables its participant members to learn to use effective coping devices so that homeostasis can be maintained. The therapeutic environment assists people to meet basic needs and also to grow and increase their potential for more effective and satisfying life or death processes. For example, a therapeutic relationship with one patient may be to assist him to a peaceful death. A therapeutic relationship with another patient may be to help him learn how to speak after having had a stroke.

CHARACTERISTICS OF A THERAPEUTIC ENVIRONMENT

To promote a therapeutic environment, the nurse must be aware of physical, interpersonal, and cultural stimuli and how each interacts with and influences other parts of the environment. No environment, not even a total institution, is completely nontherapeutic. In fact, in many total institutions, patients provide therapeutic care for one another when staff members are unable to provide this care. Likewise, no environment is totally therapeutic. The nurse works with other staff and patient members to attain an ideal goal of a therapeutic environment.

With the therapeutic environment approach, the nurse uses the total external environment to benefit the patient. A therapeutic environment has a number of characteristics: provision for cultural differences; provision for meeting the immediate needs of its members; acceptance of behavior without judgmental reactions; provision for choice to participate in plans for care; shared responsibility for implementing decisions; open communication; and opportunity for learning through experience. These characteristics should all be considered in the evaluation of a therapeutic environment.

Although dividing the environment into physical and interpersonal elements does create artificial boundaries, such a division does make them simpler to discuss. Figure 22-1 lists the characteristics of a therapeutic environment. It is wise to remember that on a real hospital unit, physical, interpersonal and cultural elements interact and influence one another.

THE PHYSICAL ENVIRONMENT

The design of a hospital unit will influence patient care. The therapeutic potential of an environment is decreased by: nursing stations that are un-manned, unlabelled and difficult to approach; mazes of hallways; many doors with signs that restrict entrance to staff members only; and lack of an attractive visiting or patient activity room. At present, nurses and patients are rarely consulted about the design of a therapeutic environment; it is hoped that these two groups will begin to challenge this omission, since the design of hospital units affects their activities the most.

A THERAPEUTIC ENVIRONMENT PROVIDES FOR:
- meeting the immediate needs of its members.
- cultural differences.
- acceptance of behavior without judgment.
- choice to participate in plans for care.
- shared responsibility for implementing decisions.
- open communication.
- opportunity for learning through experience.

Fig. 22-1 Characteristics of a therapeutic environment

Many patients are confined to a bed in a single room for most of their hospital stay. Some of these patients are unable to influence important aspects of their environment. In these cases, the nurse adjusts the environment to meet the patient's needs.

Maintenance of a constant room temperature is often accomplished by central air conditioning. In hospitals without air conditioning, the nurse may open or close windows according to the patient's needs.

A low noise level is useful to patient comfort and healing. The noise level can be kept low by the use of plastic utensils, rubber wheels on movable equipment, and doors that can be easily closed. The nurse can also discourage staff or visitors from congregating to talk outside a patient's room.

Light can serve as a stimulus for sensory deprived patients, an irritant for overstimulated patients, or a comfort to the elderly patient who fears the dark. The nurse evaluates the patient's need and adjusts room blinds, window shades, or light switches.

Color scheme of hospital walls and floors is usually beyond the control of either patient or nurse. On units where some rooms are furnished or painted in different colors, patients who need stimulation should perhaps be placed in rooms where sharply contrasting colors are used or where red is a major color. Other patients could be moved to rooms where the colors exert a calming influence. Blue is such a color. In many settings, nurses do not have or use this option. If color seems to be an important issue in stimulating or calming a patient, the nurse could suggest colorful gifts when approached for suggestions by the family or friends.

Furniture is an important part of the physical environment. The patient unit usually includes the patient's bed, an overbed table for eating or writing, chairs, and a bedside table for personal belongings and equipment for bathing and elimination needs. The nurse arranges the bedside and overbed table so the patient can reach both. The unit chairs are used depending on the purpose at a particular moment. A chair can be placed near the patient's bed when the patient is allowed to be out of bed. At other times, the nurse can suggest where a visitor should set the chair so that minimum exertion and strain is placed on the patient who is listening to the visitor. When the nurse teaches the patient or converses with him, the chair should be positioned so as to provide ease for the speaker and the listener. Nursing assessment of the therapeutic effectiveness of the physical environment is summarized in figure 22-2.

THE INTERPERSONAL ENVIRONMENT

One part of the interpersonal environment is the nurse-patient relationship. Nurses strive to develop an effective working relationship with their patients.

Aspects of the Environment	Assessment
Unit or room design	Is the nursing station unmanned or difficult to approach? Are ward areas unlabelled? Is there a maze of hallways? Is there an inviting visiting or patient activity room?
Room temperature	Is there central air conditioning that is operating correctly? Does the window need to be opened or closed to adjust room temperature?
Noise level	Is rubber and plastic equipment used as much as possible? Do patient rooms have doors to close out noise? Do staff or patients congregate to talk outside patient rooms?
Light source	Does the patient need more light stimulation? Is the patient irritated by the amount of room light present? Would the patient be comforted by keeping a small light on? Do blinds, shades, or light switches need to be adjusted?
Color scheme	Does the patient need colors that exert a calming influence? Does the patient need colors that exert a stimulating influence? Can the nurse suggest appropriate patient gifts by color?
Furniture	How can the nurse arrange the room furniture so as to be most therapeutic for the patient?

Fig. 22-2 Assessing the physical environment for therapeutic effectiveness

At first, the student nurse may be unsure about what a working relationship is. Through the application of basic concepts and repeated experiences with the patient, there will develop an awareness of the effects of behavior and a confidence toward establishing a sound nurse-patient relationship. Figure 22-3, page 344, suggests ways nursing staff members can provide a more therapeutic interpersonal environment.

Meeting Immediate Needs

In providing a therapeutic environment, the nurse tries to meet the patient's immediate needs. These are the essential activities of daily living such as providing for food, fluid, hygienic care and comfort, rest and activity, safety, and

Interpersonal Aspect	Nursing Goals
Nurse-patient relationship	Strives to develop an effective working relationship. Becomes aware of effect of nurse behavior on patient and influence of patient behavior on nurse.
Immediate needs	Assesses patient's need to be alone or together at mealtime. Provides personal toilet articles and wearing apparel as much as possible. Considers requests for rest and activity. Provides for physical and interpersonal safety. Requests facilities for meeting immediate needs of staff.
Accepting behavior	Works to accept behavior of patients that upsets the nurse. Works to accept behavior of staff that upsets the nurse.
Offering choice	Evaluates importance of efficiency. Works to collaborate with patients in care planning.
Sharing responsibility	Addresses the healthy aspects of the patient's behavior. Finds a level at which every patient can move toward participation in own care.
Opening up communication	Sees relationship between ineffective staff behavior and the patient. Tries to open up communication.
Learning behaviors	Helps patients become aware of their thoughts, feelings, and behavior. Assists patient to try new behaviors in a protected environment.

Fig. 22-3 Providing a more therapeutic interpersonal environment.

elimination. In providing food and fluids, the nurse assesses the patient's need to be alone or with another person at mealtimes and tries to provide the needed experience. The nurse realizes that personal hygiene and comfort includes preference for certain toilet articles and wearing apparel. The nurse assesses and intervenes in the patient's need for rest and activity and provides recreational opportunities consistent with his strength and abilities.

Consideration of the patient's safety includes not only physical interventions but also interpersonal interventions. Physical safety measures may be: assisting the patient out of bed; using siderails on beds as necessary; and testing bath and dressing temperatures prior to patient application. In addition, the nurse attempts to protect the patient from infection and injury or self-mutilation, from harming others, and from making decisions that are beyond his current capacity.

Since an environment influences all participants, there should be some provision for meeting the immediate needs of the staff also. For example, there should be adequate eating, resting, activity, safety and elimination provisions for staff members as well as for patients in a therapeutic environment.

Accepting Behavior

In a therapeutic environment, behavior of all participants is viewed as a reflection of needs and past and present experiences. It is often difficult for nurses to accept all patient behavior. Although there are individual differences, nurses seem to have particular difficulty accepting patients who are angry, demand attention, or refuse to comply with the treatment plan. If an environment is to be truly therapeutic, nurses must begin to examine their biases in these areas. Also, there must be an increased effort by all members of the health team to be more accepting of one another's behavior. At present, it is frequently difficult for nursing personnel at different levels of experience, education, and viewpoint to accept one another.

An accepting environment is one where a person's actions are not judged as good or bad or right or wrong. Each person is respected. It is agreed that each person has rights, needs, and opinions.

Offering Choice

It is widely agreed that patients should be allowed and encouraged to participate in their own care planning. At times, rigid schedules or poor planning prevents this goal from being met. With the increased interest in patients' rights, collaboration of patient and nurse in care planning will probably be more in demand. Nevertheless, patients who have high dependency needs or are less outspoken, may require extra support in participating even to a limited degree.

Sharing Responsibility

Sharing responsibility between patient, nurse and other health team members is essential for a therapeutic environment. The reason for this shared responsibility is apparent. All are involved in promoting the patient's health and well-being. The patient who threatens suicide must be told that this information will be shared with other staff members. Likewise, in any teaching endeavor, the nurse must have the patient's cooperation (and that of the other members) if the patient is to learn and apply what he has learned.

The *therapeutic community approach* was developed by Maxwell Jones.[1] This approach is used in some mental health units and focuses on shared responsibility as a major aspect of patient care. In a therapeutic community, patients and staff meet together daily to make joint decisions about patient care. All of the members of the hospital unit — the community — decide together how to deal with community problems such as a suicidal patient, a disturbed patient, the discharge of a patient, or the resignation of a staff member. The therapeutic community approach has the potential for patients and staff to learn decision-making skills.

The therapeutic community addresses itself to the health of the individual; it assumes that even the sickest patient has some strengths upon which to draw. Each patient is expected to start where he is and build from there. A patient is not permitted to say, "I'm too sick to participate." Therapeutic communities discourage regression.

Acutely ill patients in general hospital units have a limited capacity to share in the responsibility for their care and therefore may require more assistance. The nurse can reduce nonadaptive regression by encouraging even acutely ill patients to share in their care at the level of their ability. In some patients this level may be extremely low; participation may be limited to such things as helping to turn oneself or washing the hands.

Opening Up Communication

The communication network is a specific focus in the therapeutic community. Stanton and Schwartz have demonstrated that there is a direct relationship between disturbed staff behavior and disturbed patient behavior.[2] It seems that patients are quite sensitive to staff tensions and are able to sense when the staff is upset without being told about the problem. This is not an unexpected finding since it is a known fact that anxiety can be communicated nonverbally.

General hospital staff members are less likely to focus on the development of open communication. Some staff members may even deny the importance of such a focus. Hierarchical communication structures are the least open in their communication.

[1] Maxwell Jones, *Beyond the Therapeutic Community* (New Haven: Yale University Press)
[2] Alfred H. Stanton and Morris S. Schwartz, *The Mental Hospital: A Study of Institutional Participation in Psychiatric Illness and Treatment* (New York: Basic Books)

Learning Behaviors

In the therapeutic community approach, all facets of the hospital stay are seen as possible living-learning experiences. The staff works to help patients become aware of their thoughts, feelings, and behavior. Patients are encouraged to practice new behaviors in the relatively safe therapeutic community. Patients develop awareness of their skills and limitations since other patients and staff members confront them with the maladaptive aspects of their behavior. Self-esteem is raised when patients receive recognition for their accomplishments.

Although the implementation of a therapeutic community is more evident in mental health units, many of the living-learning experiences are also available to the creative nurse in the general hospital or nursing home. The learning process is more fully explored in section 5.

ADMITTING THE PATIENT

The nurse has an especially good opportunity to promote a therapeutic environment when the patient is admitted to the hospital as hospitalization may be a time of crisis for the patient. Hospital admission is often a time when the patient may not only be in pain or confusion but probably is also highly anxious. During a crisis people are open to change and there is a potential for either growth or regression.

The nurse may first see the patient after the patient has been with the admitting clerk. In some hospitals, the nurse who will work with the patient throughout his hospital stay meets the patient right away. This is called the *primary nurse approach*; one nurse is primarily responsible for the care of a patient during the entire hospitalization period. Early contact with the patient has the potential for reducing both patient anxiety and any dehumanizing aspects of hospital admission. If it is impossible to go to the admitting area, it is important for the nurse to introduce herself to the newly admitted patient as soon as possible.

The patient's room should be prepared in advance; this shows an interest in him as an individual. He feels he has a place of his own. Some anxiety is usually felt upon admission to a hospital or health-related facility. As knowledge reduces anxiety, the patient is given information which will alleviate some of the uneasiness he is experiencing. Patients who have high levels of anxiety are unable to absorb a great deal of new information. When she first meets the patient, the nurse evaluates the patient's level of anxiety. If the patient has not been hospitalized before or is anxious about his condition, the nurse must be sure to introduce herself and the patient's roommate(s) and advise the patient how he can get needed assistance (such as showing him how to use the call bell). If the patient has been in the hospital unit before, less orientation will be required. However, making the patient comfortable and introducing him to the others is part of every orientation.

After a short time, when the patient is less anxious, he should be introduced to other health team members and informed of their functions as they relate to his care. Information pamphlets which deal with hospital policies are often available to the patient, and the nurse should always be ready to explain and answer questions about its contents. Throughout the admission process, the nurse's role is to help the patient understand.

When the nurse has assessed the level of patient anxiety, she may begin to take the nursing history. This can be done in the solarium, the visiting area of the unit, or any place that provides a private and comfortable setting for both nurse and patient. Nursing histories differ but, generally, the nurse obtains information from the patient about food preferences, allergies, current medications, activity, rest requirements, and current symptoms. A nursing history can be a valuable tool in creating a therapeutic environment. While taking a nursing history, the nurse observes the patient's reactions to the nurse and to being hospitalized. She intervenes as necessary. All observations and interventions should be charted and used to provide a therapeutic environment.

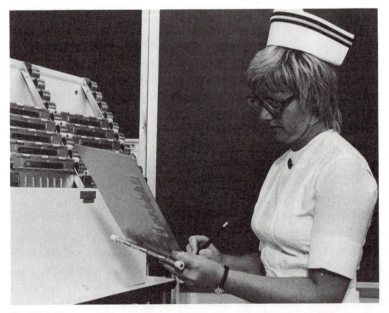

Fig. 22-4 The nurse helps to make a therapeutic environment by carefully charting relevant patient information.

Once the initial orientation is completed, the patient may be examined by the hospital physician. This examination is sometimes delayed because of the patient's condition or the doctor's schedule. Patients may also be scheduled to have routine laboratory tests. The student nurse checks with the head nurse or nursing instructor to determine what arrangements need to be made for tests which are part of the hospital admission.

The nurse also assists the patient in the care of his clothes and valuables at the time of admission. Most hospitals allow patients to keep their clothes in a closet in the room. Some hospitals still require that the patient's clothes be sent to a central clothes room. The patient should be allowed to wear his own clothes whenever possible since clothes represent a part of one's identity. There are some times when the nurse would ask the patient to wear hospital garb instead of his own clothing. For example, the patient who is scheduled for surgery should wear a hospital gown and leggings as apparel becomes soiled during the surgical procedure.

If an unconscious or very ill patient is unable to assume responsibility for his valuables, they are sent to the cashier's office or sent home with the patient's family. Eyeglasses, contact lenses, and dentures should be kept on the unit since the patient may soon feel well enough to use them. These items are also part of a person's identity and the person may feel dehumanized without them. The nurse tries to decrease the number of dehumanizing aspects of the environment.

If the patient is well enough, he can sign a statement assuming responsibility for the valuables kept at the bedside. Since hospital policies vary, the student needs to check with each head nurse to find out what procedures are to be followed. Figure 22-5 summarizes nursing interventions at admission.

ADMITTING THE PATIENT IN A THERAPEUTIC MANNER INCLUDES:

- Meeting with the patient as soon as possible after the patient comes to the hospital.

- Presenting information to the patient depending on the patient's level of anxiety and need for orientation.

- Helping the patient to understand what is happening to her.

- Providing privacy during nursing history taking.

- Intervening in patient anxiety.

- Telling patient what to expect next.

- Assisting the patient with clothing and valuables.

Fig. 22-5 Nurses intervene during patient admission.

DISCHARGING THE PATIENT

Many patients may find discharge from the hospital a happy time. Others may be extremely apprehensive about leaving the protective environment of the hospital and resuming previous responsibilities. The nurse should not assume the patient is happy or glad to be discharged. It is best not to make leading statements such as, "I'll bet you're glad to be going home!"; the patient may find it hard to share his feelings of anxiety about being discharged. The nurse can evaluate the patient's nonverbal behavior and make open-ended statements to elicit the patient's feelings. Gathering his belongings with a smile would tend to indicate the patient would rather leave than prolong his hospital stay. Being slow to get his belongings together, appearing sad or anxious, or asking to stay longer, would indicate the patient is apprehensive about being discharged.

It is important that the nurse use verbal as well as nonverbal observation since the overcooperative patient often conceals apprehensive feelings. By making statements that the patient can choose to respond to or not, the nurse gives the patient an opportunity to share feelings about discharge. The nurse can make open-ended statements such as, "You're going home today", or "It'll be quite a change for you to go home."

Discharge planning should begin when the patient is admitted. Patients who have special needs, require frequent emotional support, or teaching before discharge may require a great deal of nursing intervention prior to discharge. Early preparation, therefore, is necessary.

Some patients require referral to another agency at the time of discharge. One agency that can be especially useful to patients is the visiting nurse service located near the patient's home. Visiting nurses are frequently quite interested in talking with hospital personnel before the discharge of the patient and will often make at least one visit to the patient's home for the purpose of evaluating the need for their services. Visiting nurses also make home visits to evaluate the home environment if the hospital nursing staff is concerned about family readiness to accept the patient's return. The visiting nurse can also help teach family members how to care for the patient.

Nurses are becoming more active in referring patients to appropriate services. Students should check into potential referral sources for each patient they work with, even if such referrals cannot be followed through by the student. By following this procedure, the student will be a knowledgeable graduate nurse who can make appropriate referrals.

At the actual time of discharge, the nurse helps the patient to gather together his clothes and valuables. Any final appointments or details can be written down for the patient. The nurse should not attempt to do any teaching at discharge since the patient will probably not be able to learn at that time.

BEFORE DISCHARGING A PATIENT, THE NURSE ASKS:

– Did I assume the patient is happy or glad to be discharged?
– Did I evaluate the patient's verbal and nonverbal reactions to discharge?
– Did I offer the patient a choice to discuss his feelings about being discharged?
– Did I do sufficient discharge planning?
– Did I evaluate each source of referral?
– Did I help the patient to gather his belongings?
– Did I write down final details and appointments for the patient?
– Did I check to be sure the discharge order had been written?
– Did I escort the patient to the door of the hospital?

Fig. 22-6 Discharging the patient.

In order to assure a smooth discharge for the patient, the nurse checks to see that the order has been written by the physican; she then notifies the business office that the patient will be discharged. The patient is accompanied to the door of the hospital and helped into the waiting car if necessary. Many hospitals require this to be done with the patient in a wheelchair. Figure 22-6 lists some questions the nurse may ask prior to discharging a patient.

SUMMARY

A therapeutic environment provides for meeting the basic needs of its members; provides for cultural differences; accepts behavior without judgmental reactions; provides for patient choice to participate in the treatment plan; shares responsibility for care; has open communication and learning opportunities. Aspects of the physical environment which the nurse considers are: design of the hospital ward or room, temperature, noise level, light stimulation, color, and furniture. Aspects of the interpersonal environment which the nurse considers are the nurse-patient relationship and staff-to-staff communication.

When admitting the patient the nurse takes steps to increase the therapeutic effectiveness of the environment. Some of the ways this is done is by evaluating and intervening in patient anxiety and giving information about the immediate environment. Throughout the admission process, the nurse helps the patient to understand what is happening to him.

Discharge planning should begin many days before discharge. When discharging a patient, the nurse does not assume the patient is glad to leave the hospital. Rather, the nurse observes verbal and nonverbal signs that can reveal patient feeling. The nurse is especially active in learning about and suggesting referral sources outside the hospital that may be useful to the patient.

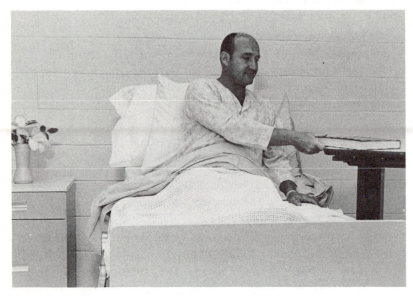

Fig. 22-7 The effectiveness of the therapeutic environment is also influenced by the physical aspects of the hospital room.

ACTIVITIES AND DISCUSSION TOPICS

- Choose one unit of a hospital or institution. Evaluate the therapeutic effectiveness of the physical and interpersonal environment. Figures 22-2 and 22-3 may be helpful in doing this evaluation.

- Find out the admission process on a hospital unit. Ask a nurse if you can go with her as she admits a patient. After the admission, talk with the nurse about your observations and questions.

- Talk with several patients about their admission to the hospital or nursing home. Find out what they liked best and disliked most about being admitted.

- Study the discharge process of a hospital unit. Make arrangements to observe a nurse who is discharging a patient. After the discharge, talk with the nurse about referral sources for patients and problems she has had with patient discharges.

- Several students may visit referral agencies which provide health care services. After making an appointment with the director, find out what kinds of services are offered. Keep notes and share your findings with the class.

REVIEW

A. Multiple Choice. Select the best answer(s). Some questions have more than one answer.

1. The purpose of a therapeutic community is to

   a. use the total external environment to benefit the patient.
   b. enable its members to use effective coping devices to restore homeostasis.
   c. make joint decisions about patient care.
   d. make joint decisions about problems on the hospital unit.

2. Staff members can provide a more therapeutic interpersonal environment by

   a. accepting the patient's behavior.
   b. encouraging the patient to participate in planning his care.
   c. adjusting the light source.
   d. sharing responsibility between patient, nurse, and other health team members.

3. The therapeutic potential of an environment is decreased by

   a. an attractive patient activity room.
   b. unmanned nursing stations.
   c. bright colored rooms.
   d. many hallways.

4. The people involved in a therapeutic community are

   a. all patients and staff on the ward.
   b. doctors and nurses on the ward.
   c. patients on the ward.
   d. all members of the health team.

5. The therapeutic community approach was developed by

   a. Alfred H. Stanton.
   b. Morris S. Schwartz.
   c. Erving Goffman.
   d. Maxwell Jones.

B. Match the interpersonal aspects of the therapeutic environment in Column II with the appropriate nursing goal in Column I.

Column I	Column II
1. Help patient become aware of his thoughts, feelings and behavior.	a. immediate needs
	b. learning behaviors
2. See the relationship between ineffective staff behavior and the patient	c. nurse-patient relationship
	d. offering choice
	e. opening up communication
3. Consider requests for rest and activity.	f. sharing responsibility
4. Become aware of the effect of nurse behavior on the patient and the influence of patient behavior on the nurse.	
5. Collaborated with patient in care planning	
6. Find level at which patient can .participate in care	

C. Briefly answer the following questions.

1. Name six elements of the physical environment that should be assessed for therapeutic effectiveness.

2. List four ways the nurse can enhance the therapeutic environment during patient admission.

3. List four ways the nurse can enhance the therapeutic environment during patient discharge.

4. What is the purpose of a therapeutic environment?

chapter 23
MIND-BODY
RELATIONSHIPS

STUDENT OBJECTIVES

- Explain the holistic approach to patient care.
- Identify causes of illness.
- List 5 sources of information for assessing mind-body relationships.
- List 4 goals for nursing intervention in mind-body disturbances.

Modern health practice claims to be founded on the principle that a person is an organized, whole, interacting system. Practitioners have been slow to use this integrated approach, however. Many health professionals still avoid either their patients' psychological, social, economic, or physical difficulties. On a medical ward, the patient with primarily psychological or social problems is often referred to a mental health specialist or transferred to a phychiatric unit; the patient with a physical condition is usually referred to a professional specialized in that area. Consequently, one professional treats the patient's body while another treats the patient's mind or social relationships. As a group, nurses are more likely to treat both mind and body. Therefore, it is important that the student learn how body and mind interact.

THE HOLISTIC APPROACH

In recent years, there has been an increased effort to learn about the interplay of the body and the mind. A *holistic approach to patient care* attempts to

356

consider the total patient, not merely the mind or the body of the patient. A unified concept of health attempts to understand the interrelationships of physiological, psychological, social, and cultural processes. People are viewed as open systems where there is a continuous interchange between the internal environment of the person and the external environment. People not only react to changes in the environment but also create changes within it. The nurse assumes that any function or malfunctioning of either mind or body effects changes in the other.

If a malfunction occurs, there has been a breakdown in adaptation and homeostasis. Illness is not only an attack by destructive forces in the external environment but may also involve the person's protective reactions to stressors.

Sometimes illness occurs due to unsuccessful adaptation to an external stressor. Sometimes it results from an ineffective internal regulatory mechanism. Illness can result from an inherited defect.

Social factors can also contribute to illness. For example, cigarette smoking is a factor in lung cancer. Peer group pressure becomes a strong influence when friends and parents smoke. Thus, the initial push to smoke cigarettes can be a social one. Another example concerns a disease like poliomyelitis. Polio is more likely to occur in individuals who have not obtained immunity either naturally or through vaccination. Persons who are involved in community life (a social process) are more prone to accept free vaccination. In polio, then, as in lung cancer, social factors may be involved in the illness process.

Sociocultural factors also contribute to disease. For example, cigarette smoking, diet, obesity, and exercise are important factors in heart disease. All four are embedded in an individual's sociocultural background and personality style.

Unsuccessful adaptation can lead to either physical or mental difficulties, or both. Symptoms such as chronic shortness of breath indicate a failure of the body to adapt. Symptoms such as chronic anxiety also indicate adaptive failure. Figure 23-1 depicts factors that may lead to unsuccessful adaptation which, in turn, results in physical-emotional difficulties.

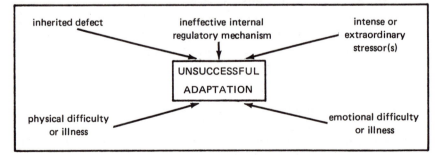

Fig. 23-1 Unsuccessful adaptation – causative factors and results

Homeostasis

All levels of adaptation can be viewed from the point of homeostasis. On all levels, there is an attempt to maintain homeostasis. Physiological levels have been well studied; it is relatively easy to examine the blood sugar level for diabetes or the blood pressure level for hypertension.   ·

On the psychological level, there is less agreement about what variables to study. Self-esteem, security, anxiety and mood are regulating devices that are more difficult to examine. Accumulation of chronic fear or resentment is one sign that homeostasis is or has been threatened. People may attempt to maintain homeostasis through the use of a number of psychological or social processes: avoidance, denial, rationalization, neurosis are some examples. If the person departs from a situation, the device of *avoidance* is used. If he ignores the fact that the situation even exists, he is using *denial.* If there are attempts to explain the situation away, *rationalization* or *intellectualization* is being used. If the patient isolates the impaired emotional view of a situation, he may be fleeing into a *neurosis.* Withdrawal from all activities is accomplished through *depression.* If withdrawal from contact with reality is used, the person is called *schizophrenic.*

Breakdown of homeostasis can begin at any level but one level always influences the other levels of homeostasis. For example, a spreading infection indicates a breakdown in the mechanisms of immunity. Such a breakdown could be due to stressors such as inadequate nutrition, chronic high anxiety, genetic defect, or other stressors that make it impossible for the person to deal with that infectious process at that time. If the patient becomes very angry because of this infection, he may experience a breakdown in homeostasis at the psychological and social level and consider killing himself. It is possible that the patient may become so angry and depressed that he may commit suicide before he can be adequately treated for the infectious process.

A chronic rage or anger reaction can also affect physiological functioning. The body responds to rage or anger feelings by continuous arousal of the emergency and alarm systems. Various hormones and chemicals are released during these alarm reactions. Continual arousal creates marked changes in various organs of the body. Although the initial threat to homeostasis may have been at the emotional level (anger or rage), the secondary, physiological disturbance may result in a bleeding ulcer or in excessively high blood pressure. What is a homeostatic or protective device in emergency situations becomes an illness process when used to excess by the person in chronic rage, guilt or anxiety.

Maladaptive Functioning

It is helpful if treatment is directed toward both the physiological and psychological levels of adaptation. Some conditions seem to involve beginning maladaptive functioning at the mind level. Examples of such conditions are *pseudocyesis* (false pregnancy) and conversion hysteria. In pseudocyesis, the woman may influence her hormonal system to produce symptoms of pregnancy because in her mind she wishes to be pregnant. In conversion hysteria, the person may become unable to see or move one or more of his limbs due to strong feelings that inhibit sight or movement. In both cases there will be physiological changes as a result of thoughts or feelings; these thoughts or feelings, in turn, will influence physiological functioning. Figure 23-2 diagrams the interplay of factors in one mind-body disturbance.

Some conditions seem to begin in physiological maladaption and then become influenced by emotional or thought disturbance. The study and treatment of physical handicaps and disabilities and their effect on emotional processes is called *somatopsychology*. The patient with diabetes can be thrown into a diabetic crisis if there is an emotional upset. A patient with epilepsy can have an epileptic seizure precipitated by strong emotions. The patient who has multiple sclerosis or chronic heart disease is likely to have emotional reactions to changes in his physiological functioning due to the illness process.

A person's response to disability or handicap is a function of that person's perception of the condition. It should not be assumed that all patients will respond to the same handicap or disability in the same way. The condition takes on a meaning for each individual person. It is possible to assume, however, that all patients will respond in some way to a disability or handicap.

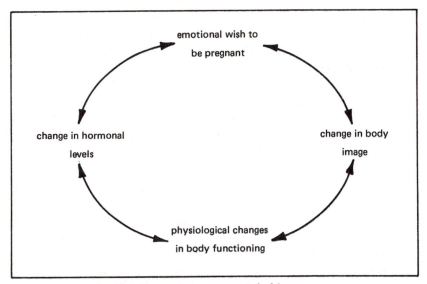

Fig. 23-2 Factors that may operate in false pregnancy.

Some disorders cannot be classified as being caused by either physiological or psychological maladaption. Conditions such as ulcers, migraine headache, bronchial asthma, and essential hypertension seem to result from a nearly equal interplay of physiological, psychological, social, economic, and cultural factors. These conditions are referred to as *psychosomatic* or *psychophysiological* disorders because there is an application of both psychological and physiological principles in the study and treatment of these conditions.

Most recent theories of psychosomatic medicine recognize the complexity of the factors that interact in illness and disease. The body organ(s) that becomes the site of the illness process is probably determined by both genetic and experience factors. Extraordinary stress may or may not produce an illness depending on the intensity and kind of stress as well as the capacity of the person to resist the stress. Emotional conflict may not produce illness by itself but it seems to lower the person's resistance to stress.

BIOLOGICAL RHYTHMS AND HEALTH

Human beings have developed elaborate biological time clocks to maintain health and homeostasis. A 24-hour daily cycle of rhythm is influenced by changes in sunlight, darkness, moonlight, atmospheric pressure, and electromagnetic forces. For example, body temperature fluctuates throughout the day. People are best able to perform tasks that require close attention or muscle coordination when body temperature is highest.

Body processes are biologically timed. The mouth, stomach and intestines are sites for the secretions of saliva, gastric juice, pancreatic and intestinal juices. These secretions are available when food is ready to be digested. Illness processes can occur when body processes go out of rhythm. For example, hydrochloric acid (present in gastric secretions) helps to digest food. When there is no food available for digestion, the presence of this acid can create an ulcer.

Insomnia (inability to sleep) is often a clue that an illness is beginning. Depressed people may report insomnia before and during their depression. Another homeostatic device that can be upset if sleep is infrequent is that of dreaming. Drugs such as barbiturates, hypnotics, tranquilizers and narcotics interfere with dreams. Dreaming seems to be necessary for emotional learning and memory. The nurse evaluates the patient's need for sleep and dreaming and whenever possible uses nursing measures other than giving medications to provide for these needs. Patients who take drugs to sleep may complain of a "hangover" effect the morning after having taken the drug. These disadvantages of medications should be weighed against the advantages of a drug approach to sleep.

A number of stressors such as interpersonal upsets, infections, allergies, surgery and physical overexertion can disrupt the coordination of biological rhythms and cycles. Disruption of these rhythms can lead to recurrent symptoms and illness. Mind-body relationships, then, are in turn influenced by external environmental processes.

FEELINGS AND THE BODY

Emotions are often experienced in body parts. A person may "feel" surprise in the back of the neck or in the abdomen. The body area where emotions are experienced varies from person to person. What begins as a mental reaction is experienced in a body area. Happiness could be felt as a lightness in the chest. Sadness could be a heavy feeling in the same place. Patients may report anxiety as "butterflies in my stomach" or "a tight feeling in my chest." The nurse should be aware that patients may communicate their thoughts and feelings via body sensations.

Body and emotion interact with each other throughout the life cycle. The infant learns to use body language before action or verbal language. He shows distress by increased breathing and reddened skin. The prefix *soma* refers to the body. A person who *somatizes* or uses the process of *somatization* converts feelings into body sensations or symptoms. Diarrhea prior to exams or developing a headache after an angry interchange are examples of somatization.

Emotional tension, anxiety, or fear can lead to chronic muscular tension. A chronic state of muscle tension can lead to bone changes and a characteristic posture that conveys feelings of hurt, hate, prudishness or guilt.

THE BRAIN AND THE BODY

In most people, the left hemisphere of the brain controls the left side of the body above the neck and the right side of the body below the neck. This effect is due to the crossover of the corticospinal or pyramidal nerve. In right-handed persons, the left hemisphere is responsible for voluntary movements of the right side of the body. The left hemisphere may be responsible for what is called *conscious thought*; this includes logical thought, especially in verbal and mathematical functions.

The right hemisphere of the brain controls the right side of the body above the neck, and the left side of the body below the neck. The right hemisphere of the brain is responsible for voluntary action on the left side of the body. In right-handed adults, the right hemisphere is probably responsible for intuitive thought, orientation in space, artistic endeavors, crafts, body image and recognition of faces. The right hemisphere may be responsible for what is called *the unconscious mind* and may be related to varying levels of awareness such as daydreaming.

Both modes of operation seem to be important to psychological, social, economic and cultural functioning. Generally speaking, American society tends to esteem logical, sequential, analytical thought. Figure 23-3 summarizes how the brain may influence thought and activity.

NURSING ASSESSMENT

In assessing patients with disturbed mind-body relationships, the nurse uses both factual information from the patient and observations about the nurse-patient relationship. Information is obtained about the symptoms, life concerns, major body systems involved, life situation, attitudes toward living, and the number, nature, and intensity of life stressors. The nurse also evaluates the patient's level of anxiety. Quiet listening and observation techniques are used. Appearance, posture, gestures and manner of speaking convey impressions about the patient as a unique individual.

The holistic approach examines the multiple causes for the patient's condition. This includes *precipitating factors*, situations which seem to bring on the condition; and the interrelationships between the patient's life situation and his condition. The patient's history is complete only when it incorporates both physical and psychological or interpersonal data. Since the physician is apt to focus on physical data, the nurse concentrates on psychological and interpersonal data.

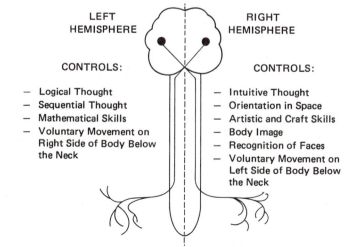

LEFT HEMISPHERE

CONTROLS:

— Logical Thought
— Sequential Thought
— Mathematical Skills
— Voluntary Movement on Right Side of Body Below the Neck

RIGHT HEMISPHERE

CONTROLS:

— Intuitive Thought
— Orientation in Space
— Artistic and Craft Skills
— Body Image
— Recognition of Faces
— Voluntary Movement on Left Side of Body Below the Neck

Fig. 23-3 The brain influences the body.

A nursing assessment includes information about the patient's current symptoms; his past health and his family's health; the patient's perception of himself; attitude toward and perception of the conditon and hospitalization; perception of changes in his life-style; and patient losses and changed relationships.

History of Symptoms

In finding out about symptoms, the nurse asks for a description of their location, quality, intensity, onset, precipitating factors, what relieves or intensifies them, and what other symptoms or occurrences are associated with each symptom.

Using growth and development theory, the nurse realizes that many symptoms may have appeared earlier in the patient's life and are now recurring because of present stress. She tries to establish the relationship between the time the symptom first occurred and the time(s) when there were recurrences.

Family Health History

A history of family health may be of great value. Disturbed mind-body relationships often recur in families, probably due to inherited genetic weakness. This weakness leads to a *predisposition* or tendency for certain disturbances to occur. Disturbed mind-body relationships may also occur in families where the patient has learned to pay more attention to and worry about symptoms which affect certain body areas.

Attitude and Perception of Self

Information about events which occurred at or near the onset of the condition is especially helpful in nursing assessment. Such information can be used to determine why the patient became unable to adapt at that time. An attitude of surrender or giving up may have preceded the onset of the condition. If the patient thinks he is no longer able to cope effectively with changes in his environment, he may give up and succumb to a condition or relapse to a previous illness condition.

This giving up period has been described as one where the person feels helpless or hopeless, is denied past satisfactions, and seems to be unable to think of past and future goals. This state may be brief or intermittent. During its presence, the person's ability to maintain homeostasis is altered and the ability to resist *pathogenic* (disease-producing) processes may be decreased. Knowledge about these periods can direct treatment plans. Such knowledge can also be used to detect potential problems and prevent illness through early intervention.

Attitude Toward Hospitalization

The patient's present environment — the hospital or institution — can increase or decrease the patient's ability to re-establish homeostasis. For this reason, the nurse is concerned about his perception and attitude toward his condition and hospitalization. An assessment is made about whether the patient is angry, resentful, sad, anxious, or fearful. The nurse finds out what the patient knows about his condition and what he expects from the hospital staff, his friends, and his family.

Changes in Life-Style

Changes in the patient's life-style may have precipitated or influenced his condition. The nurse asks what disruptions have resulted because of his condition. For example, has the patient had to change his daily routine, work, social relationships, or leisure activities? Has the patient been able to establish substitute activities for these changes?

Losses and Changes in Relationships

Changes in or loss of significant interpersonal relationships can precipitate or influence a patient's condition. The nurse could evaluate the number of patient losses within the past year. Figure 23-4, page 364, gives guidelines for nursing assessment in disturbed mind-body relationships.

NURSING INTERVENTION

There are four goals of nursing in mind-body relationship disturbances:

- Reduction of stress and anxiety.
- Maintenance of psychophysiological functioning.
- Restoration of homeostasis.
- Maximization of individual potential.

The nurse directs her actions towards meeting these goals.

Assessment Area	Questions the nurse asks the patient or herself
Patient symptoms	Where is the symptom located? What does the symptom feel like? How intense is the symptom? When did the symptom begin? What changes in the symptom have occurred since it started? What situations seem to affect the symptom? What makes the symptom better? What irritates the symptom? What other symptoms do you associate with this symptom?
Family health history	What symptoms have you noticed in other members of your family? What conditions do they have that require treatment?
Patient's attitudes toward self and condition	Did you ever feel like giving up? If *yes*, when did you have this feeling? Did you ever feel like giving up right near the time you got this symptom?
Patient's reaction to treatment or hospitalization	Is the patient angry, sad, anxious, or fearful? What does the patient know about his condition? What does this patient seem to expect from me?
Changes in life-style	What things have changed for you since you got this condition? Has there been a change in your social relationships? Has there been a change in your leisure activities? If *yes*, have you been able to find substitutes for these changes?
Losses within the past year	Have you lost any family members or special friends due to separation or death?

Fig. 23-4 In a nursing assessment of patients with disturbed mind-body relationships, both factual information and observations about the nurse-patient relationship are utilized.

Reduction of Stress and Anxiety

The nurse provides a therapeutic environment for the patient by adjusting temperature, lighting, and noise in the unit, and by seeking out resources for ventilation of staff and patient feelings. The nurse prepares the patient for procedures, orients the patient to his surroundings, decreases pain, and gives honest reassurance. Honest reassurance differs from false reassurance by conveying a sincere intent to help the patient and to understand his concerns. False reassurance is not a useful nursing intervention; the nurse gives false reassurance when she tells the patient "everything will be all right." This reassurance is false because the nurse has no guarantee of what will happen in the future. Honest reassurance is given by the nurse when she stays with the patient, leans toward him, maintains eye contact, and tells the patient verbally and nonverbally that the nurse is interested in hearing about his concerns.

Although high levels of anxiety are disruptive, mild anxiety prepares the patient for learning. Patients who appear too comfortable before surgical or diagnostic procedures should be approached by the nurse and engaged in a conversation about what to expect in the way of pain and procedures. This is a good approach regardless of patient anxiety, but is especially important as a way to focus patient attention on the upcoming event. Focusing on detailed technical information about the surgery or procedure is not helpful. However, leaving the patient alone because he appears comfortable may create problems of overreactions afterwards. The nurse tries to open up communication in a way that keeps anxiety levels from getting too high or too low. The nurse's physical presence, short comments relating to the patient's thoughts and feelings, brief orientations and information are used to decrease patient anxiety.

Maintenance of Psychophysiological Function

The nurse investigates baseline information that was placed on the medical-nursing history, physical exam findings sheet, and the initial laboratory reports. This baseline information provides a measure with which to compare ongoing patient functioning. For example, the baseline information is checked if the nurse is concerned about whether the patient has gained or lost weight during hospitalization or has increased or decreased blood pressure.

Baseline information enables the nurse to carry out procedures which help to re-establish homeostasis. Other nursing interventions which help to maintain psychophysiological functioning include: health teaching of patients and their families; therapeutic admission and discharge procedures; observation of psychophysiological functioning on an ongoing basis; and making encouraging statements about the patient's successful coping attempts.

Restoration of Homeostasis

Some patients arrive at the hospital in an acutely ill state. Nursing interventions can be made while obtaining information about the patient's condition. Crucial determinations that need to be made immediately are: Is the patient alive or dead? Is he conscious or unconscious? Is the patient in acute distress? If so, what kind of distress? Is the patient restless, confused, unable to respond or concentrate?

Data about why the patient came to the hospital is gathered very quickly by asking:
- What problem brought you here?
- What led you to come to the hospital for help?
- What difficulties are you having?
- Besides breathing (bleeding, anxiety, pain, etc.), what else is bothering you?

Vital signs need to be taken; a quick physical assessment is done to make sure brain, heart, lung and kidney functions are being maintained. When the nurse observes vital signs, skin and level of consciousness, she evaluates the need to restore homeostasis. Other health personnel such as the physician are alerted to assist if homeostasis is not being maintained.

In assessing the patient's level of consciousness and brain functioning, the pupils of the eye are observed to see if they are *dilated* (open) or if they react unequally to the light of a flashlight. Swelling in any body area, absence of breath sounds, unusual chest sounds, area of special tenderness or lack of ability to void are all signs of danger that homeostasis is or has been upset. Panic or severe levels of anxiety can also lead to loss of homeostasis. Whenever any of these signs and symptoms are observed, the nurse takes immediate steps to restore homeostasis. CAUTION: Student nurses or beginning nurse practitioners will require practice and adequate supervision prior to making assessments and interventions with acutely ill patients.

Maximization of Potential

Maximization of patient potential is encouraged through verbal and nonverbal communication with the patient, his family, and other health personnel. Effective solutions to problems can be supported through communication, and ineffective solutions can be re-evaluated. Talking with the patient about needs and wishes can lead to appropriate patient teaching. He can be taught problem-solving by describing, exploring, and validating his thoughts and feelings about the problem at hand. Figure 23-5 shows nursing interventions for disturbed mind-body relationships.

SUMMARY

The holistic approach to patient care is used by the nurse to consider the total patient, not merely the mind or the body. If a disturbed mind-body relationship results in an illness process, the nurse considers all aspects of physiological, psychological, social, and cultural mechanisms that help to maintain

Maladaption due to:	Intervention
High stress and anxiety	Adjust temperature, light, and noise levels. Provide for expression of patient and nurse feeling. Prepare patient for procedures. Orient patient to environment. Decrease pain. Give honest reassurance. Decrease anxiety.
Improper psychophysiological functioning	Investigate baseline information. Teach patient and family. Admit and discharge patient using therapeutic principles. Make statements of encouragement about patient's successful coping attempts.
Homeostasis imbalance	Determine crucial area of malfunction. Determine reason for admission. Make quick physical and interpersonal exam. Alert other health personnel to assist as necessary.
Minimal use of potential	Communicate effectively with patient, his family, and other health personnel. Explore patient needs, thoughts, feelings, and behavior. Assist patient to define goals. Encourage self-awareness and acceptance of patient by himself and acceptance of others by the patient.

Fig. 23-5 Some nursing interventions for disturbed mind-body relationships

homeostasis. Biological rhythms and their effect on health are also considered. The nurse is aware of how brain, feelings, and body are interrelated in patient behavior.

A nursing assessment includes information about the patient's symptoms, life concerns, major body systems involved, attitudes toward living, and the number, nature, and intensity of life stressors. Nursing intervention includes reduction of stress and increase or decrease of anxiety, maintenance of psychophysiological functioning, restoration of homeostasis, and maximization of each patient's potential.

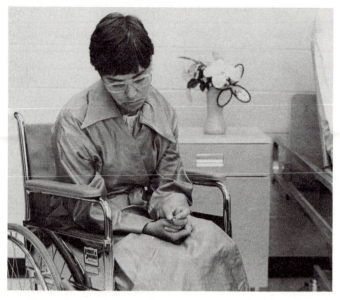

Fig. 23-6 Unsuccessful adapation can lead to both physical and mental difficulties.

ACTIVITIES AND DISCUSSION TOPICS

- Read the charts of several patients. Decide whether a holistic approach to assessment and intervention was made. What additions or changes can you think of that would improve the approach?

- Find a patient who is willing to talk with you about his or her psychophysiological condition. Examples of patients you might talk with are those with ulcers, essential hypertension, bronchial asthma, colitis, or migraine headache. Assess the patient's condition using figure 23-4.

- Observe five people for the feelings their postures convey. How do you convey feelings through use of your posture?

- What ways do you convert your feelings into body symptoms or sensations?

- Which part of your brain is dominant? Are you a person who is analytical and who uses a logical, sequential type of thinking? Are you a person who is more intuitive, with artistic and creative skills? How does your dominant brain influence what you value or expect from patients?

- What disturbed mind-body conditions recur in your family? What have been the precipitating factors and stressors involved in these conditions? How could you decrease the possibility of incurring these conditions yourself?

REVIEW

A.   Multiple Choice. Select the best answer(s). Some questions have more than one answer.

1.   Nursing interventions for patients experiencing high stress and anxiety are

   a. adjusting temperature, light and noise levels.

   b. providing for expression of the patient's feelings.

   c. investigating baseline information.

   d. assisting the patient to define goals.

2.   Illness can occur due to

   a. an unsuccessful adaptation to external stressors.

   b. a maladaptive functioning at the mind level.

   c. an inherited defect.

   d. an ineffective internal regulatory mechanism.

3.   The left hemisphere of the brain controls the

   a. left side of the body above the neck.

   b. right side of the body above the neck.

   c. right side of the body below the neck.

   d. left side of the body below the neck.

4.   In right-handed adults, the right hemisphere of the brain is responsible for

   a. artistic endeavors.

   b. logical thought.

   c. body image.

   d. orientation in space.

5.   Situations which seem to bring on a disturbed condition are called

   a. predispositions.

   b. pathogenic processes.

   c. precipitating factors.

   d. sociocultural factors.

B.   Match the items in Column II with the correct definitions in Column I.

Column I   Column II

1. Disorders that cannot be   a. avoidance
    classified as being caused by   b. denial
    either physiological or   c. depression
    phychological maladaption.   d. intellectualization
                                       e. neurosis
2. The study and treatment of
    physical handicaps and dis-   f. psychosomatic
    abilities and their effect on   g. schizophrenia
    emotional processes.   h. somatopsychology

3. Isolation of an impaired
    emotional view of a situation.

4. Departing from a situation.

5. Withdrawal from all activities.

6. Ignoring the fact that a
    situation exists.

7. Trying to explain a situation.

8. Withdrawal from contact with
    reality.

C.   Briefly answer the following questions.

1. Explain the holistic approach to patient care.

2. List five sources to be considered in assessing mind-body relationships.

3. State four nursing objectives to help re-establish balance in mind-body
    disturbances.

4. Name three ways the nurse can give the patient honest reassurance.

chapter 24
STAGES OF ILLNESS
AND THE SICK ROLE

STUDENT OBJECTIVES

- List six factors that affect the way a person views his state of health or illness.

- Match four nursing interventions to problems in the illness stage.

- Name three tasks the patient needs to accomplish in order to effectively progress through convalescence.

- Name four aspects of the sick role.

- Explain how illness can be a way to respond to social pressure.

No person is either completely ill or completely healthy. It is useful to think of the stages of illness as a continuum, figure 24-1. Homeostasis is upset as the patient begins to question whether he might be ill. At the healthy end of the continuum is the stage of wellness. In the center of the continuum is the stage

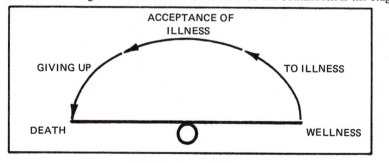

Fig. 24-1 Stages of illness

of acceptance of illness. At this point the patient can either give up and move toward death, or move toward the health end of the continuum, wellness. If the patient moves toward wellness again, he passes through the transition stage and back to wellness. Finally, at the health end of the continuum is the recovery stage where the patient resumes his well role.

At one time, health was thought to be the absence of disease. Illness was thought to "descend" on the person. Today, social and cultural factors are considered important to any definition of health or illness. Illness can be viewed as one way to respond to social pressures. Escape into illness relieves the person of his responsibilities as family member, religious participant, political influencer, economic wage earner, and so on.

TRANSITION TO ILLNESS

The transition to illness is often obscure. A person may experience only vague discomfort or the sense that something is different. Familiar coping devices are used to deal with the discomfort. Frantic escape into working overtime or increased emphasis on social activities may be attempted to convince oneself and others that the symptoms are not serious.

At the same time that the individual is trying to convince himself and others that the discomfort is not important, he is also searching for the meaning of the symptoms. Could the headache be a brain tumor? Does the bleeding mean cancer? Is the loss of memory a sign of senility? Is the hallucination a sign of madness? These reactions of overtly trying to convince oneself and others through behavior and asking internal nagging questions can exert a strong pressure toward illness; both add additional stress.

During the transition-to-illness stage, people may seek the help of trusted others. Depending on social and cultural values, family, clergy, tribal medicine men or others that are perceived as helpers may be consulted. While seeking this help, other feelings beside anxiety may be experienced. Guilt is not uncommon in people who feel illness is a punishment. Anger and irritability that illness should occur or relief that one can now relax and be sick are other expected responses.

When symptoms are first noticed, self-treatment may be attempted. If family and friends discount the symptoms there may be less effort by the symptomatic person to seek help. If self-treatment is ineffective and family and friends pressure the person to seek further help, medical or nursing assistance may be sought.

A number of factors affect the way a person may view his state of health and illness:

1. The number and persistence of symptoms.
   A minor symptom that disappears rather quickly may be discounted.
2. The person's ability to recognize symptoms.
   This factor may account for the failure to seek help when a symptom may seem minor or chronic.
3. The perceived severity of the symptom(s).
   To a concert pianist, any discomfort in the hands or fingers may be perceived as serious while in other people the same symptom may be ignored.
4. The extent of social and physical disability.
   In the American culture, the very young or very old people are expected to be less responsible and less active; therefore, a marked disability may be overlooked in these groups.
5. The cultural background.
   Some cultural groups teach their members to "grin and bear it." Other cultural groups teach their members to complain or to seek help when certain body systems are involved and not to seek help when certain other body parts are affected.
6. The access to and knowledge of the meaning of symptoms.
   Nurses and doctors may have more knowledge of the meaning of symptoms but may not seek help for themselves because of some other factors.
7. The availability and accessibility of help.
   People may be unaware of available health facilities. Other people may be put off by having to wait for treatment or by having to present payment prior to admission.

The degree of disruption in their lives is a major determinant for seeking help. If a person can no longer carry on the activities that family, friends, or employer expect of him, he is more likely to accept help. Figure 24-2 summarizes factors that influence a person's willingness to define himself as ill or well.

PEOPLE DEFINE THEMSELVES AS ILL DEPENDING ON:

 – The number and persistence of their symptoms.
 – Their ability to recognize symptoms.
 – How serious they perceive the symptoms to be.
 – How socially and physically disabled they are.
 – What their cultural background is.
 – How much knowledge they have about the meaning of their symptoms.
 – How available and accessible help is.

Fig. 24-2 Factors influencing the person's willingness to be defined as ill.

Problems in the Transition to Illness Stage	Nursing Intervention
Need for information	Gives information about the possible meaning of symptoms. Tells patient about sources of diagnosis and treatment.
Anxiety	Stays with patient. Encourages ventilation of thoughts and feelings.

Fig. 24-3 Nursing intervention in the stage of transition to illness

The nurse can be of help to people in the transition to illness, figure 24-3. By giving accurate information about the possible meaning of the symptoms and discussing available care, the nurse can assist in decision-making about seeking care.

The nurse who works in a clinic or doctor's office should realize that patients are often extremely anxious about the possible meaning of their symptoms. In this situation, interventions are used which have been found effective for decreasing anxiety. The nurse can provide assistance to individuals who seek diagnostic tests or come for an annual physical exam. Sometimes a patient may complain of not feeling well but the doctor can find no visible signs of illness. Such a patient might be accused of malingering; this refers to pretending one is ill. However, patients may have their own ideas about illness and may be quite sure they are ill. Being defined as a malingerer can present further problems for the patient. Malingerer has a negative connotation and once the patient is so defined it is difficult for him to receive care for an illness process. It must be realized that vague physical complaints are sometimes presented because they are thought to be more legitimate than the intense emotional or interpersonal difficulties being experienced by the patient. Many times depression is presented as a vague, physical complaint. Also, vague complaints may be expressed because the illness process is often not obvious in the early stages.

The nurse can be of assistance to the patient who feels well but whose routine physical exam reveals signs of illness. She can intervene in such situations by staying with the patient and utilizing communication skills to encourage discussion about the seeming contradiction between feeling well and having diagnostic signs of illness.

Acceptance of Illness

Once a person accepts support from significant other people that illness is present and a diagnosis is made, he becomes a patient and assumes the sick role.

The *sick role* is a dependent stage during which the patient is not expected to be a useful and productive member of society.

According to Parsons in *Patients, Physicians and Illness*, the sick role has four aspects:

1. The patient is excused from normal social role responsibilities.

   For example, the patient who is a father is no longer expected to help raise his children, and the patient who is a teacher is no longer expected to teach.

2. The person definitely needs help.

   There is no expectation that he will get well merely by deciding to do so; he must be treated and taken care of. This leads to enforced dependency; the patient must be dependent on those who give him care.

3. The person must accept the responsibility to get well.

   This leads to the expectation by many nurses and doctors that all patients should want to be cooperative.

4. The person seeks technically competent help.

   This leads to cooperation and involvement in his care.

Since the sick role has four aspects, it is possible for some patients to accept only one or two aspects of the role. Some patients may allow themselves to be excused from normal social responsibilities but may not accept enforced dependency or cooperate with health personnel. The nurse remembers that the way the patient socially defines his position may or may not coincide with the medical diagnosis of the patient. Nurses can become frustrated and angry when the patient does not live up to their expectations. If this occurs, it is up to the nurse to re-examine her expectations.

The sick role is an exchange process. Individual freedom and control are exchanged for care, protection, and freedom from responsibility. The sick role can be unhealthy if the person adopts it throughout life. This is often done by patients who have been hospitalized for several years such as those in long-term institutions. They see themselves in the role of patient rather than as a person who may become a patient at times.

Patients may receive secondary gain or satisfaction as a result of the way health personnel and others respond to their illness. The wheelchair patient who receives sympathy and a "poor you, let me help you" approach is receiving secondary gain from his disability. *Secondary gain* is gratification that results when patients seek or get extra attention or favors because of their conspicuous symptoms. Like the sick role, secondary gain is an exchange; the patient must give up certain independent acts in order to receive sympathy or attention from others.

If health personnel see only the secondary gain the patient is enjoying, the patient may be accused of being a malingerer who is "just trying to get attention."

Actually there is an underlying patient need which must be assessed and met. The nurse assesses both primary and secondary needs. In a therapeutic environment, the sick role is discouraged. Seeing patients as completely sick presumes that the difficulty lies within them. In fact, internal, social, and cultural factors seem to interplay in the process of being defined as sick.

The nurse can intervene in the acceptance of illness. Encouraging some form of independent action in even the sickest patient is one way to intervene. Thinking through one's own expectations for patient behavior and being clear in the communication of these expectations is another way.

Talking with the patient about what his illness experience means to him is another useful intervention. If the patient's body functions or parts have been altered by illness, losses must be grieved and resolved. With this resolution, coping devices can be reorganized and the patient can enter the convalescent stage. Figure 24-4 deals with problems common to illness.

Disability and the Sick Role

With increased knowledge about how to control acute disease, health personnel have turned their concern to chronic disease and long-term incapacity. In many cases, the major therapeutic task is rehabilitation. Great strides have been made toward restoring or minimizing the effects of lost function.

The psychosocial outcome of rehabilitation efforts is uncertain. In general, there needs to be a greater emphasis on the development of new patterns of behavior. Often there is little correlation between the degree of physical disability, the success of physical or environmental modification, and the social functioning of the patient.

The important distinction to communicate to patients with chronic diseases and long-term incapacities is that they are not sick but are different as a result of their disease or incapacities. As long as the disabled person views himself (and is viewed by others) as sick, he will continue to act the sick role and will have expectations of getting well.

Problems in the Illness Stage	Nursing Intervention
Self-Actualization	Encourage independent patient action.
Communication	Clearly express the nurse's expectations to the patient.
Grief	Assist patient to grieve loss of body part, organ, or function.

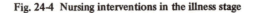

Fig. 24-4 Nursing interventions in the illness stage

Disabled people who can accept that they are no longer sick, but are different in some of their abilities can begin to function according to their distinctive needs, problems, and ways of adapting. Because this is so, an important element in rehabilitative nursing is a clear picture of how the patient views himself. Self-concept and body image will be discussed in more detail in chapter 26.

The Transition to Wellness

In the stage of convalescence or transition to wellness, the patient returns to health. If there has been a permanent disability, the patient must reorganize his self-image and expectations so they are realistic in light of his current capabilities.

As the patient is able to move out of his room, master activities of daily living, and assume a less dependent role, he develops an increased sense of worth. Anxiety, except perhaps discharge anxiety, is likely to decrease since the patient is used to the hospital environment by this time; also, the patient usually will not have to endure painful or unusual treatments.

Patients vary in their convalescent roles. In some, physical convalescence occurs prior to emotional convalescence. The nurse is aware that physical healing does not mean the patient has resolved feelings of loss or decreased self-worth. Patients who have found the sick role provides secondary gain may be less likely to be emotionally prepared for return to wellness.

To progress through convalescence effectively, the patient needs to accomplish three tasks. One of these tasks is to redirect energies toward the full potential for living. This is accomplished by the nurse and patient talking about what meaning this illness experience has had for the patient. Feelings can be resolved as they are discussed, examined, and clarified. Without such discussions there is more likelihood that the patient will try to push these feelings out of his mind. Even though the patient tries to do this, strong unresolved feelings will continue to haunt his thoughts and behavior.

Another task of convalescence is to move from the dependent role to an independent role. Patients who have experienced changes in body image due to surgery or trauma must resolve these losses and accept some degree of ongoing dependency.

A third task of convalescence is to resolve changes in roles. The patient does not immediately stop using patient behaviors on the day of discharge. The family may have to continue helping with some activities of daily living for some time. In assessing the patient's ability to move smoothly through convalescence, the nurse considers the following questions:

- Is the patient prepared physically *and* emotionally for discharge?

- Are there rewards for the patient to encourage him to leave the sick role?

- Does the patient's family, friends, and nurse encourage independent, well behavior?

The family may be unprepared for the gradual resumption of independent action by the discharged patient. The family may expect that things will be like they always were. If the family expectations are not in line with the patient's behavior, there is likely to be frustration on both sides.

The tasks of convalescence can best be accomplished when the nurse includes the patient and family in planning and care. With shorter hospitalization, many feelings about the illness process are no longer resolved during the hospital stay. The family can be quite helpful in the resolution of these feelings once they are aware of the need and have been counseled about how to encourage such resolutions. This part of discharge planning is as important as the plans for physical adaptation and self-care. This nurse should include all of these considerations when teaching the patient and his family.

Achievement of the tasks of convalescence can be evaluated through follow-up home visits or interviews with the patient and his family during clinic visits. One clue that the patient has not resolved the tasks of convalescence is his constant discussion and anxiety in relation to the illness experience.

If the nurse is unable to help the patient resolve these feelings, she may suggest that the visiting nurse make a home visit to evaluate the need for further counseling or therapy. Sometimes such treatment can be provided in the home by mental health nursing specialists. Figure 24-5 summarizes nursing interventions in the convalescent stage of illness.

Problems in the Convalescent Stage	Nursing Intervention
Redirect energies toward full potential for living	With the patient, discuss the meaning of this illness experience for him.
Move from dependent to independent role or grief	Encourage gradual, planned independent action. Help patient talk about thoughts and feelings; about loss or continued dependency.
Resolve changes in roles	Prepare family and patient for expected patient behaviors and tasks. Include patient and family in discharge planning. Tell family how they can help patient adjust to living at home. Teach patient and family appropriate self-care. Evaluate achievement of well state through home visits, aftercare clinic interview, or referral to visiting nurse service.

Fig. 24-5 Nursing interventions in the convalescent stage of illness

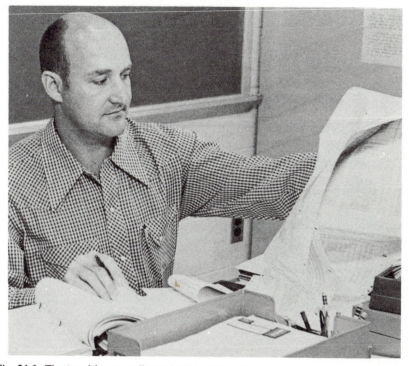

Fig. 24-6 The transition to wellness should promote independence and a successful change in roles when necessary.

SUMMARY

The relationship between illness and health can be thought of as a continuum of stages from health, to transition to illness, to illness (the sick role), to convalescence, and back to health. This continuum can be interrupted by death or a long-term disability.

Transition to illness and transition to wellness are both stages that are affected by social, cultural, economic, and knowledge factors. The nurse intervenes in both transitional stages by providing information, helping the patient to explore his thoughts and feelings, and by collaborating in treatment planning with the patient and family.

ACTIVITIES AND DISCUSSION TOPICS

- Evaluate several patients' process of defining themselves as sick. Use figure 24-2 for this evaluation.

- Use figure 24-2 to evaluate the times when you did or did not define yourself as sick. What factors encouraged you to seek help? What factors discouraged you from seeking help?

- Talk to several patients who are in the acceptance stage of illness. Find out what aspects of the role they have accepted by asking them to tell you what they think about their hospital stay.

- Locate a patient who the nursing staff thinks is "just trying to get attention." Try to figure out how the concept of secondary gain might be operating with this patient.

- Talk with several patients who have long-term illnesses or disabilities. Which ones consider themselves to be sick and which ones consider themselves to be different as a result of their illness or disability? Which patients have better rehabilitation potential?

- Make a home visit to a patient who was unable to complete convalescent tasks in the hospital. Prior to your visit, make a nursing care plan which focuses on convalescent tasks.

REVIEW

A. Multiple Choice. Select the best answer(s). Some questions have more than one answer.

1. Some responses to illness are
   a. anxiety.
   b. anger.
   c. guilt.
   d. relief.

2. In assessing the patient's ability to move smoothly through convalescence, the nurse considers:
   a. Is the patient able to discuss the meaning of his illness experience?
   b. Is the patient prepared physically and emotionally for discharge?
   c. Are there rewards for the patient to encourage departure from the sick role?
   d. Does the patient's family, friends and nurse encourage well behavior?

3. Transition to illness and transition to wellness are stages that are affected by
   a. social factors.
   b. cultural factors.
   c. economic factors.
   d. knowledge factors.

4. The sick role can be defined as
   a. a situation where the person considers himself to be ill but health personnel do not.
   b. a dependent state where the patient is not expected to be a useful and productive member of society.
   c. the return to health that requires passage through certain stages.
   d. an imbalance that occurs when a person is unsuccessful in adapting to stressors.

5. Gratification that results when patients seek or get extra attention or favors because of their conspicuous symptoms is called
   a. the convalescent role.   c. malingering.
   b. the sick role.   d. secondary gain.

B. Match the nursing interventions in Column I to the problems in the illness stage of Column II.

   Column I   Column II

   1. Give information about the possible   a. anxiety
      meaning of symptoms.   b. communication
                                                 c. need for information
   2. Encourage ventilation of thoughts   d. self-actualization
      and feelings.

   3. Encourage independent patient
      action.

   4. Clearly express the nurse's ex-
      pectations to the patient.

C. Briefly answer the following questions.

   1. Name three tasks the patient needs to accomplish in order to effectively progress through convalescence.

   2. Name four aspects of the sick role.

   3. What is one clue that indicates the patient has not resolved the tasks of convalescence?

   4. List six factors that affect the way a person may view his state of health or illness.

   5. Explain how illness can be a way to respond to social pressure.

chapter 25
COPING DEVICES

STUDENT OBJECTIVES

- Define coping devices.
- Match mental mechanisms with their definitions.
- Give three examples of avoidance feelings used when actual feelings are unacceptable.
- List four common actions used to cope with stress.

People cope with stress in a number of different ways. Stress that is primarily psychological or interpersonal can be dealt with by thought or mental mechanisms through feelings or by behavior that can be observed. *Mental mechanisms* are internal processes which can only be assessed through observing outward behavior. Coping devices include mental mechanisms, as well as actions such as pacing the floor, talking with a supportive person, and listening to music. *Coping devices* include thoughts, feelings, and behaviors that help people to deal with stress. Because coping devices assist patients to reduce stress or anxiety, the nurse does not prevent the patient from using any devices unless the patient is first presented with an alternative way to cope.

MENTAL MECHANISMS FOR COPING

There are many mental mechanisms that people use to alleviate stress and increase their own comfort. Most of these mechanisms are used in varying degrees by all people at some time in their lives.

Although there is an inclination to classify some mental mechanisms as more sophisticated than others, people tend to use those coping devices they have learned to use and are familiar with. Difficulties may occur if a person limits the number of coping devices to one or two because there are many situations that may require the use of other devices as well. When a person is confronted by a situation and the use of preferred coping devices is restricted, additional problems will further vex the patient.

Mental mechanisms will be discussed individually so the student can learn to identify them one by one. In real life, these mechanisms are not used singly. Many of them are related and tend to be used in combination. The way the nurse assesses the mental mechanisms being used is through observation of the patient's verbal and nonverbal behavior. By listening to his words, and by watching his nonverbal behavior, the nurse can speculate about the mechanisms which are operating to help the patient cope.

Repression or Dissociation

All people function at various levels of awareness at different times. Situations which are pleasant or nonthreatening are more apt to be remembered. Traumatic situations and situations that are associated with extreme anxiety may automatically be put out of conscious awareness by the mechanisms of *repression* or *dissociation*. Dissociated or repressed material is treated as if it does not exist or is unrelated to the situation on hand.

If the nurse tries to use logic to convince a patient who has repressed an anxiety-provoking situation, the patient will not believe her assertion that the situation has occurred. The nurse may be apt to think the patient is not telling the truth when in fact the patient has repressed or dissociated the experience as a way to decrease anxiety. Examples of situations that may be repressed by patients include hospital admission, the time prior to and immediately after surgical procedures, painful experiences and any other experience that created severe anxiety. Since it is not always possible to know what is highly anxiety-provoking for each patient, the nurse takes the patient at his word if he claims he does not remember. It is never wise to argue with the patient, try to convince him, or act as if the patient is not being truthful. Such nurse behaviors may be perceived as a further threat to the patient; as a result, he may deal with the discomfort by dissociating or repressing the nurse-patient interactions.

Unconscious thoughts or feelings continue to influence conscious behavior although the person exerts no control over them. For this reason, the person who is less threatened by situations uses the mental mechanism of repression or dissociation less frequently. People who are open to their experiences and do not repress or dissociate them can exert more control over their lives. They generally experience more satisfying relationships with others.

Denial

Denial is a mental mechanism that also indicates a lack of awareness. The range of denial is great. The person who uses denial acts as if the current or past situation is not occurring or did not occur. In denied situations that are close to awareness, the patient may actually have an inkling that the situation did occur. In denied situations that have been repressed or dissociated, the patient may have disowned the experience and really believes the event did not occur.

Denial is similar to repression but it is not the same. The term denial is usually used when the patient makes implied or direct statements that the situation has not occurred. For example, the patient may say, "Put a stocking on my left toes" after the toes have been amputated; or the patient may say "it didn't happen" after a loved one has died. On the other hand, events that are repressed are not mentioned by the person unless repressed feelings and thoughts begin to come into awareness; this may be precipitated by another traumatic experience or a therapeutic encounter.

Denial serves the purpose of protecting the patient from extreme anxiety. When the nurse has talked several times with a patient about a denied experience, it is appropriate to begin to express neutral doubt. For example, if a patient states he was hospitalized on a psychiatric unit for breaking a window, the nurse can express doubt by saying, "People get admitted here for breaking a window?" When the nurse does express doubt, she is careful not to make fun of the patient by using a teasing or unbelieving tone of voice. Doubt is expressed matter-of-factly so the patient can continue to maintain denial if he needs to do so.

Identification

Identification has several distinct meanings. One meaning is to model oneself after another person. Identification is a coping device that can be used when life seems incomplete. This mechanism is used in all children when they imitate parents or others. In identification, another's behavior is imitated. Dressing like a favorite movie star, developing prejudices like one's parents or trying to live like a fictional hero are ways to identify with others. Statements such as, "My father said. . ." or "My mother did it this way" imply that identification has taken place.

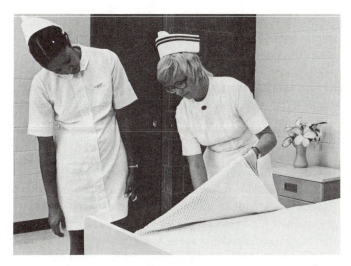

Fig. 25-1 The student nurse identifies with the graduate nurse.

Student nurses learn to identify with other nurses by wearing uniforms and by acting like other nurses. At times, patients may come to trust the nurse and identify with her. When a patient who has established a relationship with a nurse says, "I want to be a nurse like you," the patient has identified with the nurse.

Identification is sometimes used in a second sense; that is, one may respond to a person in thought, feeling, or action as though he were like some third person. *Transference* is the term that is used when the patient attributes characteristics to the therapist or nurse that really belong to significant other people in the patient's life. It can be said that a patient usually identifies the nurse with another significant person in the patient's life. Some transference occurs in all significant relationships. The nurse-patient relationship is often an intimate one so the patient may distort the nurse-patient interactions. For example, since both nurse and parent perform functions that meet physical needs of the patient, the patient may identify the nurse with his parent. A patient may also see the nurse as an authority figure like his father and transfer the feelings he has toward his father. Transference goes beyond the limits of age, sex, and situation. Although the patient may be elderly or middle-aged, he may react toward the nurse as if the nurse were a parent. As long as the patient sees some similarity between the nurse and a significant other person, transference can occur.

Patients may remark, "You remind me of my granddaughter" (or father, mother, sister, brother, husband). Although these clues are conscious recognitions, they are signals that transference may be occurring. Transference can be either positive (affectionate) or negative (hostile and angry).

The nurse uses her knowledge about transference to understand the significance of patient behavior. If a patient tells the nurse — on first meeting — how kind and good the nurse is, transference is probably in existence. The patient cannot possibly know what kind of person the nurse is in such a short time. He is probably transferring thoughts and feelings from previous relationships.

The nurse does not give the patient her interpretation of the unconscious meaning of such statements. Rather, she uses the statements to help the patient explore problems or concerns he has on his mind. The nurse does not deny or ignore the importance of the patient's unconscious processes. To do so is to deny or ignore the patient as a whole person. Experienced nurses and psychotherapists are more skilled in interpersonal relationships; however, the beginning nurse can develop skills to recognize forces which affect communication.

Countertransference is another form of identification. Countertransference refers to the primarily unconscious emotional reaction of the nurse to the patient. The nurse attributes to the patient characteristics that really belong to a significant person in the life of the nurse. When the nurse describes a "personality clash," "becoming too involved" or feeling "really uptight" with a patient, countertransference is probably occurring.

Countertransference can be a useful experience if the nurse uses it to further understand self and patient. It is not helpful to the nurse-patient relationship if the nurse refuses to examine her own behavior. Countertransference is likely to occur whenever the nurse has unresolved feelings toward significant people in her own life. Students who are resolving feelings toward their parents, husbands, friends, sisters, brothers, grandparents, or children are prone to have countertransference feelings toward patients who remind them of these significant people. Situations where the nurse becomes romantically involved with a patient may be due to transference and countertransference reactions. The student is cautioned not to label all strong emotional reactions of patient or nurse as transference or countertransference. Complaints or affection by nurse or patient can be legitimately due to the present nurse-patient situation.

Regression

Regression means "to go back." When a person regresses, he goes back to earlier interests, modes of satisfaction, and problems. People often regress during periods of high stress. Hospitalization, loss of a loved one, or any high anxiety situation can lead to regression.

In the hospitalized patient, regression may take the form of trying to control what the nurse does, becoming more concerned about one's body and basic needs, and showing a need to be taken care of both physically and emotionally.

When under physical or emotional stress, children show regression by going back to earlier patterns of speech or behavior. A tired child will suck her thumb although she has given up thumbsucking in general. Adults show regression too. An anxious patient may make demands and act in ways he would never act if he were not under stress.

Displacement

Displacement occurs when feelings about an object or person are shifted to another object or person. This transfer often allows for more socially acceptable or comfortable behavior. For example, when a man is angry with his boss, he may go home and argue with his wife. The patient who is angry with the doctor for not explaining a treatment may yell at the nurse. The student who is anxious about passing a course may scream at a trusted instructor who is not responsible for passing the student. In each of these situations of displacement, the person who shifted feelings let them out on more socially acceptable or less threatening people. Objects can also be used to displace feelings. Breaking a vase when one is angry at a spouse or slamming the door after an argument with a loved one may both be examples of displacement.

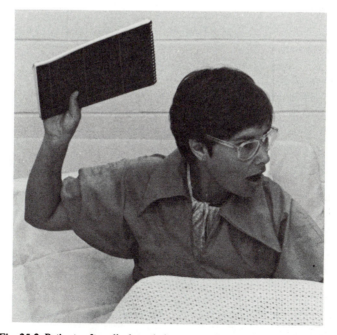

Fig. 25-2 Patients often displace their anger on handy objects or people.

Affectionate or lustful feelings toward another may be shifted if the other conveys rejection of these feelings. Children can displace affection to pets or playthings if parents refuse their affection. Feelings or thoughts which are extremely frightening may be displaced by dreams. In the dreams, people and feelings may represent other people and feelings.

It may be an unexpected and uncomfortable experience for the nurse to be screamed at. Being the object of ridicule and discourtesy is never pleasant. If the nurse can view this behavior as the way the patient can best deal with the stress of the moment, she may be less likely to retaliate with anxiety or anger.

Suppression

Suppression is a conscious decision not to act. The unpleasant is dealt with by simply ignoring it. Saying, "I don't want to think about it" implies suppression is being used. Suppression is effective while another task or event is occurring. For example, a student nurse who is hungry before classtime may forget about it if the class is interesting. When the class is over, the hungry feeling will probably return. Patients who have pain may use activity to suppress the pain. When the activity is over, the experience of pain will recur.

Reaction Formation

Reaction formation occurs when a person develops an attitude or action directly opposite to the actual wish or desire. It means doing the opposite of what one really feels like doing. The real feeling is repressed in reaction formation and its opposite is exhibited in the behavior. Reaction formations differ in acceptance and value by the various cultures. People from a culture that tends to value the clean, tidy person may develop clean, tidy attitudes or actions, even though they would really like to be messy or irresponsible.

Individuals who are fighting hardest against their own impulses or wishes are apt to use reaction formation. The person who has just given up smoking is the greatest reformer of others who smoke. The one who would like to overeat may be most critical of those who do overeat. The person who is angry but fears admitting the anger often over-reacts by being extremely charming and agreeable. People who never appear angry or irritated and always try to cheer others up may be using reaction formation to protect themselves from their own angry feelings.

Sublimation

Sublimation is the redirection of an unacceptable tendency and the substitution of a more acceptable tendency. Both sublimation and reaction formation are ways the person diverts forbidden and dangerous impulses. Games and sports are socially acceptable sublimations of aggression. People who love to eat may become great cooks as a way to sublimate urges to eat. Sexual drives may be diverted to contact sports such as basketball or to art forms such as painting or sculpture.

Compensation

Compensation is the process by which a person excels in one area in order to overcome or substitute for a real or imagined weakness in another area. Compensation cannot be used as a coping device unless the person is aware of the real or supposed defect. A patient who denies having a problem would be unable to use compensation as a coping device.

Compensation serves two purposes. The first purpose is to free the person from feelings of inadequacy. The second purpose is to gain approval from other people. For example, a deaf person may become an outstanding golfer in order to compensate for his deafness. A paralyzed person may turn to teaching to compensate for lack of physical mobility.

Rationalization

Rationalization is use of an excuse to justify behavior while disguising an unconscious motive. In this way, the person tries to make his action appear reasonable, honorable, or successful. The person usually admits to the act; however, he gives a socially acceptable reason rather than the real reason for acting as he did. Sometimes the person who uses rationalization stumbles and halts in the verbal attempt to explain his actions.

A patient may say, "I'm too tired to get out of bed" when actually he feels depressed and worthless. Other examples of rationalization are saying, "It's all for the best" or "I didn't care anyway" when something goes wrong. Explanations such as "I can't," "I couldn't help it" or "Just this one time" are probably rationalizations. The nurse who explains her behavior to the patient by saying, "I forgot" is probably using rationalization.

Projection

Projection is the process in which unacceptable thoughts or feelings are attributed to others. Patients who say their hospitalization is all the fault of

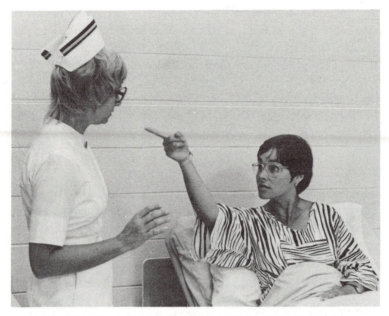

Fig. 25-3 This patient is projecting her own thoughts and feelings.

their family are using projection. Projection is used when the person finds it too anxiety-provoking to recognize his own unpleasant characteristics. Patients who blame divorces, arguments, or other interpersonal situations all on the other person are using projection because they refuse to acknowledge their part in the difficulty.

Extreme projection occurs in some forms of hallucination. An *hallucination* is a false perception; it has no relation to reality and there is no exterior stimuli. A person who has auditory hallucinations (hears voices) usually is unable to accept his thoughts, feelings, and desires so they are projected out to the external environment and are perceived by the patient as "voices." The patient with auditory hallucinations refuses to acknowledge his own thoughts or feelings and so is using projection.

Intellectualization

Intellectualization is a coping device that is frequently used by well-educated people. The person who uses intellectualization is often afraid of his own feelings and uses technical terms to explain an experience. The patient who uses intellectualization will answer with detailed impersonal statements when asked what he is feeling.

Delusion

A *delusion* is an extreme explanation a person develops for a seemingly unexplainable occurrence. It is a false, fixed thought that is based on an element of truth. In a delusional process, the element of truth is expanded and interpreted in an illogical manner. People who develop delusions cannot be talked out of them through logical reasoning. A delusion is the product of an illogical thought process that develops to protect the person from a threat. For example, a woman who perceives her husband is withdrawing from her may develop the delusion that he is having an affair with another person. The delusion may be a lesser threat than the actual fact that the husband is withdrawing; it protects the wife by allowing her to place all the blame on him for whatever takes place.

The type of delusion or explanation a person develops is related to the protection needed by that person. If the person feels insecure and insignificant, delusions of grandeur, such as believing he is Jesus Christ or the President of the United States, may be developed. In *delusion of grandeur*, the insecure person copes by thinking he must be a great person. If the person fears intimacy, he may develop delusions of persecution. For example, he may believe his employer is overcritical and treats him unfairly or he may believe someone is trying to poison him. In *delusion of persecution* one's own angry feelings are projected to others so that the anxiety which accompanies intimacy need not be faced.

Conversion

Conversion is the act of transforming feelings into a physical disability or symptom. In our society, some feelings require restraint and control. Feelings such as lust or anger can be controlled by developing physical symptoms that limit activity. A woman whose right arm becomes paralyzed yet shows no organic impairment may have taken this way to prevent herself from striking a friend with whom she is angry. During wartime, conversion hysteria is frequently encountered; a soldier's right arm may become paralyzed.

Depersonalization

Depersonalization is a sense of being someone else; a loss of personal identity. The person may report that his body does not seem to belong to him. Depersonalization is a common reaction to stress. It is likely to occur when one is forced to change his or her body image due to accident, surgery, implants, artificial appliances or dialysis, chronic disease, or hospitalization. Psychiatric patients may feel alien toward their bodies. Depersonalization, like the other mental mechanisms, protects the person from undue stress. Figure 25-4 summarizes information on mental mechanisms. The student should remember that the use of mental mechanisms is necessary for adjustment to life. All persons use them. Only when they are used in extreme are they considered unhealthy.

FEELINGS USED AS COPING DEVICES

Feelings are fleeting mood states which can be pleasant, uncomfortable, or painful. Feelings include such experiences as anxiety, disgust, fear, guilt, anger, isolation, helplessness, hope, inadequacy, joy, love, sadness and suspicion.

Mental Mechanism	Action Definition
Repression or Dissociation	Traumatic situations are automatically put out of conscious awareness
Denial	Acting as if the current or past situation is not happening or has not happened
Regression	Going back to earlier interests, modes of satisfaction and problems
Identification	Taking in parts of others' behavior and making it part of the person
Displacement	Feelings about an object or person are transferred or placed on another person or object
Suppression	Making a conscious decision not to act
Reaction Formation	Developing an attitude or action directly opposite to the actual wish or desire
Compensation	Overcoming or substituting for a real or imagined weakness
Rationalization	Using an excuse to disguise an unconscious motive
Projection	Attributing one's own unacceptable thoughts or feelings to others
Intellectualization	Using technical terms when asked for feeling responses
Delusion	False fixed explanation as a way of dealing with seemingly unexplainable occurrences
Sublimation	Redirecting an unacceptable drive into an acceptable channel or substituting an acceptable tendency for an unacceptable tendency
Conversion	The act of transforming feelings into physical symptoms or disabilities
Depersonalization	Feelings of unreality about one's own body; loss of personal identity

Fig. 25-4 Mental mechanisms

When a feeling is unacceptable to a person, another one may be substituted. For example, as stated earlier, anger may be used to avoid intimacy. Sometimes an engaged couple may argue and quarrel just when they are becoming emotionally close to one another. The anger and quarreling may protect both from becoming too close or intimate. A patient and nurse may react to one another with anger when they are threatened by a closer relationship. Anger is also used to protect a person from the discomfort of anxiety. The energy generated by the anxious feelings can be converted into anger. Anxiety is a vague, uncomfortable state; anger is less vague and may be more bearable for some people. Often when people think they are being criticized by others, they will convert the anxiety into angry retaliation.

Depression is a mood state that can be used as a coping device to avoid sadness. The person who is unable to grieve because he feels unable to tolerate sadness may become depressed. Elation is another coping device that is used to avoid feelings of anxiety or sadness.

The nurse assumes all patient feelings are legitimate. Feelings expressed by the patient are never denied or ridiculed. Rather, the nurse helps the patient to describe and explore feelings so they can be placed in proper perspective. Some of the frightening qualities of the feeling experience are reduced; being able to talk about them helps the patient to understand how the feelings began and what brings them out. Figure 25-5 shows how feelings are avoided and replaced by others.

ACTIONS USED AS COPING DEVICES

All behavior has meaning. The way a person acts serves an adaptive purpose. The goals may not be easily understood but there is a purpose for individual behavior.

Feelings	Examples of feelings that are used to avoid actual feelings
anxiety	anger; elation
intimacy or tenderness	anger
sadness	depression; elation

Fig. 25-5 Feelings used as coping devices.

Behaviors that are appropriate coping devices for one culture may be inappropriate in another culture. Some common ways to cope with stress in the middle-class American culture are:

- Listening to music or other rhythm forms

- Talking it out with another person

- Participating in oral activity such as eating, chewing gum, or smoking

- Using alcohol or drugs

- Sleeping

- Relaxing, vacationing, or engaging in other nonwork activity

- Using emotional releases such as crying, swearing, fighting, singing, laughing, or whistling

- Looking for new information to think the problem through

- Being touched, stroked, or having sexual experiences

- Releasing energy through physical exercise (cleaning, dancing, sport), pointless activity (tapping finger or toes, scratching, or pacing the floor), or work

When the patient is hospitalized, use of these common coping behaviors may be greatly restricted. Patients who would use physical action when under stress may now have only withdrawal and verbal methods available. Because their usual method of physical action is not available, patients may become extremely irritable and even openly hostile when they are under stress.

The nurse can help by channeling the excess energy into constructive exploration of the patient's thoughts and feelings. Support may be necessary for the patient who is learning to express his feelings openly. Support can be provided by listening attentively to patient remarks and making encouraging statements such as "Go on" or "Tell me more."

Another nursing intervention is that of suggesting acceptable tension outlets. These activities may include knitting, sewing, kneading, reading or watching adventure stories, keeping a journal or diary, walking, hitting an object (such as a punching bag, Ping-Pong ball, etc.) typing, cutting, cleaning, and structured exercise. Ambulatory patients can be directed to activities that provide the most appropriate actions. Immobilized patients can benefit from passive exercise such as watching an emotional movie or sporting match; active exercise such as punching a pillow; or participation in a preferred activity that is not otherwise contraindicated.

Destructive activitiy is clearly not useful as a source of decreasing tension or anxiety. The nurse should clearly state this to patients who attempt to hurt themselves, others, or valuable objects. Other activities the patient finds to release tension should be allowed and encouraged.

SUMMARY

Coping devices include thoughts, feeling, and behaviors that help people to deal with stress. Thoughts or mental mechanisms are usually seen in combination. People who use primarily one or two mental mechanisms are less equipped to deal with stress. Mental mechanisms include repression or dissociation, denial, regression, identification, displacement, suppression, reaction formation, sublimation, compensation, rationalization, projection, intellectualization, delusion, conversion, and depersonalization. Transference and countertransference are forms of identification that are of special importance to the nurse. The nurse never takes away the patient's mental mechanisms or tries to talk the patient out of using a certain device unless the patient is first presented with an alternate way to cope.

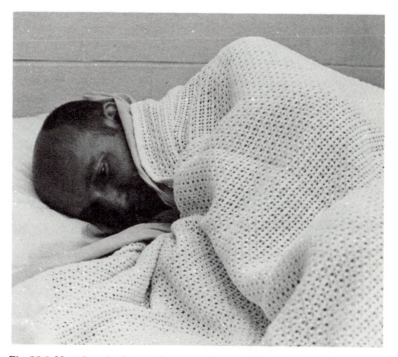

Fig. 25-6 Mental mechanisms such as regression are devices for coping with stress.

Feelings can be used to avoid other feelings. The nurse treats all patient expressions of feelings as legitimate. She helps the patient to cope by discussing and exploring his feelings so they can be understood and dealt with constructively.

Hospitalization may severely restrict coping actions that are generally used by the patient. The nurse suggests alternatives and provides appropriate outlets for patient tension and anxiety.

ACTIVITIES AND DISCUSSION TOPICS

- Make a list of the mental mechanisms you use most frequently. Which ones are most helpful in decreasing your stress?
- Read several patient charts and see if you can discover which mental mechanisms are being described.
- Describe the type of patients with which you would most likely get "overinvolved," feel "uptight" or have a "personality clash."
- Recall an incident where you were involved, or observed another nurse, in a transference or countertransference reaction. What exactly took place and how could the situation have been handled differently?
- Discuss how patients you have cared for used one feeling to avoid experiencing another feeling. List ways to help patients cope more directly with their feelings.
- List ten activities you could suggest to patients who are immobile yet need to decrease tension and anxiety.

REVIEW

A.   Multiple Choice. Select the best answer(s). Some questions have more than one answer.

1.   In the hospitalized patient, regression may take the form of
    a. trying to control what the nurse does.
    b. believing the nurse is one's mother.
    c. becoming more concerned about one's basic needs.
    d. showing a need to be taken care of both physically and emotionally.

2.   It is true that denial
    a. protects a person from extreme anxiety.
    b. is similar to repression.
    c. indicates a lack of awareness.
    d. is a conscious decision not to act.

3. Using an excuse to disguise an unconscious motive is
   a. displacement.
   b. reaction formation.
   c. rationalization.
   d. projection.

4. The nurse never tries to talk the patient out of using certain coping devices unless the patient is
   a. projecting his anger to the hospital staff.
   b. repressing a situation.
   c. convinced the nurse is his mother.
   d. first presented with an alternate way to cope.

5. An example of countertransference is:
   a. The patient is angry with the doctor and so he yells at the nurse.
   b. The nurse feels a strong attraction to the patient because he reminds her of her father.
   c. The student strives to be like her nursing instructor.
   d. The patient is hostile to the nurse because she reminds him of a former teacher.

B. Match the mental mechanisms in Column II to their definitions in Column I.

Column I	Column II
1. Developing an attitude or action directly opposite to the actual wish or desire.	a. compensation
	b. conversion
	c. delusion.
2. Using technical terms when asked for feeling responses.	d. depersonalization
	e. displacement
3. Overcoming or substituting for a real or imagined weakness.	f. intellectualization
	g. projection
4. Feelings about an object or person are transferred or placed on another person or object.	h. reaction formation
5. Attributing one's own unacceptable thoughts or feelings to others.	
6. False fixed explanation as a way of dealing with seemingly unexplainable occurrences.	
7. The act of transforming feelings into physical symptoms or disabilities.	
8. Feelings of unreality about one's own body.	

C. Briefly answer the following questions.

1. Define coping devices.

2. List four common ways to cope with stress in the middle-class American culture.

3. Explain why a hospitalized patient may become extremely irritable and openly hostile when under stress.

4. Define sublimation and give an example of it.

5. Give an example of the avoidance feeling that may be used when the following actual feelings are unacceptable to the person:

    sadness:

    anxiety:

    intimacy:

chapter 26
BODY IMAGE
AND SELF-CONCEPT

STUDENT OBJECTIVES

- Define body image.

- State the relationship between body image and self-concept.

- Match developmental difficulties that can affect body image and self-concept with the appropriate developmental period.

- List three areas for nursing assessment in body image difficulties.

- List four nursing interventions used to enhance body image and self-concept.

The mental picture a person develops of his or her physical self is called *body image*. Body image begins to develop in early infancy. The infant begins to get a sense of what belongs to him by moving parts of his body, looking at it, smelling it, tasting it, listening to its sounds, touching it, and observing what happens when he places his body in contact with other objects in the external environment. For example, the infant discovers that the nipple which provides him with food can be taken away and that it does not feel or taste the same as his own fingers. He learns that it is not part of his body.

Parental anxiety about body exploration may be interpreted by the child as "my body is bad," or "I am bad." If severe anxiety or panic is aroused, the child may repress or dissociate a part of his body. He may not include it in his mental image of himself.

As the infant passes through childhood to adulthood, other objects become part of the body image. The way clothes are used to cover the body and convey messages becomes part of the mental picture too. The nurse's cap and uniform may become part of the body image held by some nurses. Deciding whether to use jewelry or makeup is part of the development of body image. In disabled people, the use of such things as glasses, a cane, a wheelchair, or a prosthesis (artificial body part) can be incorporated into the body image.

Body image is also developed through posture. Dancers and athletes experience and identify movements and feelings related to their bodies that others may not. The patient who lies in bed most of the time may develop a different body image simply because he does not receive stimulation to many body areas.

Body image includes perceptions, attitudes, feelings and reactions relative to one's body. The degree and type of feeling each person has about his body is learned through social, environmental and cultural interactions. There are some

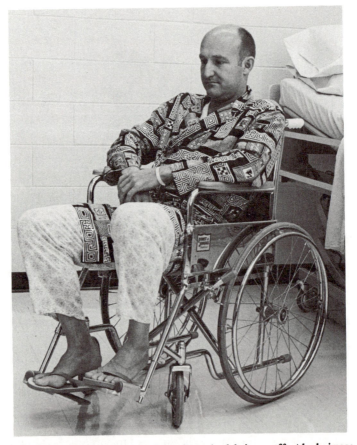

Fig. 26-1 Spending long periods of time in a wheelchair can affect body image.

stereotyped ideas about what is considered an attractive body. People whose bodies do not fit within these stereotyped dimensions may have negative feelings about themselves. Those with physical defects may have body image problems not only because of the way they feel about their bodies but because of the way others react to the defects.

The body image that people develop may or may not be the same as the actual body structure. A time lag exists between body changes and the change in the mental picture. Friends who meet each other after many years are more aware of the change in their friend than they are in the change in themselves. Elderly psychiatric patients frequently report they are young adults. People who become blind in their youth may always carry around a mental picture of themselves based on their last view of themselves. Frequently, a person who loses a limb or body organ continues to experience a sensation that the part is still present. Because the sudden loss may be too radical a change to accept, the mind continues to include the lost part in its body image. As adaptation takes place, the body image is more likely to be closer to the actual body structure.

Both children and adults need to have a relatively stable, definite concept of their bodies. A consistent body image helps to maintain homeostasis; a realistic body image requires positive social feedback from others. To a large extent, people become what others tell them they are. Certain characteristics are attributed to people on the basis of how they look. These characteristics may differ depending on the culture. For example, in American society, slimness is considered a positive attribute while in other cultures obesity is a positive attribute as it may indicate wealth and power.

The child or adult who does not have a stable and definite body image can experience severe anxiety and difficulty in relating to other people. In order to develop a stable, definite concept, it is necessary to recognize the boundaries between the self and others. If people can perceive themselves accurately, they are more likely to perceive other people accurately.

SELF-CONCEPT

Body image can influence self-concept; the reverse is also true. *Self-concept* is based on the total collection of feelings a person has about the self. If the body image is definite and consistent with reality, the person is likely to feel satisfied about the self. A person's unfavorable body image can lead to feelings of inferiority or intense anxiety. Likewise, if a person has negative feelings about himself, he is apt to have an inconsistent or poorly defined body image.

Self-concept includes feelings about one's social, moral, and spiritual self. It develops only through social interaction with significant other people. The self-concept exists to protect the person from anxiety. In turn, protection from anxiety promotes feelings of security when relating with other people. Experiences are organized so as to avoid disapproval of others and so avoid anxiety. Without such a way to view the self and experiences, the person would be overwhelmed by having to recall various ways to act in certain situations. The individual's self-concept guides behavior because it organizes experience and behavioral reactions that are useful for promoting security in various interpersonal situations.

The self-concept may not protect the person from anxiety and low self-esteem when the stress levels are high. In such situations, repression may take place; experiences that could correct the faulty self-concept are cut off. By providing a consistent and accepting relationship, the nurse can help the patient to use less repression and to correct his faulty self-concept.

Another aspect of the self-concept is the moral self. The moral self develops as a way to obtain approval from parents and avoid any disapproval. Parents and other authority figures such as nurses tend to withhold affection following behavior which does not please them. Affection or pleasurable responses are bestowed after behavior that is approved. Before long, the child or patient may learn that being good means to do what is approved, and being bad is the result of doing what is disapproved. Goodness is then associated with the feeling of being loved or liked while badness is associated with a feeling of being unworthy, unloved, disliked, and rejected.

As a rule, the spiritual or religious self has early beginnings in church or other organized experience. Some experiences that might influence the self-concept are teachings such as people are "guilty sinners," "blameless lambs," or "created in the image of God." As people mature they may continue to build the spiritual self based on organized church-related experiences, nonorganized religious experiences, or scientific beliefs. For example, many scientists do not believe in a personal God but do believe in a Higher Order to the universe. All of these experiences have an effect on how the person comes to think of himself as a social, moral, and spiritual person.

BODY IMAGE AND SELF-CONCEPT DIFFICULTIES

Some changes are more problematic than others. Body defects that are present from birth or those which occur in early infancy seem to have less emotional significance and require less adaptation than changes that occur later in life. Abrupt body changes are often more difficult to handle because they

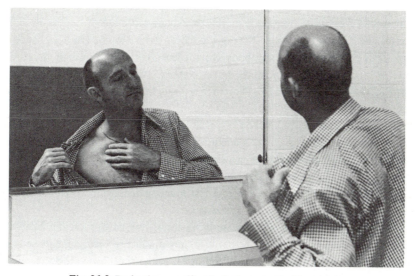

Fig. 26-2 Body changes affect body image and self-concept.

impose greater stress and require quicker adaptation. Changes to the face or head, genitals, and female breasts may be more stressful than changes in other areas. As in other potential crises, the individual's perception of the change is the deciding factor in whether homeostasis is disturbed and/or healthy adaptation occurs, figure 26-2. As with crises, body image and self-concept difficulties can be divided into developmental and situational changes.

DEVELOPMENTAL CHANGES AND BODY IMAGE

Developmental changes are expected physical, social, economic and emotional changes that occur at specific intervals in a person's life history. Important periods for expected change are infancy, childhood, adolescence, adulthood, middle age, and later years. Changes in body image can occur at some or all of these crucial periods.

Infancy and Childhood

The child who does not develop a sense of trust related to significant other people will often have a poor self-concept. The infant who does not receive adequate body and sensory stimulation has a poor base for developing (1) a stable, consistent body image and (2) sense of body boundaries. When parents devalue or do not accept their child, it is difficult for the child to place appropriate value on his body or himself. The child who feels his body fails to come up to parental expectations frequently develops a poor self-concept, indefinite body image, and feelings of shame. Young children who are not given a chance to explore their environment and body, cannot learn definite body boundaries or develop a stable, consistent body image. A child whose body does not conform to the body build or behavior that is thought to be appropriate for his or her sex may have some body image confusion.

School age children who have physical impairments such as defective vision and hearing may show signs of inadequacy and inferior feelings. Children who are within the normal range of physical development, yet cannot accept themselves for emotional reasons, will often show excessive interest in their bodies. This interest probably occurs because their strong feelings become focused or projected to some aspect of their appearance.

Children who have a negative body image often have a greater need for physical stimulation. This may be because they did not receive adequate sensory or body stimulation as infants. Children who strike their hands together, twirl, or rock constantly may be attempting to provide themselves with the physical stimulation needed for development of an adequate body image.

Adolescence

Growth is one factor that leads to change in one's body image. Growth is very rapid during preadolescence and adolescence. Since it is difficult to ignore this growth, the adolescent is forced to change his body image. Physical changes in height, weight, and body build lead to a change in (1) the body image, (2) use of the body, and (3) the self-concept. Awkwardness due to rapid growth may lead to feelings of insecurity and inadequacy. Peer pressure to conform to body size and shape may lead to poor self-concept and a distorted body image in those who cannot conform.

Adulthood

A significant task of adulthood is intimacy. People attempt to further define themselves and their bodies through sexual experimentation. Intimacy can be accomplished without sexual relationships, however. When sexual union is not fused with psychological union, problems of body image and self-concept may develop.

Parenthood is a time in adulthood when body image and self-concept can be reaffirmed or threatened. Throughout pregnancy, the female must cope with the progressive changes in her body. First may come nausea and mood changes, altered sleep and voiding patterns, an enlarging abdomen, heartburn, enlarged breasts, increased weight, pigment changes and hemorrhoids.

When *quickening* occurs (first felt movement of the fetus) the female may have other problems; she may wonder if she can stretch enough to deliver the baby or if she can produce a healthy infant. The expectant father, too, can experience self-concept difficulties if his mate withdraws from him, becomes self-involved, or gives him less attention.

Middle Age

The middle-aged adult begins to notice body changes related to the *climacteric* or menopausal period. The climacteric is due to a decrease in estrogen production in the female, and physical changes leading to loss of strength, energy, and stamina in the male. The previous image of the self as young, strong, energetic, and attractive may become inadequate. Due to physical changes, the middle-aged person may feel inadequate in comparison to the young adult. Depression, irritability, and anxiety about sex roles often develop at this time. Feelings may be more related to sex role reactions than to actual physical changes. Attempts to try youthful cosmetics, clothes, hair styles, or plastic surgery may all be efforts to adapt to body changes.

At this time, the self-concept can be shaken when the middle-aged adult is unable to provide for others; for example, when children no longer need financial assistance from the parent. If job or work is unsatisfying, the person may suffer a decreased sense of self.

Later Years

The later years of life bring physical, social, economic, and emotional changes. Retirement and loss of a spouse and/or other significant people can influence self-concept. The decline of physical powers heightens fears of death and isolation. Wrinkles, loss or gain of hair, loss of teeth and taste, decreased strength, and misshapen knuckles, feet and nails can lead to a subjective view of ugliness.

Because of these changes, the elderly person may feel despair, frustration, or anger. Such feelings are especially common in persons whose self-concept is related to independence, strength, or attractiveness. Figure 26-3 summarizes some developmental changes that could influence body image and self-concept.

SITUATIONAL CHANGES AND BODY IMAGE

Situational changes include a wide range of experiences and can result in a changed body image. Some changes which will require nursing intervention

Developmental Period	Possible Body Image and Self-Concept Difficulties Can Develop Due to:
Infancy	Lack of adequate body and sensory stimulation. Lack of parental acceptance of body form or movement.
Childhood	Defective vision or hearing. Emotional conflict.
Adolescence	Rapid growth. Peer pressure to conform to body size or shape.
Adulthood	Fusion of sex and psychological aspects of intimacy. Pregnancy and motherhood. Fatherhood.
Middle Age	Psychological and physiological changes of the climacteric. Inability to provide for others. Unsatisfying job or work.
Later Years	Retirement. Loss of spouse. Decline of physical powers. Effects of aging.

Fig. 26-3 Developmental changes that could influence body image and self-concept.

include those changes due to accident and trauma; surgery; implants, artificial appliances and dialysis; chronic conditions; and hospitalization. Although other situational changes will not be dealt with here, the nurse is wise to remember that experiences such as divorce, graduation, and even promotion can also affect body image.

Accident and Trauma

Sudden blows or collisions such as car accidents can result in abrupt body changes; for example, severed legs or arms, scars, and bleeding are physically and emotionally stressful. Burns are especially traumatic; they occur unexpectedly and can lead to real difficulties. Accident or trauma can force adaptation to a new life-style. Body parts may be changed or deformed. The reactions of others to these body changes must also be dealt with by the victim. Even if there are no major body changes due to accident or trauma, body image and self-concept can be affected by the abrupt shock of the event.

Surgery

Planned surgery creates anxiety in most people. The idea of being out of control while under anesthesia, the fear of death, the anticipation of being cut and stitched or of losing a body part are all sources of anxiety. Unplanned surgery presents additional difficulties such as awaking after surgery to find a changed body.

Implants, Artificial Appliances, and Dialysis

Being given another person's heart or kidney is sure to bring about physical and psychological stress. Artificial appliances may be difficult to incorporate into the body image. People who require artificial limbs, hip pinnings, ileostomy or colostomy bags and drains may react negatively, not only to the new smells, sensations, and movements, but also to the necessary change in body image. Patients who require kidney dialysis or other procedures on a regular basis may have severe emotional reactions to these procedures. Body image is affected when the person requires constant help to maintain body processes. Once an artificial appliance becomes part of the body image, the patient may become quite anxious if the appliance is removed. Whenever the nurse removes a patient's false teeth, artificial eye or limb, or bowel or bladder appliance, it is important to remember that such losses may create anxiety because the change threatens an established body image.

Chronic Conditions

Coronary heart disease, stroke, multiple sclerosis, arthritis, and cancer are long-term processes that may require constant adaptation to body changes. Many long-term illnesses bring more and more restrictions to daily activities as their course progresses. In addition, some chronic illnesses may seem to improve and allow more activity, only to recur and restrict movement again. Such changes require constant body image adaptations.

Obesity is another chronic body state that can create a disturbed body image; when it occurs in adolescence, especially, body image disturbances are more likely to take place. Besides adjusting to viewing oneself, an obese person must also contend with the reactions of other people.

Hospitalization

The enforced dependency of hospitalization and the intrusive physical procedures such as enemas and bedpans can create guilt and embarrassment.

Procedures or interpersonal relationships that create negative feelings in the patient are prone to disturb body image and self-concept. Restriction of activity and enforced immobilization remove the usual channels for emotional discharge through motor activity. Therefore, the child and adult patient must find other ways to express their feelings. A variety of coping devices may be used, depending on the personality and the interpersonal situations which are available. Figure 26-4 summarizes some situational changes that can influence body image and self-concept.

NURSING ASSESSMENT

Nursing assessment is based on an effective nurse-patient relationship. The assessment should include:

- The significance of body image alteration
- The stage in grief process and failure to grieve
- The expected male and female reactions to body changes
- The Draw-a-Person test

Situational Change	Examples
Accident and trauma	sudden blow or concussion car accident severe burns
Surgery	fear of being out of control while under anesthesia fear of death fear of being cut or stitched fear of losing a body part awakening after surgical amputation of a body part
Implants, Artificial Appliances and Dialysis	heart or kidney transplant artificial limb ileostomy colostomy kidney dialysis removal of appliance which has been incorporated into patient's body image
Chronic conditions	coronary heart disease stroke multiple sclerosis arthritis cancer obesity
Hospitalization	enforced dependency intrusive physical procedures

Fig. 26-4 Some situational changes that can influence body image and self-concept.

The Nurse-Patient Relationship

Establishing a therapeutic relationship involves the nurse's ability to give of self without expecting anything in return. There are a number of factors which can interfere with this relationship. The major factor is often the nurse's own fears, dread, and feelings of anxiety about developmental and situational body changes. When the nurse is unaware of her own feelings, disgust, revulsion, sadness, or anger may be communicated nonverbally to the patient.

Anxiety can be aroused by feelings of inadequacy and helplessness when viewing the patient with major body changes. If the nurse deals with anxiety by using anger, sarcasm, teasing, joking, or withdrawal, the therapeutic relationship cannot be maintained. Forcing the patient to be pleasant and cooperative or interfering with the patient's attempts at independence are measures that meet the nurse's need, but not necessarily the patient's.

There is a tendency for some health personnel to ignore the patient with a long-term illness because his symptoms are no longer interesting. As a result, he is likely to feel rejected. Rejection often leads to withdrawal or to increased demands for care. Patients who become more demanding may run the risk of being called problem patients. A study of the patients who are ignored or considered to be problems may help to identify those who have difficulties with body image and self-concept.

The nurse can also assess her own reactions to body changes which are the result of developmental or situational experiences. Talking about such thoughts and feelings with other trusted health personnel can provide a release. Feelings can also be constructively expressed through artistic productions such as poetry, painting or writing. Physical action such as jogging, doing a task, or walking will also afford an outlet.

The use of open-ended questions and observation of overall behavior will furnish the nurse with insight about the patient's self-concept. Discussion topics that are brought up frequently by the patient and his omission of important topics are both clues for the nurse.

The patient will also be watching the nurse. He will observe to see how she reacts to body changes he has undergone. The patient may wonder whether the nurse thinks he is still a worthwhile person despite his body changes. Lack of eye contact from the nurse to the patient, stares, wrinkling the nose, and other nonverbal communications that convey unworthiness can decrease the patient's self-esteem.

Significance of Body Image Alteration

In order to evaluate the effect of the alteration or change, several factors must be considered. The developmental stage, the onset, and the location are aspects to consider in the assessment. Body image alterations are assessed in a number of ways.

The nurse evaluates whether the alteration occurred at birth or very early in the patient's life. Such alterations generally present fewer body image difficulties than alterations that occur at adolescence or later.

The nurse evaluates whether the body alteration was gradual or abrupt. Abrupt changes challenge homeostasis more seriously than do gradual ones.

The nurse evaluates the location of body changes. Changes on the body surface are more visible and thus are more apt to create body image problems. Body changes which affect the patient's social, sexual, or economic roles are more likely to upset homeostasis than body changes which are unrelated to important role performances.

Stage in Grief Process and Failure to Grieve

Common reactions to a change in body function or loss of a body part include sadness, anger, disgust, guilt, and revulsion. The change or loss may be generalized and the patient feels *he* is unable to function just because part of him is malfunctioning.

There are individual differences in the degree of reaction to a body change. The amount of hurt experienced by the person depends on the value the person has placed on the body part. Not everyone will perceive the same loss or change in the same way.

Feelings may be generalized and then projected. If the patient feels he is repulsive because he has a colostomy, he will probably feel that others are repulsed by the colostomy also.

The patient reacts to a change or loss by passing through the same stages as a person who grieves the loss of a significant other person or who grieves his own upcoming death. The nurse must assess whether the patient is in the shock, disbelief or denial stage. The anger or guilt stage may be evident by the patient's statements such as "Why me?" or "I must have done something bad to deserve this."

When the stage of acceptance begins, the patient may begin to peek at the dressing or surgical site, or to feel the amputation stump. The patient may also repeat his perceptions of the loss or change over and over; this is an effort to resolve his feelings. The patient will probably ask the same questions over and over about what happened to him, what is happening now, and what to anticipate in relation to healing, family relationships, work, sex, and leisure activities.

The nurse is especially careful to study those patients who do not outwardly react to body changes or losses. Failure to grieve can hinder recovery and the patient's ability to resolve losses. The grieving process is necessary if the patient is to develop a stable, consistent body image and self-concept.

Expected Male and Female Reactions

Generally, females have a more stable body image than males. Females have a more definite sense of body boundaries than males; perhaps they devote more attention to their bodies.

It is culturally more acceptable for the middle-class white male to control the expression of his feelings yet he probably has greater anxiety about situations that may threaten body image. Because male patients may control their open expression of anxiety more carefully, the nurse must be even more observant of nonverbal behavior and act accordingly.

The Draw-a-Person Test

With children, the Draw-a-Person Test may be the most useful way to evaluate body image disturbances. The child is given a piece of paper and drawing materials and told to "draw yourself." The picture can then be compared with self-drawings to determine if a body image disturbance exists. Several books of children's self-drawings are available at college libraries and psychology departments. Students and new nursing practitioners are wise to share their thoughts about self-drawings with more experienced personnel before making any definite formalized assessments. Observe figures 26-5 and 26-6, page 412, and decide which drawing indicates a body image disturbance.

NURSING INTERVENTION

Major nursing interventions which may be successfully used include:

- Provide anticipatory guidance
- Assist with grief work
- Counteract effects of deprivation and immobilization
- Demonstrate respect for the patient as a person
- Help the patient to understand and learn from his experiences

Patients who have difficulties in body image and self-concept respond to interventions which are directed toward achieving adaptation to change and acceptance of the self.

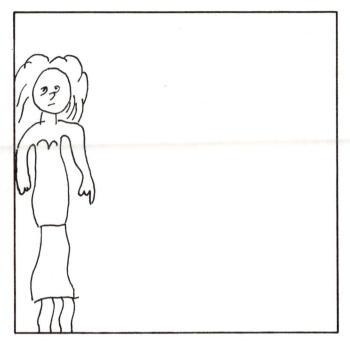

Fig. 26-5 Simulated drawing by 12-year-old girl. What does the picture
tell you about body image clarity and boundaries?

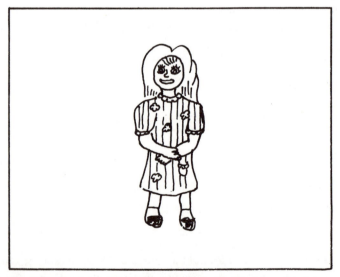

Fig. 26-6 Simulated drawing by 9-year-old girl. What does the picture
tell you about body image clarity and boundaries?

Anticipatory Guidance

Anticipatory guidance is a preventive intervention in potential crisis situations. People are prepared to cope with upcoming situations through discussion and problem solving before the situation actually occurs. Anticipatory guidance can be helpful not only for the patient but also for the expectant father, the family of a patient about to have surgery, and the friends of an adolescent involved in a car accident. Anticipatory guidance may provide a good foundation for effective grief work.

Assisting With Grief Work

The nurse allows the patient to deny his loss and to refuse to look at the changed body part. Continued acceptance is conveyed to the patient through direct eye contact; interest in talking about the patient's concerns when he is ready is also conveyed.

In the anger stage, the nurse accepts the anger. She realizes that although the patient sometimes directs anger toward the nurse, the anger is really about the body change. When the patient begins to show signs of accepting the body change, the nurse can assist him to examine and become familiar with the change. For example, the nurse might say, "Your stoma is clean and healing well," or "The line where your stitches were is right here below your arm."

Counteracting the Effects of Deprivation and Immobilization

Sensory deprivation or sensory overload can both lead to body image difficulties. One of the ways people know *who* they are is by knowing *where* they are in relation to their external environment. Overstimulation or understimulation can lead to feelings of unreality. The nurse can help provide the necessary stimulation to maintain a consistent body image by giving backrubs and asking the adult patient to participate in his care. Play activities can furnish children with important sensory stimulation and information about their bodies. Simple games like "Where is your nose? Here is your nose!", or "Where is your toe? Here is your toe!" can be carried out when bathing the child. Mirrors and verbal feedback can provide other useful information the patient needs to maintain a stable body image. Contact with the self is an important means of developing and maintaining body image. Patients should not be discouraged from touching or viewing themselves unless these behaviors are contraindicated for some other reason.

Treating the Patient as a Person

Nurses are likely to overemphasize physical malfunction and focus attention on it; this may cause the patient to feel fragmented and unwhole. When a series of doctors and nurses examine the same malfunctioning aspects and ask the same questions, there may be a greater sense of fragmentation. One way to avoid this sensation by the patient is to assign one nurse to his care. She should write the nursing history and be primarily assigned to that patient throughout his stay.

Children deserve respect and explanations for procedures just as adults do. Nurses should treat them with the same consideration shown to adults.

Area of assessment	Examples of questions to consider
Nurse-patient relationship	Does the nurse expect certain returns that have not been communicated to the patient? Is the nurse aware of his or her own fears, dread, and anxiety about developmental or situational changes? What outlets does the nurse use for these feelings? Does the nurse use anger, sarcasm, teasing, joking, or withdrawal to deal with anxiety? Does the nurse ignore the patient with a chronic condition? What topics does the patient omit and overfocus on? What nonverbal clues does the nurse convey to the patient about body changes?
Significance of body image alteration	Did the alteration occur at birth or after adolescence? Is the body alteration gradual or abrupt? Where is the body change located?
Stage in grief	Is there a failure to grieve? Is the patient in shock, denial, anger, guilt, or acceptance? Does the patient assume the nurse is repulsed by body changes?
Expected male-female reactions	Is the patient male or female? Does the male patient show less expression of feeling?
Draw-a-Person Test	Does the child draw an age appropriate figure drawing of himself?

Fig. 26-7 Nursing assessments for body image and self-concept difficulties

Intervention	Examples
Anticipatory guidance	Discuss upcoming situations with patient and family. Assist with problem solving.
Grief work	Give acceptance through direct eye contact, and by being available to talk with patient. Accept anger of patient. Help patient to explore and discuss body changes.
Counteracting effects of deprivation and immobilization	Give backrubs. Ask patient to participate in own care. Play body exploration games with children. Provide mirrors and verbal feedback about patient's body. Allow self-contact with body unless contra-indicated.
Treating patient as person	Assign one nurse to work with a patient. Give explanations of procedures to both adults and children.
Helping patient to learn	Observe for need to clarify or re-explain procedures or experiences. Participate with child in structured play experiences. Demonstrate procedures using appropriate methods and materials. Provide successful role models.

Fig. 26-8 Nursing interventions for body image and self-concept difficulties

Helping the Patient to Understand and Learn From Experiences

Patients need to have clear explanations of past, present, and future treatments. Explanations can be told to the patient, written down for him, shown to him through pictures, or equipment can be used to demonstrate information. During these learning experiences, the nurse observes for evidence that the patient needs clarification or is anxious about some aspect of the experience.

Children can learn through play. Dolls can be used to demonstrate surgical procedures or body changes. Materials that the child is familiar with, such as facial tissues or tape, can be used to demonstrate more complicated procedures in a simple way.

Children who seem upset can also use dolls, clay, or other materials to express their anxiety or anger. The student or new graduate nurse may require additional learning and supervision in play therapy with children.

Patients with visible handicaps can be offered the opportunity to talk with or observe others who have successfully dealt with the same handicap. Such opportunities should be available only when the patient is capable of learning. When signs of acceptance and a decrease in anxiety are apparent, the patient is ready to learn from a successful role model. Figures 26-7 and 26-8 summarize nursing assessments and interventions for body image and self-concept difficulties.

SUMMARY

Body image is the mental picture a person develops of his biological self. Self-concept is a term used to refer to the feelings and attitudes a person has towards his social, moral, and spiritual self. Definite and consistent body image and self-concept seem to be related to positive mental and physical health.

Any body change can result in problems with defining the body image and self-concept. These changes can be either normal developmental changes or unexpected situations such as accidents, surgery, chronic conditions, or hospitalization.

Nursing assessment is based on a therapeutic nurse-patient relationship. It includes assessing the significance of body image alteration, stage in the grief process, sex of the patient, and the Draw-a-Person Test. Nursing intervention includes providing anticipatory guidance, assisting with grief work, counteracting effects of deprivation and immobilization, treating the patient as a person, and helping the patient to understand and learn from his experiences.

ACTIVITIES AND DISCUSSION TOPICS

- Write down a list of at least five characteristics that you think describe you. Try to think of how this concept you have of yourself has developed.

- Draw a picture of yourself. What does the picture tell you about your body image and self-concept?

- Spend several hours pretending you have one of the following body image changes:

  (1) blindness – wear dark glasses and use a cane.

  (2) inability to walk – use a wheelchair or crutches.

  (3) deafness – place earplugs in your ears.

  (4) loss of important body possessions – if you usually wear jewelry, makeup, or a certain type of clothes, wear no jewelry or makeup and wear a different type of clothing to your next important social activity.

  (5) lisp or use another speech impediment – practice speaking only with the speech impediment chosen.

  Observe how others react toward you, and what your thoughts and feelings are during these hours.

REVIEW

A. Multiple Choice. Select the best answers. Questions have more than one answer.

    1. Situational changes which affect body image include
       a. surgery.   c. menopause.
       b. graduation.   d. divorce.

    2. The child who feels his body fails to come up to parental expectations frequently develops
       a. an indefinite body image.   c. a feeling of shame.
       b. a stereotyped body image.   d. a poor self-concept.

    3. A person who does not have a stable and definite body image can have
       a. difficulty maintaining homeostasis.
       b. severe anxiety.
       c. difficulty in relating to other people.
       d. low self-esteem.

    4. A person's body image may include his
       a. clothing.   c. eye glasses.
       b. posture.   d. artificial appliance.

    5. In order to maintain a therapeutic relationship with the patient who has experienced a major body change, the nurse must not
       a. interfere with the patient's attempts at independence.
       b. force the patient to cooperate.
       c. use inappropriate body language.
       d. tease or joke about the situation.

B. Match the developmental period in Column II with the developmental changes that could influence body image and self-concept in Column I.

Column I	Column II
1. Lack of adequate body and sensory stimulation; lack of parental acceptance of body form or movement.	a. adolescence b. adulthood c. childhood
2. Defective vision or hearing; emotional conflict.	d. infancy e. later years f. middle years
3. Rapid growth; peer pressure to conform to body size or shape.	
4. Fusion of sex and psychological aspects of intimacy.	
5. Psychological and physiological changes of the climacteric; inability to provide for others.	
6. Decline of physical powers.	

C. Briefly answer the following questions.

1. Define body image.

2. State how body image is related to self-concept.

3. List four nursing interventions used to enhance body image and self-concept.

4. List three areas of nursing assessment in body image difficulties.

5. Explain the purpose of anticipatory guidance.

D. Prepare nursing care plans focused on the problem of body image, for the following patients.

1. Mrs. A., who went to surgery for a removal of what was thought to be a benign cyst in her left breast, is returning from surgery after having had a radical mastectomy.

2. Johnny R., an infant, whose mother supports him incorrectly when holding him, never makes eye contact with him, and constantly finds flaws in his appearance.

3. Elizabeth C., a two-year-old who lost her sight yesterday as a result of a car accident.

4. Hector G., age 14, who has one undescended testicle.

5. April R., a teenager who is pregnant but is not married.

6. Mrs. R., a mother whose children are all in college, is entering menopause.

7. Mr. G., age 48, who tells you he is "gay, but happy" despite the fact that his male lover recently left him "for a younger guy."

8. Samantha U., age 15, who lives in a communal setting with other lesbian mothers.

9. Mr. B., age 42, is admitted for vague physical complaints. He tells you he wonders if he has chosen the right profession; he wonders if his marriage will work, and asks for advice on how to "meet young chicks."

10. Mr. W., age 62, is in the hospital for a prostatectomy. He confides in you that he suspects this will be difficult for his love life. He also tells you he will be retiring next week from a job he has held for 30 years.

11. Mr. C., age 21, refuses to participate in Lamaze classes with his pregnant wife. He has started to drink excessively. You meet him in the emergency room of the hospital where he has been brought by the police after a fight in a bar. He keeps insisting the pregnancy was his wife's fault and that he doesn't "want any little brats in my house!".

SECTION 5
THE
LEARNING
PROCESS

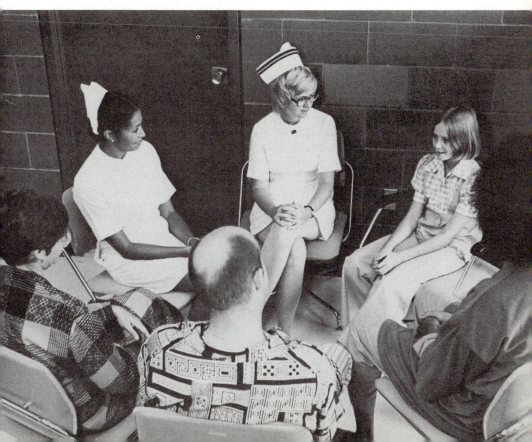

chapter 27
NURSING
CONFERENCES

STUDENT OBJECTIVES

- List four purposes of the preconference.
- List five purposes of the postconference.
- Identify ways that evaluation conferences are used effectively as learning tools.
- List four reasons that adequate clinical supervision and supervised clinical nursing conferences are important to the new graduate nurse.
- Match nursing skill evaluation examples with the appropriate evaluation area.

Nursing conferences span a wide range of activities. The student nurse will probably be involved in conferences before and after giving patient care. These conferences are held with the instructor and fellow students. Other conferences which may be attended by students are evaluation conferences and patient planning conferences with other nursing personnel.

The graduate nurse will participate in nursing conferences to plan and evaluate patient care. Conferences which teach and supervise new graduate nurses in the care of patients is an example of this kind of nursing conference.

THE PRECONFERENCE

Prior to giving care to patients each day, the instructor and students gather for a *preconference.* This nursing conference combines group discussion with planning of nursing care. One purpose of such a conference is to provide the specific focus for learning based on the objectives set up by the instructor. For example, if lectures that week have been presented on orientation to the hospital environment or on the need for food and fluid, the clinical conferences and learning experiences should focus on those areas.

Another purpose of the preconference is to begin to analyze nurse-patient experiences. The instructor might ask questions about possible situations that may be encountered on the ward or may provide students with written objectives for the day.

A third purpose of the preconference is to define the limit and scope of nursing practice. Medical orders and interventions may be separated from nursing orders and interventions at this time. The student may be cautioned not to go ahead with some nursing measure unless the doctor has written a specific order to give that care (for example, giving fluids to a patient who has been vomiting). Another purpose of the preconference is to reinforce the idea that nursing care must be based on nursing process. Nursing care is analyzed and organized based on scientific principles and theory. Nursing goals are based on needs such as improving circulation, not on tasks such as giving a bedbath.

Preconferences are most effective when they are prepared for in advance. Students are often given their assignments the day before they are to give patient care. During this time, the student can read, think, and plan for the next day's care.

Sometimes it is impossible for the instructor to plan objectives that can be met by all students. For example, there may be only two patients available who have the health problems that fit well with the current learning objectives. However, students should prepare for the objectives as if they will be met in the next day's clinical experience. This activity will enhance learning in three ways: (1) the student will learn scientific principles and theory that are applicable to other clinical situations, (2) the student will be better prepared to contribute to the postconference discussion, and (3) the student will be better prepared for examinations which test professional knowledge.

THE POSTCONFERENCE

The *postconference* is a purposeful discussion that follows the clinical laboratory experience.

- Scientific principles and theory are correlated with actual clinical practice in the care of patients.
- Constructive discussion about the clinical experience will enhance learning.

- Guidelines for providing nursing care are identified during the postconference.

- The students' thoughts and feelings are clarified.

- Focus is kept on patients, staff, students and instructors as people with needs.

A postconference is not just a report of what happened on the ward. The postconference is an attempt to understand the meaning of the clinical experience. Some questions that are useful to ask in postconferences are shown in figure 27-1. The student may notice that the questions are very similar to the *who-what-when-where* questions used in therapeutic communication with the patient. This is because the process used by the nurse is the same; its purpose is to develop understanding. The correct answer is not the important part of the discussion. How the response is obtained and what the answer means is the primary aim of postconferences, as it is in nurse-patient communication.

While on the ward, it may be useful to jot down examples of experiences that could be discussed later. Three factors which have been found to be dealt with most effectively in postconferences are:

- The nursing care given to a patient or to a group of patients.

- The role of the nurse or student nurse in relation to other members of the health team.

- Any highly emotional reaction that occurred while the student was on the ward.

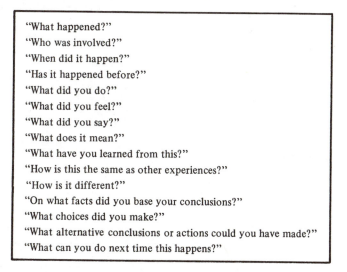

"What happened?"
"Who was involved?"
"When did it happen?"
"Has it happened before?"
"What did you do?"
"What did you feel?"
"What did you say?"
"What does it mean?"
"What have you learned from this?"
"How is this the same as other experiences?"
"How is it different?"
"On what facts did you base your conclusions?"
"What choices did you make?"
"What alternative conclusions or actions could you have made?"
"What can you do next time this happens?"

Fig. 27-1 A postconference can be more productive by asking these questions.

Strong emotional reactions to ward experiences are best brought up at the beginning of the postconference. If the student is preoccupied with strong feelings, it will be impossible for her to learn from the experiences of other students. There is a tendency for students to be anxious or shy about these emotional reactions and to think that others will not understand or be interested. Actually, the other members of the group are supportive and interested because they, too, have had strong emotional reactions to the same or a similar episode. As with other experiences, it is important not only to verbalize the feelings but also to understand what happened. The questions in figure 27-1 will also be helpful in understanding emotional reactions.

At first the student may experience anxiety when participating in preconferences and postconferences. In time, the initial anxiety about sharing experiences will pass and the student will realize that this type of nursing conference can be useful.

Figure 27-2 is a sample laboratory guide which may be used for clinical experiences. Such guides can help to focus goals in preparing for clinical assignments as well as assist in postconference discussions.

SAMPLE LABORATORY GUIDE
NURSING DEPARTMENT

Laboratory #1

Orientation to the Hospital Ward

Objectives:
1. To become familiar with objects and people on the hospital ward.
2. To develop beginning priorities for patient care.
3. To practice communication techniques.

Learning Experiences:
1. Participate in orientation to the hospital ward.
2. Talk informally with nursing staff members about their roles
3. Assignment to a patient to work with this week.
4. Read patient chart and Kardex.
5. Begin to develop a nursing care plan for the patient.
6. Do a ten-minute process recording with the patient.

Questions for Postconference:
1. What experiences created anxiety in you today?
2. What satisfying experiences did you have?
3. What resources were used to help to orient you to the ward today?
4. What objects or people do you still have questions about?
5. What parts of the patient's record and communication helped you to become aware of patient needs?
6. What aspects of the nurse care plan did you have difficulty with?

Fig. 27-2 A laboratory guide can help the student to prepare and learn from clinical experiences.

EVALUATION CONFERENCES

While the student is obtaining clinical experience, the instructor continues to take notes to assist in the evaluation of student progress. These detailed notes with specific examples will also help the student to know where further learning is necessary. Students are usually asked to participate in evaluating what has been learned for particular experiences or courses. Most of the time evaluation conferences are held between the student and the clinical instructor on a one-to-one basis. These conferences should be held several times during a semester so the student will have a chance to improve needed nursing skills. If the student does not receive adequate feedback about her performance, she should actively seek out such evaluations. Student nurses may be evaluated on nursing skills and abilities such as: observation, perception and communication skills; nursing process and nursing care planning skills; health team member skills; and learning abilities. Figure 27-3, pages 428 and 429, illustrates a sample evaluation form.

PATIENT PLANNING CONFERENCES

Part or all of the nursing staff may hold patient planning conferences to plan for total patient care. Attendance at such conferences can be a beneficial learning experience. Some patient planning conferences include the patient. Often, the nursing staff will meet before the patient is included in their discussion in order to discuss patient care problems and nursing interventions. When the patient is asked to join the nursing conference, valuable information may be obtained about patient needs which were overlooked, unexpressed or unavailable. Participation by the patient can contribute to the effectiveness of the conference by providing:

- Feedback for the evaluation step in the nursing process
- Identification of nurse feelings or stereotyped attitudes toward the patient
- Observation of the patient's interpersonal skills in a group setting
- Opportunity for the nurse to practice group skills
- An increase in self-esteem and self-actualization through joint planning
- A sharing of needs that may have been overlooked
- Opportunities for nurses to learn more about specific nursing care and patient needs

Figure 27-4, page 430, shows how patient participation in nursing conferences can aid in both patient and nurse learning.

SAMPLE STUDENT NURSE EVALUATION FORM

Student _____ Nursing Course _____ Date _____ Instructor _____

Nursing Skill or ability	Instructor's evaluation				
	functions independently	needs some help	needs moderate supervision	needs intensive or frequent supervision	was not observed
Observation, perception, and communication					
Separates observations from perceptions example:					
Makes pertinent observations example:					
Records clearly, completely, accurately example:					
Focuses on patient during conversation example:					
Identifies communication skills and blocks to communication example:					
Participates in pre and postconferences example:					
Reports errors or omissions in patient care example:					
Reports off to nurse in charge example:					
Nursing process and nursing care plan					
Identifies patient's needs example:					

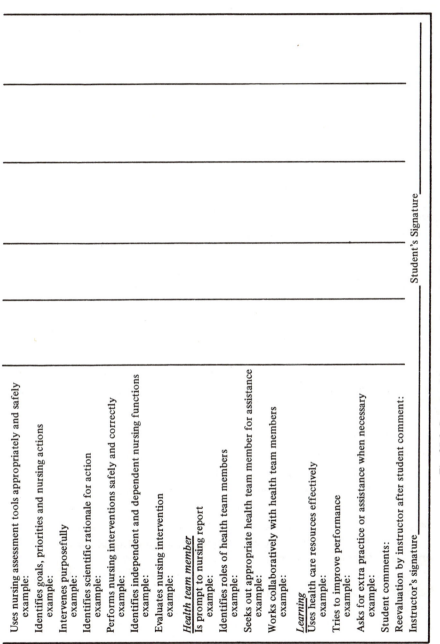

Uses nursing assessment tools appropriately and safely
example:
Identifies goals, priorities and nursing actions
example:
Intervenes purposefully
example:
Identifies scientific rationale for action
example:
Performs nursing interventions safely and correctly
example:
Identifies independent and dependent nursing functions
example:
Evaluates nursing intervention
example:

Health team member
Is prompt to nursing report
example:
Identifies roles of health team members
example:
Seeks out appropriate health team member for assistance
example:
Works collaboratively with health team members
example:

Learning
Uses health care resources effectively
example:
Tries to improve performance
example:
Asks for extra practice or assistance when necessary
example:

Student comments:
Reevaluation by instructor after student comment:
Instructor's signature

Student's Signature

Fig. 27-3 Sample of form to use for evaluating student progress.

NURSE-PATIENT CONFERENCES	
How the patient can help or be helped	Examples
Provide feedback to the nurse	Shares patient perceptions of nursing care, such as, "That nightlight really helped me."
Help identify nurses' stereotyped attitudes or feelings	Disproves ideas that the patient is too weak, shaky or noncommunicative to participate by actually participating
Observe interpersonal skills	Gives the nurse important clues about how the patient might function in family, work, learning, therapy, or social groups
Practice group skills	Allows the nurse to practice leading or participating in a group
Teach	Tells the patient how nurses can be of help to patients; for example, "Mr. Smith will spend 10 minutes with you twice a day to discuss your pain."
Increase self-esteem and promote self-actualization	Allows the patient to feel competent to help the nurse, such as, "You've told us some things we didn't know before."
Share needs	Tells the nurses about needs and preferences that were overlooked or have just emerged, such as, "I just started to have trouble sleeping."

Fig. 27-4 Patients and nurses can work together in conferences to improve patient care.

IN-SERVICE EDUCATION CONFERENCES

In-service education is a term used to describe on-the-job learning experiences that are structured to meet the needs of the employed nurse. The associate degree nurse usually requires more technical supervision than other nursing graduates. This is because associate degree nursing students have only two years to become proficient in nursing skills while other nursing students have three or four years. All new nursing graduates require some in-service education and supervision. Although some hospitals provide in-service education there are many that do not. When seeking employment, graduate nurses should ask about and express strong support for adequate clinical supervision and clinical nursing conferences.

Some of the reasons adequate supervision and structured clinical nursing conferences are important are:

- All needed nursing skills have not been developed to their highest level of performance.

- In order to increase the nurse's self-esteem and confidence, new graduates must be adequately prepared before attempting to carry out unfamiliar procedures.
- New graduate nurses who attempt procedures without adequate training and supervision are legally liable for the outcomes.
- Theory will become more clearly related to practice when adequate practice is accompanied by discussion of theory application.

SUMMARY

Nursing conferences span a wide range of activities. Students participate most actively in preconferences and postconferences. Preconferences prepare the student for learning in the clinical practice area. Postconferences help the student to understand and solve problems about clinical experiences. The student will participate in self-evaluation on a one-to-one basis with his or her instructor. Students may be allowed to attend nursing conferences held by the nursing staff. Some of these nursing conferences include patients as active participants in planning and evaluating care. Graduate nurses can continue to learn by asking for and participating in the in-service program; learning experiences and adequately supervised clinical nursing conferences should be planned for maximum benefit. Such on-the-job experiences are important for personal, professional, and legal reasons.

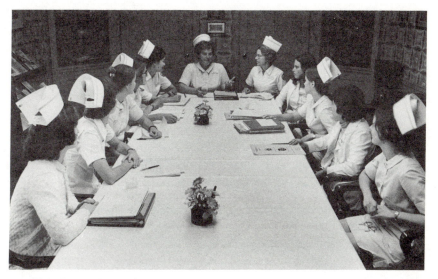

Fig. 27-5 The nursing conference combines group discussion with the planning of nursing care.

ACTIVITIES AND DISCUSSION TOPICS

- After participating in several preconferences and postconferences with your instructor and fellow students, answer the following questions.

    a. Were any or all of the purposes you read about carried out? If not, what do you think prevented them from being carried out? What could you do to make the preconference or postconference a more effective learning experience?

    b. What strong emotional reactions to clinical experiences did you have but did not share with the group? What prevented you from sharing? What can you do differently next time?

- After taking part in student-instructor evaluations of your clinical experience, think of ways you could have participated more openly or constructively in the evaluation. What might have prevented you from doing so?

- Talk with several nurses regarding their thoughts and feelings about including patients in their planning conferences. Discuss benefits that might be gained from including patients.

- Talk with one or two nursing personnel about their in-service experiences. What can you learn from them about the kind of job setting you might want to choose?

REVIEW

A. Multiple Choice. Select the best answer(s). Some questions have more than one answer.

1. Participation by the patient in a patient planning conference can provide

    a. feedback for evaluating the nursing process.

    b. opportunity for the student to discuss strong emotional reactions.

    c. opportunity for the nurse to practice group skills.

    d. increased self-esteem and self-actualization.

2. Evaluation conferences are effective learning tools when the

    a. instructor hands out student evaluations before class.

    b. student evaluates what has been learned from particular experiences.

    c. instructor gives detailed examples of areas in which the student needs practice.

    d. conference is held on a one-to-one basis.

3. An on-the-job learning experience that is structured to meet the needs of the nurse is
    a. an evaluation conference.
    b. an in-service education conference.
    c. a patient planning conference.
    d. a postconference.

4. A laboratory guide can help to focus goals in preparing for
    a. clinical assignments.
    b. postconference discussions.
    c. both of the above.
    d. neither of the above.

B. Match the evaluation *area* in Column II to the appropriate nursing skill evaluation *example* in Column I. Each area in Column II is used more than once.

Column I	Column II
1. Focuses on patient during conversation.	a. health team member skills
2. Uses nursing assessment tools appropriately and safely.	b. learning abilities
3. Asks for extra practice or assistance when necessary.	c. nursing process and nursing care planning skills.
4. Tries to improve performance.	d. observation, perception and communication skills
5. Records clearly, completely, and accurately.	
6. Identifies roles of health team members.	
7. Identifies scientific rationale for action.	
8. Seeks out appropriate health team members for assistance.	

C. Briefly answer the following questions.

1. List four purposes of the preconference.

2. List five purposes of the postconference.

3. List four reasons adequate clinical supervision and supervised clinical nursing conferences are important to the new graduate nurse.

4. Name three factors that are dealt with effectively in postconferences.

chapter 28
LEARNING
THROUGH TEACHING

STUDENT OBJECTIVES

- Identify the relationship between learning and health.
- List eight areas of learning to be assessed.
- List the five steps included in the teaching-learning process.
- Differentiate between positive reinforcement and negative reinforcement.

Teaching has always been a part of nursing. With the increase of scientific knowledge and demands from a better-informed public, nurses need to be even more adept at teaching than ever before. Teaching and learning can be thought of as a process. In order to teach, one must first learn. Nurses teach what they have learned. Likewise, patients who have learned may teach other patients, family members, and, in some cases, nurses. In short, nurses and patients teach one another. The process is not limited to the nurse as instructor and expert in all things.

There is an expanded interest in the importance of learning as related to health. Some communication and behavioral difficulties appear to be based on faulty learning. Many psychiatric patients have apparently never learned appropriate ways to interact with others.

LEARNING AND HEALTH

Learning can influence preventative health measures. Learning about factors which seem to be associated with heart conditions may influence decisions about inactivity, inappropriate diet and whether to continue smoking. Learning about genetic factors can influence the decision of parents to risk producing a physically imperfect infant.

Learning can be used to influence biological functions that were previously thought to be under involuntary control. Through biofeedback, people have been taught to slow down the pulse and respiration, to lower blood pressure, to end a migraine headache, and to minimize menstrual difficulties.

The nurse has the potential to influence the health status of people because she is considered an expert in this area. People can be influenced by formal teaching and by the informal comments made to patients and families. The nurse also teaches by setting an example in the way she acts, looks, and communicates. A nurse who is overweight, smokes, uses alcohol or drugs unwisely, or is unable to communicate clearly cannot hope to reinforce healthy behavior in others. By practicing healthy behavior, the nurse serves as a *role model* for patients. Role models demonstrate through their actions how to act effectively; they do not necessarily have to talk about the matter.

ASSESSING LEARNING STATUS

Everyone has strengths, weaknesses, and difficulties which should be considered and utilized if the learning process is to be truly effective. Therefore, when preparing to teach or learn, the student assesses the level of readiness, prior learning, meaningfulness of material, need for repetition, degree of participation in learning, and how self-pacing, feedback and reinforcement might be used.

Readiness

No matter how crucial the instructor's assignment is or how important it is for the patient to learn a task, no learning will take place unless the learner (either student or patient) is ready to learn. It is not unusual to overhear nurses making comments such as, "I taught Mr. Nelson to care for his colostomy but he never does it." Until the learner – in this case, Mr. Nelson – is ready to recognize that it is important to learn, no learning occurs. The instructor or nurse may attempt to teach but the student or patient must be ready to learn.

One of the factors that influences readiness to learn is strong feeling. If the student or patient is highly anxious, fearful, guilty, angry, or depressed, his readiness is decreased. The student who tries to study when experiencing strong feelings will often have difficulty learning the material. When trying to teach patients, the nurse can assess the level of strong feeling in the patient and use appropriate communication skills to reduce the intensity and then establish a working nurse-patient relationship.

Another factor that influences readiness is debility. Examples of debilitating circumstances are pain, weakness, fatigue, thirst, and lack of oxygen. If the patient or nurse suffers from any of these problems, learning is unlikely to occur.

Prior Learning

Before attempting to teach a patient, the nurse finds out what the patient already knows about the subject. More patients now read about illness processes and some are more sophisticated about medical and nursing treatment. Spending long periods of time reviewing material the patient already knows is not only a waste of valuable time but can also be boring. Bored learners often stop listening to the teacher. Once the learner has lost interest it may be difficult to regain it.

Prior learning can be assessed in a number of ways. If the material to be taught includes learning a task, the nurse can ask the patient to demonstrate the task. For example, the nurse might say, "Show me how you irrigate your colostomy and I'll help you if you need it." By observing the patient, the nurse can decide what the patient knows and what the patient needs to be taught.

Another way to assess prior learning is to ask the patient to tell the nurse what he knows. For example, the nurse might say to a patient with diabetes, "Tell me what you know about your diet," and then amplify the particular point which needs further clarification; for example, food exchange.

Still another way to assess prior learning is to use a written method to evaluate what has been learned. As a student, your instructor may give you a *pretest* to determine if you already know the material about to be taught. Pretests can be checklists or fill-in the blanks, multiple choice or essay type questions. The idea is to find the simplest, most efficient way to discover what the learner already knows. Nurses can use written pretests to evaluate what the patient already knows. Some patients may have difficulty reading or writing. The nurse should evaluate the patient's ability in this area so as not to embarrass him.

Meaningful Data

People learn more easily when the material to be learned is meaningful to them. Highly technical terms and unexplained complex tasks are apt to lack meaning for the patient. The nurse must use words that fit the patient's educational level and cultural group.

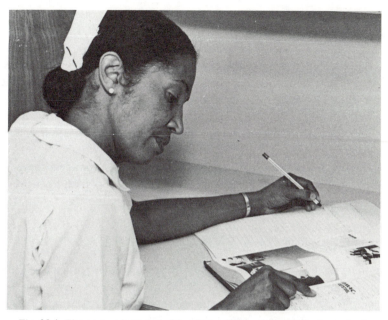

Fig. 28-1 The nurse selects materials which will be meaningful to the patient.

To be meaningful, the material should be related to prior learning. Material to be learned is most likely to be remembered if it continues on where the previous learning left off. The way material is presented can increase its meaning for the learner. The nurse assesses the method or methods of learning most appropriate for the learner, figure 28-1. For example, people who cannot read would not be given written materials. Likewise, people who have hearing or visual problems would probably not be given audiovisual materials. The nurse can also ask the patient what learning method he has found works best for him.

Repetition

Repetition enhances the ability to learn. This can be illustrated by examining how anxiety, newness, or complexity make repetition necessary. In cases of anxiety brought on by their current experience, patients and students may miss the information being taught for the first time; they are thinking about or responding to anxiety-provoking elements in their current situation. For example, a patient who is about to have surgery may require teaching about what to expect after surgery. This patient may be so anxious about the surgery, though, that he does not really hear what the nurse is trying to teach. In such situations, repeating the material at specific intervals increases the chance the patient will hear what the nurse is saying.

Repetition also enhances learning when new material or a complex task is to be learned. Since many people can only learn a certain amount of information at one time, repetition may be necessary. Other people seem to benefit from repetition by using more than one method of learning. For example, the nurse may talk with the patient, then show a filmstrip, and then demonstrate a task. In this way, the talk, filmstrip, and demonstration promote learning because material is repeated in three different ways.

In assessing the patient's need for repetition, the nurse considers how new or complex the material is for the patient. The nurse can also ask the patient what areas of learning seem to be most difficult for him.

Degree of Participation

Learning seems to occur more rapidly when the learner participates actively in the learning process. Lectures or talking to the patient may not result in learning. The more actively the nurse can involve the patient in the learning task, the more likely it is that he will learn. Through discussion, the nurse can involve the patient in planning the objectives, in choosing the methods, and in evaluating the outcome of the learning that has taken place. The more the patient can handle and physically use equipment, talk with other patients about how they dealt with a problem, and make decisions about his own learning, the better are the chances for mastery of the subject matter.

Nurses often talk about motivating the patient. Usually, the best way to motivate the patient is to increase his degree of participation in his own care.

Self-Pacing

Everyone learns at his own pace. Some people learn quickly, others more slowly. *Self-paced learning* is learning that occurs at the rate most comfortable for that person. It is important that the nurse assess the rate at which the patient is most likely to learn. Sometimes nurses assume the patient can learn a task quickly because they are familiar with the task. To the patient, though, the task may be quite new and even frightening. In other situations, nurses may think the patient needs to go over the material when, in fact, the patient already knows the material.

During the teaching-learning process, the patient may learn some things very quickly and other things very slowly. As the process proceeds, the nurse continually assesses whether the pace of learning should be increased or decreased.

The patient is probably the best gauge for pacing his learning. The nurse can ask the patient, "Is this too fast for you?" or "Take your time, I'll wait until you're ready."

If the nurse has chosen to teach a group of patients, it may be difficult to pace learning for each patient in the group. Although group teaching has the advantages of using the nurse's time more efficiently and providing peer support for the patients, it may not be possible to provide self-paced learning for each patient.

Feedback

Learning is more likely to occur when the learner receives feedback about his progress. Some people have a greater need for feedback than others do. The nurse can assess the learner's need for feedback by observing the responses to the nurse's statements of evaluation. The nurse gives the patient feedback by making statements such as "You're able to walk more smoothly now" or "You can draw up the insulin but you need some more practice in giving the injection."

Reinforcement

Positive reinforcement occurs when one person verbally or nonverbally communicates interest in, concern over, or approval of another's behavior. Positive reinforcement usually leads to the continuation of the behavior. *Negative reinforcement* occurs when one person does not respond to or conveys disapproval of the other person's behavior. In common terms, this type of learning is called reward and punishment. In fact, what is reward or punishment for one person is not always reward or punishment for another.

When teaching patients, the nurse uses both positive and negative reinforcement to increase learning. Whenever the patient is able to perform all or part of a learning task, the nurse can comment on the performance. Such comments will not only provide feedback to the patient but will also increase the likelihood that the patient will continue to behave in the approved manner. In a simple conversation, the nurse can increase the potential for discussion of certain topics merely by commenting on the topic after the patient mentions it or by asking the patient to say more about the topic. This technique of commenting on patient statements is used quite often in psychiatric nursing; it helps the patient to learn more about his thoughts and feelings.

Reinforcers are used by the nurse to help to continue or decrease the occurrence of specific patient behaviors. *Behavioral modification* is the term used to describe the process where the patient's behavior is changed or modified in relation to positive or negative responses by the helping person. Not all patients respond positively to the same reinforcers. There is a specific assessment process used to increase or decrease patient behaviors. For this reason, nurses who intend to use this method of changing patient behavior must receive special training and education in this method. Some books that may increase the student's knowledge in this area are given in the bibliography for this chapter. Figure 28-2 summarizes areas to consider for assessing the status of the learner.

THE TEACHING-LEARNING PROCESS

The teaching-learning process includes a number of steps: (1) assessing the needs of the patient, (2) developing the objectives, (3) selecting materials and method, (4) participating in instructional activities, and (5) evaluating the outcomes.

Area	Considerations
Readiness	Is the patient ready to learn? Is strong feeling decreasing patient readiness? Is debility decreasing patient readiness?
Prior learning	What does the patient already know? What can the patient demonstrate to show how much he already knows? What does the patient say he knows?
Meaningfulness of material	Is the material too technical or complex? What method of learning does the patient express a preference for?
Repetition	Is the patient highly anxious? Could repetition through several methods of learning enhance learning? How new or complex is the material?
Degree of participation	How actively can this patient be in the learning activities? Can the patient be involved in planning learning objectives? Can the patient be involved in choosing learning methods? Can the patient be involved in evaluating learning?
Self-pacing	Does the pace of learning need to be speeded up or slowed down?
Feedback	How much feedback does this patient seem to need? How does this patient respond to feedback?
Reinforcement	How can the occurrence of positive behaviors be increased? How can the occurrence of nonconstructive behaviors be decreased?

Fig. 28-2 Points to consider when assessing learning status.

Assessing Learning Needs

Part of the assessment process is to consider the learning status just discussed; that is, readiness, prior learning, meaningful material, repetition, degree of participation, self-pacing, feedback and reinforcement. However, the patient's immediate short-range and/or long-range needs must be assessed also.

The nurse includes the patient when developing the list of learning needs. At times, the patient's ideas may conflict with the list of learning needs developed by the nurse or doctor. As the patient will only learn what is important to him, the nurse starts the teaching at the point where the patient feels the need. In other words, teaching begins at the level where the patient expresses a felt need. Learning the needs of the patient may begin as early as the time of admission. When taking the nursing history, the nurse can begin to observe and assess the patient's learning needs.

Orientation to the hospital environment is required by most patients. The amount of teaching directed to this need is based on the patient's previous experience with hospitalization, previous illness, and the level of anxiety.

The geriatric resident who is confused may have additional learning needs for orientation to his environment. The nurse can assess his needs by listening to what he says and by observing if he recognizes his surroundings and seems to know who the nurse is.

Children, too, have learning needs. The nurse uses information about growth and development to assess a child's need to learn. Age is not the only indicator used, however. The child's response to what the nurse says and does can help the nurse to assess things the child may need to be taught.

Developing Learning Objectives

The nurse develops learning objectives or goals based on the needs of the patient. Learning objectives guide the selection of the materials to be presented and the method by which the information will be presented. To choose appropriate objectives, the nurse becomes familiar with the steps in the learning process:

1. Get the facts
2. Relate the facts
3. Analyze
4. Synthesize
5. Evaluate

The first step in any kind of learning is to become familiar with the facts of a situation. In teaching about coronary heart disease, the facts might include knowledge of how the heart functions. In teaching about distorted interpersonal relationships the facts might include the nurse's and the patient's observation of a specific interpersonal situation.

The second step in the learning process is to put these facts into a new context by relating facts to observations. In teaching about coronary heart disease, the interrelationships might include how the behavior affects heart functioning. In teaching about distorted interpersonal relationships, the interrelationships might include exploring one interpersonal situation where a distortion might have occurred.

The next step in the learning process is to analyze. Analysis helps people to cope with complex situations once the parts of a complex situation can be understood. In teaching about coronary heart disease, the patient might be asked to explain how his behavior at various times relates to his heart condition. In teaching about distorted interpersonal relationships, the patient might be asked to compare or contrast different interpersonal situations.

The next step in the learning process is to decide on a meaning. This meaning or *synthesis* is a bringing together of the many parts of a task or experience and arriving at a new fact or conclusion. In teaching about coronary heart disease, the patient might be asked to demonstrate and explain how to function in a new stress situation. In teaching about distorted interpersonal relationships, the nurse uses validation. When the nurse validates, she checks with the patient to see that they both agree on the meaning of an interpersonal situation.

The final step in the learning process is evaluation. Evaluation can be done verbally or it can be demonstrated through testing the new method or action. In teaching about coronary heart disease, the patient might be asked to identify proper foods, show appropriate exercises, and return in three weeks to have vital signs checked. In teaching improvement of distorted interpersonal relationships, the patient might be asked to try out a new communication skill with his family and, in the next session, report how the new skill worked.

Objectives should be chosen for each step in the learning process. Objectives are stated using action verbs such as: maintain, administer, increase, provide, establish, demonstrate, list, compare, modify, walk, choose, translate, and test. Figures 28-3 and 28-4 show some possible learning objectives for the patient with coronary heart disease and the patient with distorted interpersonal relationships.

A PATIENT WITH CORONARY HEART DISEASE: SOME LEARNING OBJECTIVES

1. Describe how the heart functions.
2. List four ways that behavior affects heart function.
3. Describe three situations where the patient's behavior can affect his heart condition.
4. Explain how to decrease heart stress in three given situations.
5. Select foods to make up an appropriate diet.
6. State the purpose of a return clinic visit in three weeks.

Fig. 28-3 Sample learning objectives for patient with a medical disorder

A Patient With Interpersonal Difficulties: Some Learning Objectives

1. Describe her thoughts and feelings while talking with the nurse.
2. Describe at least one interpersonal situation, telling who was involved, what was said, what happened, and what the patient felt and thought about what happened.
3. Compare one interpersonal situation with another similar situation, listing three similarities and three differences.
4. List one conclusion about the meaning of the interpersonal situation.
5. State one alternate way to handle the situation.
6. Report what happened when the alternate method was tried out.

Fig. 28-4 Sample learning objectives for patient with distorted interpersonal relationships

Selecting Methods and Materials

Basically, there are three types of learning tasks. The nurse is interested in all three types. One type of learning task is giving or receiving information. Another is the acquiring or teaching of a skill. A third type is providing or obtaining basic knowledge in order to problem solve. Figure 28-5 shows some problem-solving questions the nurse can use in teaching patients.

Depending on the objectives, the nurse chooses an appropriate method of teaching to enhance learning. This method may need to be modified depending on the patient's loss or problem with sight, hearing, touch, movement, attention span, age, cultural group, or anxiety level.

Teaching-learning methods that can be used to give or receive information include lecture, reading of technical or autobiographical books, audiovisual aids, counseling, play therapy, discussions with a patient who has the same condition, field trips, and creative projects. Methods that can be used to teach or acquire a skill include demonstration, return demonstration, role playing, drill, and nonverbal exercises. Nonverbal exercises are used to draw out and allow for practice in gestures, posture, and facial expression. Methods of providing and obtaining knowledge to improve problem-solving ability include the use of videotape, problem-solving discussion, and brainstorming. *Brainstorming* is a technique where one or more persons attack a problem by giving as many solutions as possible, without censoring the logic of any solution. Figure 28-6, page 444, illustrates some of these teaching-learning methods.

What is the problem?
Who can help solve the problem?
What books, references, or audiovisual aids can help solve the problem?
What has already been tried to solve the problem?
What limits are there within which to solve the problem?
What rules can be changed to solve the problem?

Fig. 28-5 Questions to ask to assist with problem solving

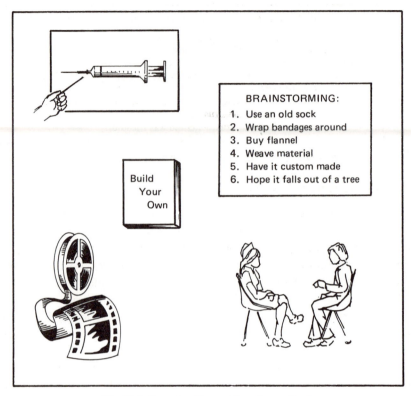

BRAINSTORMING:
1. Use an old sock
2. Wrap bandages around
3. Buy flannel
4. Weave material
5. Have it custom made
6. Hope it falls out of a tree

Build
Your
Own

Fig. 28-6 Some teaching and learning methods

Participation in Instructional Activities

The nurse sets the atmosphere so that learning can occur. A room that is overcrowded, noisy, poorly ventilated, or uncomfortable in other ways is not used. Enough time should be allotted to allow for unexpected questions or events. The time chosen for the session must be one that is agreeable to both nurse and patient. If group teaching is to take place, it may be more difficult to find a time period that is the most suitable for all concerned. Long teaching-learning periods often decrease the potential for learning. Patients who are weak or ill will benefit most from short, frequent teaching-learning sessions.

If printed or audiovisual materials have been chosen, time should be planned for discussion. If the nurse uses the demonstration method of teaching, materials should be exactly like the ones the patient will use later at home, figure 28-7. All equipment is shown to the patient and the purpose and use of each piece is explained.

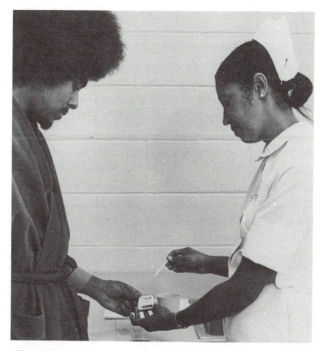

Fig. 28-7 Teaching materials should be exactly like the ones the patient will use at home.

It is wise to make a special effort to give information in a slower speaking voice than is used for everyday conversation. The patient needs time not only to hear and interpret what is said but also to associate information with the equipment and its use. An unobstructed view of the instructor and the visual aids is necessary. The patient also needs to be close enough to see and hear what the nurse is saying and demonstrating. In order to teach well, the nurse must be knowledgeable about her subject. Planning should take place before any teaching session. Preparing an outline of key points will help focus attention on points to be stressed and will avoid the omission of important information. The nurse can profit from a practice session with a friend or family member role playing the patient. Unclear teaching by the nurse can frequently be clarified in the practice session before attempting to teach the patient in the real life situation.

Evaluating the Outcomes

Judging how much was learned is part of the teaching-learning process. Evaluation may lead to feelings of frustration because it is not always possible to measure the actual results of a teaching session. For example, psychiatric patients may have learned some valuable principles but it may not be possible to see the results immediately.

Evaluation is an attempt to measure how many of the objectives the learner has met and the degree of mastery achieved. The more clearly the learning objectives have been stated, the more easily the teacher and learner can evaluate whether the objectives were met.

Every person involved in a teaching-learning program is involved in evaluation. The methods of evaluating learning outcomes differ according to the type of learning needed by the patient. If the purpose of the learning task was to relay information, the patient can be questioned to find out if he knows the information. If the purpose was to acquire a skill, a return demonstration by the patient will establish whether the skill has been acquired. If problem solving was the objective of the learning task, observing the patient and/or getting a report of what happened in a given situation is the only way to measure whether learning has occurred. Follow-up home visits or follow-up visits by the patient to the hospital or clinic may be necessary to help evaluate the application of problem-solving techniques. Figure 28-8 shows the nursing process used in patient teaching.

SUMMARY

The teaching role of the nurse has increased as knowledge has expanded and patients have become more interested in understanding about health. Faulty learning may be directly related to illness and interpersonal difficulties.

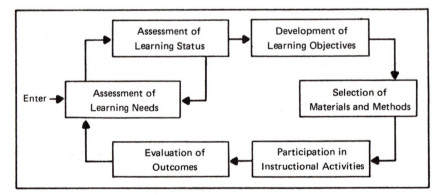

Fig. 28-8 The teaching-learning process

In preparing to learn or to teach others, the student assesses the level of readiness to learn, prior learning, meaningfulness of material, need for repetition, degree of participation, and how self-pacing, feedback, and reinforcement might be used.

The teaching-learning process is a nursing process that includes assessment of learning needs, development of learning objectives based on learning needs, selection of materials and learning methods based on the level of learning, teaching, and evaluation.

ACTIVITIES AND DISCUSSION TOPICS

- Develop a teaching-learning plan for two different patients. Consider the following questions in the development of your plans.
  a. What are the patient's learning needs?
  b. Is the patient ready to learn?
  c. What does the patient already know?
  d. How meaningful is this material to this patient?
  e. How much repetition of learning might this patient need?
  f. How much can the patient participate in his own learning?
  g. How can the patient be helped to set the learning pace?
  h. How can you provide feedback to this patient?
  i. How can reinforcement be used with this patient?
  j. What learning objectives may be useful for this patient?
  k. How do the learning objectives relate to what you know about the learning process?
  l. What methods of learning should be used with this patient? Why?
  m. What factors need to be considered when you actually begin to teach this patient?
  n. How will you evaluate how much learning has occurred?

REVIEW

A. Multiple Choice. Select the best answer(s). Some questions have more than one answer.

  1. The relationship between learning and health exists because
     a. faulty learning can lead to decreased health.
     b. biofeedback can influence biological functions.
     c. learning has no affect on health.
     d. learning health factors can influence healthy behavior.

2. Factors that influence a person's readiness to learn include
   a. depression.   c. pain.
   b. anger.   d. thirst.

3. The best way to motivate a patient to learn is to
   a. increase his degree of participation in the learning process.
   b. use visual aids.
   c. repeat the instructions several times.
   d. use technical terms when explaining the procedure.

4. An attempt to measure how many of the objectives the learner has met and the degree of mastery achieved is called
   a. feedback.   c. evaluation.
   b. prior learning.   d. validation.

5. In addition to formal teaching, the nurse also teaches by the way she
   a. looks.   c. communicates.
   b. acts.   d. does all of these.

B. Match the items in Column II to the appropriate definition in Column I.

Column I	Column II
1. Learning at the rate most comfortable for the learner.	a. brainstorming
	b. pretest
	c. role model
2. Demonstration of how to act effectively through action.	d. self-paced learning
	e. synthesis
3. A problem is attacked by giving as many solutions as possible, without considering the logic of the solution.	f. validation
4. A means of determining how much the learner knows about a particular subject.	
5. Bringing together the many parts of a task or experience and arriving at a new fact or conclusion.	
6. The nurse checks with the patient to see that they agree on the meaning of a situation.	

C.   Briefly answer the following questions.

    1.   List eight areas of learning to assess when the student is preparing to teach or learn.

    2.   Differentiate between positive reinforcement and negative reinforcement.

    3.   List the five steps included in the teaching-learning process.

    4.   List the five steps in the learning process.

    5.   Name the three basic types of learning tasks.

chapter 29
GROUP PROCESS
AND LEARNING

STUDENT OBJECTIVES

- List four purposes of groups.
- Define the group process.
- Name four reasons for group apathy.
- Match group processes with appropriate definitions or examples.
- State five steps in the group decision-making process.

Nurses are involved with many different groups of people. Nurses interact with groups of patients, families, other nurses, and other health personnel. Throughout the course of one day, the nurse may be part of many different groups. Participating in the nursing report is one example of a group situation. Providing care for a number of patients in one room often has elements of a group process. Staff conferences are another example of a group. Nurses who eat with a group of patients or staff take part in group process. Students and graduate nurses involved in educational experiences become part of a classroom group. Groups are formed to teach patients or to discuss thoughts and feelings that may be interfering with high levels of wellness. Therefore, nurses learn about group process and how to be effective group members.

GROUP PURPOSES

People are social beings who interact in groups throughout their lives. Different groups have different purposes. The family serves a number of purposes such as education in cultural values. School provides peer and pupil-teacher relationships related to learning facts but also related to getting along with other people. Eventually, people become members of play groups, work groups, church groups, political groups, and extended family groups.

Most groups serve a number of purposes. One purpose is to provide more than one source of stimulation and feedback to its members. A member of a group receives and gives information to more than one other person. Groups provide more complex interactions and practice in developing skills than does a one-to-one relationship with one other person. Because the group provides for reactions from a number of sources, a group member can receive strong validation or rejection for his ideas.

Receiving strong validation from the rest of the group can encourage a patient to try out new behaviors in situations outside the group. Self-esteem can be increased and the self-concept enhanced when the rest of the group strongly agrees with one group member. Group rejection of a member's idea can also exert great influence on that member. It is easy to discount the ideas of one or two others as ridiculous. When eight or nine other people strongly confront a member's ideas or behavior as suspect, there is a strong pull to agree with the group. This strong pull to go along with the group results from *peer pressure*. Peers, or members of one's own group, can pressure or influence other group members to change their thoughts or behavior through peer pressure.

A second purpose of a group is to provide support. The idea that others share the same fear or problems seems to provide support for group members. Just knowing that others are struggling with the same issue can help a group member.

A third purpose of a group is to reduce isolation. Interacting with other people can decrease the sense of loneliness or unreality that may occur in people who suffer from sensory deprivation. People in nursing homes, patients on long-term psychiatric units, and patients who have been in isolation or intensive care units may feel the most isolated from others.

A fourth purpose of a group is to provide learning experiences. Groups can provide facts such as how to irrigate a colostomy or discipline à child. Groups can also provide emotional learning experiences such as how to communicate thoughts and feelings to peers; how one person's behavior affects others; how to identify problematic interactions with others; and how to deal with anxiety, apathy, conflict, and competition. Groups can provide developmental growth experiences. People who never learned to cooperate in their own family group may learn this skill in a patients' group organized by the nurse. Groups can furnish useful experiences in decision making and problem solving. A group setting can also provide a place to rehearse new behaviors. The group can also encourage its members to discuss how to cope with situations outside the group such as how to relate to overprotective parents; how to be comfortable at a social outing in a wheelchair; or how to manage ileostomy care while travelling.

GROUP PROCESS

Group process is a term that refers to the flow and ebb of group *interaction*. Group process focuses on how things are happening; it is based on the relationships within the group that influence interaction and hold the group together. Group process is concerned with what is happening now and what is making these things happen. Group process is concerned with analyzing the here-and-now, figure 29-1.

Group process refers to the interaction not to the content. It is important to know what is being said (content). To be an effective group leader or member, how things are said, by whom, when, and what function is being served must also be clear. Figure 29-2 lists some content or themes that may be discussed.

FUNCTIONS OF A GROUP

For a group to operate effectively, both task and maintenance functions must be supplied. *Task functions* aid in accomplishing group goals. They help get the group going and keep it moving. Task functions are accomplished through clarifying what was said or done, suggesting an action, pointing out an idea, restating what has happened, refocusing the group on its task, and by giving information.

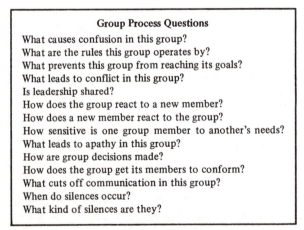

Group Process Questions

What causes confusion in this group?
What are the rules this group operates by?
What prevents this group from reaching its goals?
What leads to conflict in this group?
Is leadership shared?
How does the group react to a new member?
How does a new member react to the group?
How sensitive is one group member to another's needs?
What leads to apathy in this group?
How are group decisions made?
How does the group get its members to conform?
What cuts off communication in this group?
When do silences occur?
What kind of silences are they?

Fig. 29-1 Questions to ask when studying group process.

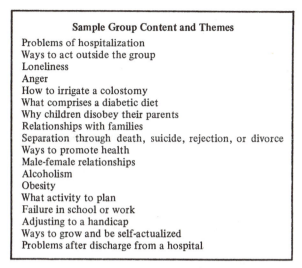

Fig. 29-2 Subjects for group discussion

Maintenance functions help improve and maintain interpersonal relationships. Maintenance functions include actions that support group members and help them to evaluate their work. Maintenance functions are accomplished by giving support and encouragement to unsure group members, relieving tension, encouraging direct communication between group members, voicing group feelings, agreeing with or accepting others' behavior, and by asking the group to evaluate its decisions, goals or procedures. Figure 29-3 illustrates the role of the group leader.

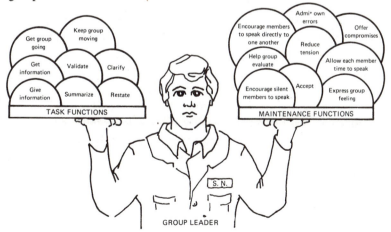

Fig. 29-3 The group leader helps to achieve the balance between task and maintenance functions.

COMMON GROUP PROCESSES

Groups exhibit common elements; some common group processes are:

- cohesiveness
- leadership
- norms
- phases of development
- scapegoating

- monopolizing
- apathy
- conflict
- decision making
- silence

Cohesiveness

Cohesiveness is a measure of how attractive the group is to its members. Cohesiveness is the sum of each member's feelings about the group. In a highly cohesive group, all members feel involved with the activities and have developed norms for the manner of operation.

Cohesive groups move together. If one of the expectations set up by the group is to be productive, a highly cohesive group will be very productive. Classroom groups with strong goals, direction, and cohesion seem to be satisfied groups.

Leadership

Leadership consists of a group of actions; it is an interpersonal process rather than a characteristic of one person. Leadership helps the group become cohesive and move toward its goals, improve interpersonal relationships between members, and make the skills of individuals available to the group. When leadership functions are distributed among group members, all participants can learn, become more self-confident, and increase their self-esteem. Effective leadership meets both task and maintenance functions of a group. The nurse who wants to influence a group positively helps to meet both task and maintenance functions, encourages all members to exert leadership, and attempts to establish a relationship with influential group members. If the nurse is able to work with a group over a period of time, she may also be able to teach leadership functions to other group members through discussion and demonstration.

Norms

Norms are attitudes or expectations shared by a group; they determine what is appropriate behavior. Norms stabilize behavior and make what happens in the group somewhat predictable. Norms that are narrow in scope and tolerate only a few behaviors are likely to occur in groups that have a punitive atmosphere. Group norms that are broader and tolerant of individual differences are likely to appear where the group climate is positive. The nurse can positively influence group norms by communicating verbally and nonverbally that (1) all members are there to work together, (2) the nurse is there to help, and (3) it is important to try to understand one another.

Phases of Development

Groups pass through *phases of development*. There are many ways to describe these phases. Generally speaking, the system that parallels the development of the one-to-one nurse-patient relationship is the easiest to understand. In this system, there are three phases that groups pass through: orientation, working, and termination. It is possible for a group to show glimpses of all three phases during one session but the major part of happenings in one session will be in one phase or another.

Orientation Phase. Common occurrences in the orientation phase of a group are:

- Concern about being accepted by the others
- Initial distrust of other group members
- Demands to be told what to do in the group and how to do it
- High anxiety levels
- Some anger at being asked to assume some responsibility for leadership
- Giving and getting information about one another and the goals to be pursued
- Formation of group norms

During this phase, there may be considerable *testing behavior* by the members of the group. This is an attempt to test the limits of acceptable behavior in this group.

Because a patient group may be similar in some ways to family groups, patients may treat each other as if they were family members. For example, one group member may see similarities between another group member and his own brother. If the group member and his brother were quite competitive, he may try to compete with the group member who reminds him of his brother. This is an example of the kind of *transference* behavior that can occur in groups.

In this case, the group member transfers thoughts and feelings he originally held toward his brother to the group member who is similar in some way to the brother.

It is difficult to predict how long the orientation phase will last. The length of this phase is related to the motivation of group members; the constant attendance of the same people in the same group; how often and for how long the group meets; and the leadership skill already held by the group members.

Working Phase. The second phase through which a group proceeds is the *working phase*. When the group enters the working phase, the norms are set, members take more responsibility for what happens in the group, conversation is more spontaneous and feelings may be expressed more directly. In the working phase, group members may spend more time on maintenance functions than they do on task functions. There may be increased positive feelings toward one another and more tolerance for others. Some groups never enter the working phase.

Termination Phase. The third phase of group development is the *termination or separation phase*. This phase is characterized by looking to the future; attempts are made to loosen relationships within the group by finding other areas of interest. Groups who have been cohesive and constructive may express feelings of grief that the group process is ending. Sadness, anger, rejection of the group, guilt, and satisfaction about accomplishments are some common reactions to the ending of a meaningful group experience. Group members who have had high levels of anxiety may experience relief that the group has disbanded.

Scapegoating

Scapegoating is a group process where one member of the group is singled out to be the target of the group hostility. The scapegoated member does not usually say, "attack me" but, nonverbally, he may set up situations which evoke the group's anger. In some patient groups, the anger shown toward one member may really be directed against the nurse. Since the nurse is considered to be an *authority figure*, the group may be afraid to show their anger. An authority figure is someone who is in command; someone who is thought to be especially powerful. Parents are seen as the first authority figures. As people grow to be adults, some continue to assume that other authority figures have the same power over them that their parents did. Group members can learn from being in a group with an authority figure that such a person is human and also has needs, limitations, and strengths.

Monopolizing

During the orientation phase of a group there may be a group member who agrees to take over and do most of the talking. This person *monopolizes* the group time. As with scapegoating, the member does not usually state, "I will do most of the talking." Rather, the person talks excessively because he or she probably feels less anxious while talking. The group allows the member to talk because they may feel more comfortable being silent. However, monopolization of group time is not constructive in working toward group goals. In the long run, the monopolizing patient will feel used by the group and the group will feel resentful.

Apathy

Apathy is a lack of interest or concern. It can be diagnosed in the group through observation of behavior. Some of the signs that apathy may be occurring are:

- Restlessness
- Frequent yawns
- Snap decisions
- Low level participation
- Dragging conversation
- Many late or absent members
- Wish to end the session
- Inability to remember the point of a discussion
- Reluctance to take responsibility for future group meetings

Some reasons for group apathy include poorly defined group goals, interest in other issues, lack of skill in problem solving, fear of the group goal or of other group members, feelings of powerlessness to influence what happens to them, or conflict between two of the group members.

Conflict

Conflict can also be diagnosed through observation of group behaviors. Conflict is probably occurring when members are impatient with each other, there is disagreement and strong feelings are expressed, members take sides and refuse to compromise, there is grumbling about not being able to accomplish the goal, and only fragments of what others say are heard. Some reasons for group

Elements of Group Process	Indicants of Process
Cohesiveness	Open, direct communication. Involvement in group goals.
Leadership	Sharing of leadership functions. Both task and maintenance functions are met.
Norms	All members know the appropriate behavior in the group.
Phases	Orientation phase: Learning about other members; striving to be accepted; being fearful and anxious about taking responsibility for what happens in the group; expressing feelings indirectly. Working phase: Norms are clear; group members take more responsibility; anxiety and fear is decreased; feelings are expressed more spontaneously and directly. Termination phase: Attempts to loosen ties to the group; looking toward the future; feelings of grief, satisfaction, or relief.
Scapegoating	One group member becomes the target for the group's hostility.
Monopolizing	One group member does most of the talking.
Apathy	Frequent yawns; inability to remember the point of the discussion; low level participation; restlessness; lateness or absences; reluctance to continue toward goal.
Conflict	Impatience, disagreement, taking sides, grumbling about inability to meet goal, not listening or hearing others' comments.
Decision Making	Orderly progression from clearly stated problem → alternate solutions → summarizing → testing solutions → deciding on one solution.
Silence	Quiet period. Atmosphere is thoughtful, sad, anxious, or angry.

Fig. 29-4 Common group processes

conflict are that the group has been given an impossible goal, group members are more concerned with status than with reaching the goal, members are loyal to people or interests outside the group, or members are involved and working toward the goal. In the last case, the conflict is a positive sign. Conflict is an expected occurrence when people are involved and trying to resolve issues. In the other cases, goals may need to be redefined or changed in order to reduce the conflict.

Decision Making

In *group decision making*, there are certain steps that must be followed in order to come to a useful decision.
1. The problem must be stated clearly.
2. Alternate solutions to the problem are stated.
3. Discussion must continue to focus on the problem with an attempt to summarize what has been discussed.
4. The solutions are tested.
5. Appropriate decision can be made.

All of these steps are necessary to make useful group decisions. Decision making is inadequate when a decision is called for without completing the preceding steps or if the group fears to make a decision.

Silence

As in the nurse-patient relationship, groups have periods of silence. Thoughtful silences can be useful after an especially involved interchange. Sad silences may follow a discussion about death or separation from others. Anxious silences will often be broken by a group member who may feel he or she is responsible for keeping the group moving. Angry silences follow angry exchanges or may be an indication that, underneath polite conversation, anger is brewing. Figure 29-4 summarizes elements and indicants of common group processes.

SUMMARY

Nurses are members of various groups throughout their lives. Knowledge of group processes can aid the nurse to be an effective participant. Groups serve several purposes that one-to-one relationships cannot provide. The focus of group process is analysis of the here-and-now; what is happening now, and

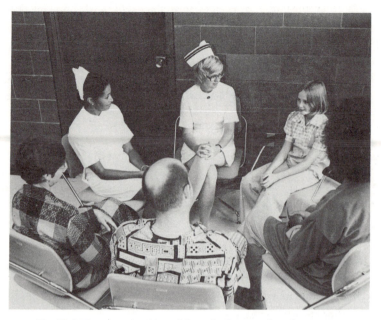

Fig. 29-5 Everyone should participate in the group learning process.

why it is happening. The topics that are discussed and themes that occur in groups are called group content. Group content is not group process, but the two are related.

Groups serve both task and maintenance functions if they are to operate effectively. Some elements of group processes are cohesiveness, leadership, norms, phases of development, scapegoating, monopolizing, apathy, conflict, decision making, and silence.

ACTIVITIES AND DISCUSSION TOPICS

Observe a group for at least three meetings. Keep a log on what occurred. Some types of groups that may be observed are social groups, teaching groups, supportive or expressive patient groups, play groups, staff groups, families, and classroom discussion groups. Community groups are: Alcoholics Anonymous, Synanon, Weight Watchers, Ostomy Club, and others.

As you observe the chosen group, ask yourself the following questions:

1. What is happening now?
2. What is making these things happen?
3. What causes confusion in this group?

4. What are the rules this group operates by?
5. What leads to conflict in this group?
6. What kind of leadership is there?
7. Is leadership shared?
8. What prevents problem solving from occurring?
9. How do the group members react to each other? To new members?
10. What leads to apathy in this group?
11. How does the group get its members to conform?
12. What cuts off communication in this group?
13. When do silences occur?
14. What kind of silences are they?
15. What topics are discussed?
16. What themes emerge?
17. Who relieves the tension? How?
18. Who breaks the silences?
19. Who helps the group to summarize or evaluate?
20. Who encourages other group members to speak?
21. Who admits their own errors?
22. Who expresses group feeling?
23. Who gets the group moving and keeps it moving?
24. Who clarifies?
25. Who validates?
26. Who restates?
27. Who gets information?
28. Who gives information?
29. Who speaks to whom?
30. How cohesive is this group?
31. What phase of development is this group in?
32. Who is a scapegoat?
33. Who monopolizes?

REVIEW

A. Multiple Choice. Select the best answer.

1. Maintenance functions of a group include
   a. validating.   c. summarizing.
   b. clarifying.   d. accepting.

2. Common occurrences in the orientation phase of a group include
   a. direct expression of feelings.
   b. initial distrust of other group members.
   c. looking to the future.
   d. attempts to loosen relationships within the group.

3. The purpose of task functions of a group is to
   a. improve and maintain interpersonal relationships.
   b. support group members and help them evaluate their work.
   c. aid in accomplishing group goals.
   d. encourage direct communication between group members.

4. Conflict is a positive sign only when group members are
   a. involved and working toward the goal.
   b. loyal to people and interests outside the group.
   c. concerned about status.
   d. not involved in the conflict.

5. The topics that are discussed and themes that occur in groups are called group
   a. process.
   b. content.
   c. development.
   d. transference.

B. Match the group process in Column II with its definition or example in Column I.

Column I	Column II
1. One member of the group is singled out to be the target of group hostility.	a. apathy
	b. conflict
	c. cohesiveness
2. One member of the group does most of the talking.	d. decision making
	e. leadership
3. A lack of interest or concern.	f. monopolizing
	g. norms
4. Impatience with others, disagreement and expression of strong feelings.	h. phases of development
	i. scapegoating
5. Attitudes or expectations shared by a group.	j. silence
6. Clearly stating the problem, then considering alternate solutions before deciding on a solution.	
7. An interpersonal process that helps the group become cohesive and move toward its goals, improve interpersonal relationships between members, and makes individual skills available to the group.	
8. Periods that may be angry, anxious, thoughtful or sad.	
9. Orientation, working and termination.	
10. Measure of how attractive the group is to its members.	

C. Briefly answer the following questions.

    1. Define group process.

    2. State five steps in the group decision making process.

    3. List four purposes of groups.

    4. Name four reasons for group apathy.

D. Read the following excerpt from a group meeting, then briefly answer the questions pertaining to the meeting.

> **You are conducting a meeting of nursing assistants in order to plan care for a patient who refuses to cooperate with them. The nursing assistants constantly complain that "we have better things to do than meet with you" and that "this patient is hopeless anyway." The group members come and go from the meeting. They blame you for not taking care of this patient yourself. You start apologizing and promise to care for the patient but they still attack you. At this point, one person starts talking on and on and the others begin to fidget. You decide to end the group stating "since you are not interested in this, we will end this meeting now."**

    1. What group process was exhibited by the complaining nursing assistants?

    2. What group process occurred when the group blamed you and you accepted the blame?

    3. What group process was exhibited when one member started talking on and on?

    4. What kind of leadership was exhibited in this group?

chapter 30
LEARNING
IN GROUPS

STUDENT OBJECTIVES

- List five qualities of a group leader.
- Name four ways a group leader can reduce initial anxiety of a group.
- List eight considerations in starting a group.
- Name three group relaxation techniques.
- Match group techniques with list of examples.

Groups provide a number of sources of stimulation so they are generally more demanding than one-to-one relationships which provide only one source. Groups are also demanding because the nurse must often switch roles; she may function as nurse, group leader, and participant.

A group meeting may be called for the purpose of discussing a topic. When the nurse conducts the meeting, questions or discussions about other unrelated topics should be avoided. Discussing medications in a group formed to teach patients about their medications and treatment would be appropriate; discussing medications in a group formed for the expressed purpose of talking about feelings toward death and dying defeats its purpose. As group leader, the nurse would be responsible for keeping the discussion focused on the main subject.

QUALITIES OF A GROUP LEADER

Leadership skills may be learned and shared. When the nurse forms a group with other nurses, patients, or families, she usually takes the responsibility for setting the direction the group will go. Each group leader develops her own style of leading the group. The attitude and expectations of the leader will influence the group process. Group members will soon learn what is expected from them by the leader's verbal and nonverbal communication. For this reason, it is important that the leader examine his or her own thoughts and feelings before beginning to form the group. This includes thinking about the group's purposes and goals and ways to use past experience and the self to constructively influence the group.

A group leader must have the ability to tolerate anxiety, frustration, and hostility. The nurse who leads a group must be flexible enough to deal with confrontation and hostility from the group members.

The leader must also be able to organize a great deal of information. Observational skills such as listening can be taxed to the fullest during a group meeting. A group leader must be willing to stop listening to the words that are being said and notice nonverbal communication in order to determine group processes. A sense of humor is another quality of a constructive group leader. Humor can help the nurse to break group tension at strategic points.

In general, a leader who shares the leadership, reduces group tensions, and promotes democratic decision making will constructively influence a group. In addition, the leader must have a firm grip on certain structural rules for forming and guiding a group. For example, the nurse as group leader must decide who will be in the group; how long the group will run; how often it will meet; where the group will meet; what attendance is expected; what will be discussed; and how to prepare individuals to enter the group.

One of the best ways to learn about being a group leader is to have a personal group experience; this experience may be in an ongoing therapeutic, task, or discussion group. Being a group leader requires an ability to expose one's weaknesses and strengths to others. The group members will soon learn what kind of person the group leader is. The nurse has to be comfortable with a number of different people at one time.

Many group leaders also seek supervision by a more experienced group leader. Group supervision enables the leader to examine group processes that he or she may have missed or could handle more effectively if given additional assistance. Reading about group process and taking additional course work in group dynamics will also be valuable.

STARTING A GROUP

Starting a group involves making all the decisions about how the group will be formed. It also includes dealing with initial problems or processes which are likely to arise. *Nurses who are inexperienced group leaders must seek supervision from a more experienced group leader before beginning a patient group.*

Early Decisions and Problems

The first decisions made by the group leader are based on the questions: "What kind of group will this be?", "Who will be included in this group?", and "What are the purposes or goals for this group?" Sometimes the goals or purposes may be set before the nurse takes leadership. At times, there will only be six or seven people available to join the group; then the nurse has no choice in deciding who should be included. Generally, groups that contain between six and twelve members seem to be best suited for frequent interaction by group members. Smaller or larger groups can be formed if the purpose is teaching.

Group purposes or goals are best stated in terms of observable behaviors. For example, a goal such as "Help the patients to understand breast feeding" is not stated as observable behavior. Understanding is an internal process that cannot be observed. A better way to state the goal would be "Have each group member state the four purposes of breast feeding."

Another point to consider when starting a group is what is to be done when members of the group leave. The leader might decide that if group members leave new group members will be added. This type of group is called an *open group.* The leader can encourage all group members to stay until the last meeting and decide not to add members when others leave. This type of group is called a *closed group.*

Next, the group leader decides where the group will meet; how long the group will last; how long each meeting will last; how often the group will meet; how the group will be seated; and what equipment must be available.

One hour should be the minimum time limit set for interactive or discussion groups. Chairs are arranged in a circle to promote interaction between group members. Teaching or activity groups may have shorter meetings and may work best in other seating arrangements.

Occasionally, two nurses may decide to work together as co-leaders of a group. The more experienced leader may head the group while the less experienced nurse observes, participates, and takes notes on group processes. Co-leading can be especially useful in working with parents or families. The two leaders can be role models for the group and demonstrate the need for cooperation. Participants can see how the leaders handle disagreements. In expressive or supportive groups, co-leaders must be especially careful to seek supervision that deals with the relationship of the co-leaders and how it might affect group processes.

Leaders who have the group's permission to record meetings may record or videotape the sessions. Additional equipment will be needed if procedures such as giving injections and bathing infants are being demonstrated and taped.

Finally, the group leader must decide how to prepare individuals for the group experience. They may be contacted singly or as a group. The leader may give potential members a lecture about the purpose of the group and the group contract. A *group contract* is a verbal or written agreement between the leader and the group members. Not all groups have clearly stated group contracts. The nurse who forms a group will often have better results if all members thoroughly understand the purposes and the expectations. The expectations and purposes will differ for each type of group. If the purpose of the group is to demonstrate insulin injections, group members should know beforehand that they will be expected to show how to give an insulin injection during the period the group is in session. Agreements governing behavior evolve from the group. Based on the purpose for which the group was formed, some commonly accepted rules may be: decisions are made by group consensus; no individual speaks for the group; undivided attention is given every speaker; and two people do not talk at once. Whatever is said in the group is to be kept confidential. Other groups may require mandatory attendance at each group meeting.

Figure 30-1, page 468, summarizes initial decisions the leader makes prior to beginning a group. Each group leader should consider the factors and make decisions about each of them. Considerable thought should be directed to this process prior to beginning a group.

An increase in anxiety and tension is one of the first problems of the newly formed group. Members are concerned about what will happen in that group. This anxiety might be conveyed to the leader in the form of a negative response to being in the group. Indirect hostility toward other members, awkward pauses, nervous laughter, or polite talk also convey anxiety and tension. Group leaders should expect a high level of anxiety in a newly formed group. Leaders have to learn to be comfortable with such reactions; the leader should understand that group members may not be aware of their feelings or may be afraid to express their feelings directly.

A problem will arise if the leader has unrealistic expectations for the group. Inexperienced nurse leaders might feel that group members should be able to work together cooperatively. Since many staff, student, and patient groups have not had constructive experiences in working together as a group, this leader expectation is an unrealistic one. It is the task of those who have worked in groups to teach each other how to work cooperatively. Experienced group members can help to encourage free expression, clarify unclear communication, and find a common ground for the discussion of differences.

Decisions	Possible Influences or Considerations
Type of group	Whether patients or families have learning or interpersonal needs.
Group composition	Personalities, diagnosis or condition, learning pace, verbal ability, availability of participants.
Group purpose or goals	Decided prior to group formation or by group decision.
Co-Leadership	Pros and cons of having two leaders.
Group size	Depends on group purposes and goals.
Leaving the group	Open or closed groups depending on group purposes, motivation of members to stick with the group, and availability of new members.
Meeting place	Comfort, availability, and seating arrangement.
Equipment	Depends on group purposes, whether recording equipment is needed, and if new materials will be introduced.
Length of meeting	Depends on group purpose and members' ability to concentrate on the task.
Recording group interaction	Group must give their permission.
Group contract or rules	Depends on group purposes and patient population; contract can be written or agreed on verbally.
Preparing members to enter the group	Individual versus group preparation; discussion, reading material, lecture, or interview can be used.

Fig. 30-1 Decisions to make before starting a group

Another early problem occurs if the group leader takes the responsibility for being the only authority in the group. There will be areas where the nurse may be the authority and giving information to the group would be considered appropriate. There are also occasions when group members can share leadership by providing and sharing helpful information.

Still another potential problem is the tendency for group leaders to develop countertransferences toward other members. When the group leader begins to notice powerful feelings of attraction to or dislike for individual members of the group, it is important that these countertransferences be examined. Another group leader who has more experience and is more objective should be contacted for discussion and supervision.

INITIAL GROUP PROCESSES:

— Increased anxiety in group members.

— Unrealistic expectations about group functioning.

— Group dependence on formal leader for answers.

— Transferences and countertransferences.

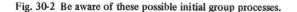

Fig. 30-2 Be aware of these possible initial group processes.

As a way to decrease anxiety, group members and leaders will frequently engage in long conversations with one other member. In such cases, the other group members may feel bored or left out of the discussion. It would be useful to the group leader to look for ways to involve more group members in the conversation. Figure 30-2 summarizes some initial group processes.

GROUP INTERVENTIONS

Communication skills that have been developed to be used with individual patients can also be used with groups of patients. Generally, a group leader poses questions for the group to answer and tries to get members interacting with each other, not just with the leader. Although many of the interventions suggested are used most often by leaders of expressive, supportive, discussion, or work groups, they are also useful in groups whose aim is to educate or encourage socialization.

Reducing Anxiety

There are a number of ways a group leader can reduce initial anxiety. One way is to let patients become familiar with the group leader before the group begins. This can be done by spending time talking to each group member prior to the beginning of the group.

Another way the leader "breaks the ice" is by sharing his or her reasons for the decision to lead this group. Also, describing any personal feelings and doubts which exist at the time relieves tension. If the nurse, as group leader, can admit to the group that she feels anxious or fearful, there is a greater chance that the others will be willing to share their opinions, wishes, and feelings. The group leader can anticipate curiosity about the leader's role; anxiety can be minimized by saying, " Some of you may wonder what I'll be doing in this group. What thoughts do you have about me and what I'll be doing?"

A group leader can also use relaxation techniques to decrease group anxiety in a beginning group. Asking group members to tell who they are and why each came to the group is one such technique. Group members might also be asked to write down what they expect from the group experience. Group members may be paired off and asked to introduce their partner to the group. In this case, each pair should be given a few minutes to find out about the other person and how he wishes to be introduced. Other group warm-ups include having members draw pictures of themselves and talk about the drawings or asking each member to shake hands with other members and state his name. Group leaders can also devise their own methods of promoting relaxation.

If the leader makes a comment such as, "I sense we're all nervous about what's being discussed," group members frequently relax and share their anxiety more openly. Humor is also a way to reduce anxiety. However, humor can be overdone or used to mask the leader's own anxiety.

Promote Interaction

During the early stages, it is to be expected that group members will be more likely to talk to the group leader than to each other. The group leader can promote interaction between members with statements such as, "I don't know. Who in the group has an idea about that?" In groups that have very little interaction, the leader might even direct one group member to speak to another by saying, "Tell Mr. Lown what you just told me," or "Mrs. Tansy, show Jimmy how to draw up the medication."

The leader can reward participation through use of verbal and nonverbal communication. The leader can comment on a member's participation by saying, "You've shared your thoughts and feelings with us today," or "Sometimes it's difficult to talk about feelings, but you tried hard today." Nonverbal rewards such as smiles, head nods, and eye contact can also be used to promote participation in the group. Some leaders serve coffee and cake or juice to patients who attend a group session. Before deciding on rewards, the leader must think about what effect they might have on the group members. Rewards or approval are never used as bribes; also, care should be taken to avoid arousing guilt feelings.

Silent group members may be encouraged to interact with the group when the leader turns toward or addresses a silent member with a comment such as, "What do you think, Mr. Towne?" This may also be done by allowing the group to handle the problem. The leader might say, "I notice there are a couple of group members who haven't talked today. Do you have any idea why?"

If everyone is silent, the group leader must first determine whether the silence is an angry, sad, thoughtful, peaceful or anxious silence. The leader can intervene to decrease excessive anxiety by saying, "Who has an idea about why silence may be uncomfortable?" With other pauses or silences, the leader waits to see how the group will handle the silence. Silence is not often a problem in childrens' groups or when the purpose of the group is to teach a procedure or task.

Share Leadership

The leader can help the group to share leadership in a number of ways. By summarizing what has occurred in the group, the leader teaches group members how to organize group events in a meaningful way. Examples of summary statements made by the leader are: "So far today we've discussed thoughts about hospitalization, but not feelings"; "We're moving closer toward a decision"; "The group seems to be angry that this is the last meeting"; "Today we've covered how to sterilize equipment." The leader can help the group to summarize by saying, "What's happened in the meeting today?"

Making statements which clarify ideas, feelings and problems helps the group to learn these skills. Examples of clarifying statements the leader might make are: "I think you're both saying you dislike noise" or "Mr. Thomas seems to be expressing anger. Am I right?" The leader can help the group to learn problem solving by clarifying the problem. This might be stated as, "The problem seems to be deciding on a free activity" or "Jenny seems to need help from the group in expressing anger" or "Mr. Todd could use group assistance in practicing the irrigation." Once the problem is clearly stated, the group can help to list alternate solutions to the problem. The leader might do this by saying, "Who can think of a way to solve this problem?" After the members have expressed all their ideas, the leader adds hers; then, the group is asked to test out or think through the result of each solution. Finally, the group decides on the best solution. It can then be tested and the results evaluated.

Guide the Group Toward Its Goals

The leader may set limits on the time allowed to discuss or decide on a minor issue. This procedure helps the group to stay focused on its goals. The leader may also place a time limit on procedure demonstrations or talks by individual members. Another way to keep the goal in focus is by not allowing the group to discuss nonrelated issues at length. To do this, the leader can comment,

"Your ten minutes to discuss are over, Tim," or "Let's get back to deciding on an activity."

A noisy pair of group members might prevent the group from reaching its goals. To deal with this problem, the leader could say, "Joe and Joan are forming their own group. What do you think about that?" In a highly structured teaching group, the problem might be handled differently. The leader might decide that the behavior of the noisy members is a sign they are involved and interested in the learning task. In a geriatric group, the leader may wonder if the two are temporarily disoriented. The leader or another group member might ask the pair to "try to listen to what's being said by the rest of the group."

Cohesiveness implies that the group members are involved and interested in group activities and goals. The leader promotes cohesiveness by encouraging members to interact with each other on an equal basis. If the leader thinks the group lacks cohesiveness, more frequent group meetings can be arranged. In planning to increase the frequency of group meetings, the leader remembers that this is a change in the group contract and cannot be implemented unless the whole group agrees to do so. Cohesiveness will probably increase with more frequent meetings since the frequency of interaction with other group members will increase.

Resolve Conflict

Conflict can be a constructive or destructive force in group interaction. The conflict that results from honest disagreement and working hard toward a goal can be a constructive experience. The conflict that results from high anxiety and unclear goals requires the reduction of anxiety and clarification of the group goals.

Conflict can arise when there is little group cohesion and various subgroups are not able to express opinions. In this case, the leader provides opportunities for all opinions to be expressed. If conflict continues, the leader can suggest a role-playing situation to assist group members to understand other points of view. Testing for agreement and observing for shifts of opinion help the leader determine how much of the conflict has decreased through understanding.

Decrease Monopolizing and Scapegoating

A group leader can deal with group members who always attempt to assume control and be the focus of attention. One way is to meet privately with the monopolizing person in order to provide support and special attention; this may decrease his frantic attempts to be the center of the group's attention.

Another way is to ask the group, "Why do you let Jack do all the talking?"

The leader can intervene in scapegoating by pointing out to the group what is happening. The following statement might be used: "One person keeps getting blamed for the group's lack of progress. I wonder why this is so?" If the group does not respond, more direct statements can be used such as, "Jack, you seem to blame Bob for never doing anything. I wonder if some of what you find annoying really comes from Glenda or me?"

Maintain Group Interest

Interest in the goals of the group may lag. At these times, the leader can vary group activities. Some suggested variations are: bringing in pictures or films, role playing, and assigning reading materials for discussion at the next meeting.

Prepare for New Members

Groups which are cohesive and have met together frequently can react strongly to the inclusion of new members. This may occur whether the groups are classroom groups, patient groups, family groups, or social groups.

When the nurse leader decides to add new members to an already formed group, she can reduce any discomfort which the group and the new members may experience. The new members can be told individually about the group contract. This prepares them to expect some lag in becoming part of the group. In addition, the group is told about the new members beforehand. The leader may also ask the group what they think about having new members and discuss the pros and cons which may appear.

Terminate the Group Relationships

When leading a highly cohesive group, the leader prepares herself and the group members for separation several meetings prior to the last meeting. Group members will need the time to summarize and evaluate the group experience and to loosen group relationships. The leader takes the responsibility for reminding the group about its end. She is also responsible for encouraging discussion about the group experience. Figure 30-3, page 474, summarizes nursing interventions with groups.

Interventions	Examples
Reducing anxiety	Meet with group members individually. Share feelings with the group. Anticipate group curiosity about the leader. Provide warm-up techniques. Express group feeling.
Promoting interaction	Ask group to answer questions and solve problems. Ask one member to talk to another group member. Comment on member participation. Approve of participation, nonverbally. Serve refreshments to group.
Sharing leadership	Role model how to summarize, clarify ideas and feelings. Ask group to summarize. Ask group to give alternate solutions to a problem. Help group to test alternatives. Ask group to decide on most constructive solution.
Guiding the group toward its goals	Set time limits on nonrelated issues and long-talking or noisy members.
Resolving conflict	Clarify group goals. Provide opportunities for all opinions to be expressed. Set up role-playing situations.
Decreasing monopolizing	Encourage group to deal with monopolizer. Meet individually with monopolizer.
Decreasing scapegoating	State observation that one member is being attacked or picked on. Ask group to figure out why scapegoating continues.
Keeping group interest	Change group activities, bring in new materials to discuss, use role playing, give between meeting assignments.
Preparing for new members	Meet with new group member individually. Tell group beforehand that there will be a new member in session. Ask for group reactions to new member joining them.
Ending the group experience	Remind members of approaching end and encourage group to summarize and evaluate group experience. In cohesive groups, encourage more discussion about thoughts and feelings regarding termination.

Fig. 30-3 Nursing interventions with groups

Type of Group	Examples
Social groups	Goes to lunch regularly with nursing staff members. Takes a group of patients on an outing. Forms a Koffee Klatch for nursing home residents. Starts a coffee hour for patients who regularly return to the clinic. Is part of a nursing class or classroom group.
Teaching groups	Asks preoperative patients to meet together to talk about surgery and postoperative care. Goes to patient's home to teach family to take over patient care. Meets with postoperative patients in a group to discuss postoperative care and future plans. Forms an ongoing group for about-to-be discharged patients to talk about preparing to go home. Calls new mothers together to teach breast or infant care. Starts a group for patients with chronic circulatory, elimination, neuromuscular or psychiatric difficulties to teach adaptive methods and preventative care. Forms a group to teach necessary nursing procedures to patients with diabetic, cardiac, or elimination problems.
Supportive or expressive groups	Gathers families of dying children together to express their feelings. Meets with dialysis patients in a group to provide support. Forms a group with patients who have a chronic condition to help them verbalize feelings and provide support for one another. Co-leads a therapeutic community meeting for staff and patients on a psychiatric unit.
Play group	At a clinic, gathers together children who regularly wait for their mothers. Forms a group for preschoolers.
Staff group	Orients new staff members through a group method. Starts a nursing group to discuss patient care. Conducts a team conference.
Activity group	Forms an activity group for nonverbal patients. Gathers patient or nursing home residents together to plan a group activity. Forms patients on a psychiatric unit into a group to repair or redecorate the unit. Begins an exercise group for patients or nursing home residents.
Nutritional groups	Forms long-term nursing home or psychiatric patients into a group to decide on and prepare a special meal. Gathers ambulatory patients to eat a meal together regularly in a solarium or available room.

Fig. 30-4 The nurse can practice leadership skills in a number of different groups.

NURSING LEADERSHIP

Nurses may begin or become part of many types of groups. Assessments and interventions for groups are useful to the nurse whether she initiates formation of a group or participates in a group. Some groups in which the nurse may become involved include: social groups for patients; teaching groups for patients or families; expressive or supportive groups for patients or families; play groups for children; staff or team conference groups; activity groups; and nutritional groups. Figure 30-4, page 475, lists some ways of exerting leadership in groups.

SUMMARY

Being a group leader requires special qualities, education, and supervision. All nurses can practice developing leadership skills in the groups of which they are part. Nurses who plan to start a group need to make the following decisions prior to forming the group: what type of group it will be, who will be part of the group, what purposes or goals the group will have, what size the group will be, what to do when members leave the group, how long the group will last, how often the group will meet, how the group will be seated, what equipment is needed, how to prepare members for the group experience, what rules or contracts there will be, and whether these will be stated as written or verbal agreements.

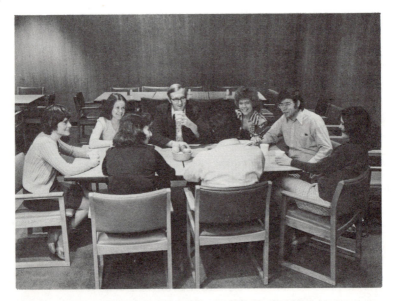

Fig. 30-5 In a cohesive group the members are involved and interested in group activities and goals.

Nurses should be aware that groups which meet regularly develop initial group processes of high anxiety, unrealistic expectations, and dependence on the leader to take responsibility for group happenings. Leaders of groups are also observant for signs of their own countertransferences. Whether nurses lead or participate, they can help the group by reducing anxiety, promoting interaction and rewarding participation, sharing leadership, guiding the group toward its goals, resolving conflict, decreasing monopolizing and scapegoating, maintaining group interest, preparing for new group members, and ending the group experience by summarizing and evaluating it.

ACTIVITIES AND DISCUSSION TOPICS

- Think of a group of which you are a member. Study the following list. How did you influence the group? Where do you need more practice? How could you develop more constructive group skills?

  1. Being realistic about what may happen in the group.
  2. Tolerating anxiety, frustration, and hostility.
  3. Organizing group information and data.
  4. Listening to others.
  5. Having a sense of humor.
  6. Sharing leadership.
  7. Promoting democratic decision making.
  8. Deciding how long the group will meet.
  9. Deciding where the group will meet.
  10. Deciding what will be discussed.
  11. Reading about group processes.
  12. Participating in a therapeutic or discussion group.
  13. Deciding on the size of the group.
  14. Decreasing anxiety.
  15. Being the group authority.
  16. Deciding on if or how to admit new members to the group.
  17. Being aware of countertransferences.
  18. Promoting interaction.
  19. Clarifying ideas and feelings.
  20. Clarifying the problem(s).
  21. Setting limits.

22. Resolving conflict.
23. Decreasing monopolizing.
24. Decreasing scapegoating.
25. Keeping group interest.

REVIEW

A. Multiple Choice. Select the best answer.

1. The group leader helps the group to stay focused on its goals by
   a. summarizing what has occurred in the group.
   b. setting time limits for discussion of minor issues.
   c. encouraging members to interact with each other on an equal basis.
   d. sharing leadership responsibilities with other group members.

2. One way a nurse can exert leadership in a staff group is to
   a. go to lunch regularly with staff members.
   b. form a group to teach necessary nursing procedures to patients.
   c. gather patients together to plan a group activity.
   d. start a nursing group to discuss patient care.

3. The minimum time limit set for interactive or discussion groups is
   a. 30 minutes.
   b. 45 minutes.
   c. 60 minutes.
   d. 90 minutes.

4. To promote interaction between group members, chairs should be arranged in a
   a. circle.
   b. semicircle.
   c. parallel line.
   d. horizontal line.

5. Before starting a group, nurses who are inexperienced group leaders must
   a. select group members who will work together cooperatively.
   b. take the responsibility for being the only authority in the group.
   c. participate in several co-leading group situations.
   d. seek supervision from a more experienced group leader.

B. Match the nursing intervention in Column II with the example of the intervention with groups in Column I.

Column I

1. Encourages discussion regarding thoughts and feelings about ending the group.

2. Asks group to give alternate solutions to a problem.

3. Provides opportunities for all opinions to be expressed.

4. Leader shares own feelings with the group.

5. Asks one member to talk to another group member.

6. Meets with new group members individually.

7. Changes group activities.

8. Encourages group to deal with member who constantly talks.

9. Verbalizes that one member is being attacked or picked on.

Column II

a. decreasing monopolizing
b. decreasing scapegoating
c. ending the group
d. keeping group interest
e. preparing for new group members
f. promoting interaction
g. reducing anxiety
h. resolving conflict
i. sharing leadership

C. Briefly answer the following questions.

1. List five qualities of a group leader.

2. List eight decisions that should be made before starting a group.

3. Name four ways a group leader can reduce initial anxiety in a group.

4. Name three group relaxation techniques.

5. What is a group contract?

GLOSSARY

Chapter 1 The Health Team and Nursing Roles

Continuity of care: The attempt to provide high level care for the patient at all times, including care from the patient's entry into a health care delivery system through discharge or transfer to another agency or facility.

Expanded roles in nursing: The assumption of new tasks as a result of physician, patient, nursing, or sociocultural demands or changes.

Health team: All personnel who are concerned with the health of the patient. In some institutions, the patient is included in health team planning.

Nursing: An interpersonal process where the patient is assisted to his or her highest level of wellness.

Nursing role of coordinator: The role the nurse assumes when planning care so as to provide the least amount of stress for the patient.

Nursing role of counselor: The role the nurse assumes when helping the patient to become aware of and deal with his feelings about what is happening to him.

Nursing role of leader: The role the nurse assumes when directing the patient to behave in a certain way or when encouraging others to be more independent.

Nursing role of liaison: The role the nurse assumes when communicating information from one source to another.

Nursing role of patient advocate: The role the nurse assumes when making sure that the patient has sufficient information to make the necessary health care decisions.

Nursing role of stranger: The role the nurse assumes when first meeting the patient and family.

Nursing role of substitute person: The role the nurse assumes when she takes on or seems to take on the role of a significant other person in the patient's life.

Nursing role of teacher: The role the nurse assumes when the nurse seeks to give information that will hopefully assist the patient to higher levels of wellness.

Nursing role of technician: The role the nurse assumes when giving smooth and calm administration of medications, treatments, and all nursing procedures.

Nursing team: A subsystem of the health team often composed of at least one registered nurse, a licensed practical nurse, and nursing aides or assistants.

Chapter 2 The Patient and the Family

Ally role: Family role where the child is asked to take sides with one parent against the other parent.

Feedback: Direct listener response to a communication message.

Messenger role: Family role where a member carries messages between two others who do not talk directly to one another.

Peacemaker Role: Family role where a member is expected to solve family arguments.

Problem child: Family role where child may be criticized for certain behaviors but indirectly allowed or supported in continuing the behaviors.

Self-esteem: A measure of how people feel about themselves and their ability to find satisfaction in life and their relationships with others.

Siblings: Brothers and/or sisters.

Chapter 3 Structuring the Nurse-Patient Relationship

Ambulatory: A patient who is able to be up and walk about without restrictions.

Nurse-Patient relationship: A professional, goal-directed relationship that is structured by the nurse to meet the expressed or implied needs of the patient or client.

Chapter 3 (Continued)

Orientation phase of the nurse-patient relationship: The first phase of the nurse-patient relationship where the nurse primarily acquaints the patient with the structure of the relationship, answers questions, listens actively, and establishes consistency.

Professional relationship: A relationship in which one person has special knowledge and skills and offers to help the other. The nurse-patient relationship is an example of a professional relationship.

Setting limits: Structuring the nurse-patient relationship in a clear and concise manner.

Termination phase of the nurse-patient relationship: The concluding phase of the nurse-patient relationship where the nurse introduces the idea of ending the relationship and assists the patient to summarize and evaluate it.

Testing limits: Patient behaviors aimed at determining whether the nurse means what she said.

Working phase of the nurse-patient relationship: The middle phase of the nurse-patient relationship; the nurse directs the patient to fill in areas of information that are unclear and assists the patient to cope with whatever the patient implies is problematic.

Chapter 4   Anxiety in the Nurse-Patient Relationship

Anxiety: A vague, unexplained discomfort usually due to unmet expectations or needs.

Fear: A feeling that occurs when a threatening object can be identified.

Panic: A very high level of anxiety where feelings of unreality occur and verbal communication with others is difficult.

Selective inattention: A protective device that people in moderate to severe anxiety use to block out parts of experiences that threaten them.

Somatization: Converting anxiety (or other feelings) into physical, bodily symptoms.

Chapter 5   The Nurse-Patient Relationship in Mental Illness

Behaviorist model of mental illness: Defines mental illness as behaviors which are reinforced and continue unchanged.

Delusion: A false, fixed thought that is based on a kernel of truth but develops into an illogical conclusion.

Hallucination: An internal, sensory perception without an external stimulus.

Medical model of mental illness: Defines mental illness as a disease like any other disease.

Process recording: A word-for-word written report of the patient's verbal and nonverbal communication and the nurse's verbal and nonverbal communication in the sequence in which it occurred, as well as an analysis and restatement by the nurse.

Psychological model of mental illness: Defines the patient's mental illness as his unsatisfying way of relating to others.

Social model of mental illness: Defines mental illness as originating in family and community relationships.

SECTION 2 HEALTH-ILLNESS RELATIONSHIPS

Chapter 6 Stability

Adaptation: Occurs when a person regulates both his internal and external environment in a successful way.

Body rhythm: An individual pattern, established by each person, that helps to maintain homeostasis through regulating performance levels, susceptibility to infection or emotional upset. An upset in body rhythm signals an illness process.

Competence: Fitness or ability to deal with the environment.

Deny or denial: Acting as if an occurrence has or is not happening as a way to cope with the discomfort of the happening.

External environmental processes: Ways in which people maintain freedom of movement and secure adequate information.

High level wellness: Maintaining homeostasis as well as pursuing goals beyond the basic needs.

Homeostasis: A healthy, more or less stable state where there is no undue imbalance between a person's internal and external environment.

Illness: An imbalance that occurs when a person is unsuccessful in adapting to complex interactions of physical, emotional, and social stressors.

Chapter 6 (Continued)

Internal environmental processes: Biochemical maintenance of body processes and defense mechanisms to meet interpersonal needs.

Level of wellness continuum: A way to evaluate level of wellness with zero health equal to death, and perfect health equal to an unknown optimum level of wellness.

Needs: Physiological, safety, interpersonal and self-actualization factors that motivate people to seek a balance between the internal state of their bodies and the external environment.

Prodromal: Relating to an early warning sign.

Stress: A condition produced by the normal wear and tear of bodily processes as well as by countless environmental demands.

Stressors: Causes of stress.

Suppress or suppression: A coping device where the person does not think about a situation or occurrence.

Chapter 7 Crisis

Adolescence: The fifth period of growth and development. Covers age 12-21 years. Major tasks are: identifying strengths and limitations of self and others; learning to be dependent, independent, and interdependent appropriately; and planning for the future.

Adulthood: The final growth and development period. Covers age 21 years to death. Major tasks are: establishing own family unit; maintaining communication with other age groups; succeeding in chosen endeavors; assessing life experiences; and facing death.

Affect: A feeling or emotional tone usually conveyed nonverbally by voice tone, facial expression and body posture.

Anger: A feeling response which can occur as a result of being restricted or as a response to anxiety.

Autonomy: A sense of self or "I" that begins to be developed when the child realizes he has some control over what happens to him.

Childhood: The second period of growth and development. It lasts from about age 1 1/2 to 6 years. Major tasks are: learning to delay satisfaction; increasing motor and verbal skill; and establishing autonomy.

Coping devices: Ways of dealing with stressors, ranging from internal thought responses to externally visible behaviors in a group.

Crisis: An upset in the balanced or stable state at which point the usual methods of adaptation are not adequate.

Delay satisfaction: After trust is established, people can learn to wait to have their needs met because their past experience has demonstrated others will respond.

Developmental crises: Periods of great social, psychological and physiological change that occur as part of the normal growth and development process and for which the person may be inadequately prepared.

Doubt: A sense of questioning and delaying satisfaction.

Guilt: A reaction to feeling incompetent.

Infancy: The first growth and development period, which occurs from birth to 1 1/2 or 2 years. Trust is one of the main developmental tasks.

Interdependent relationship: The ability of each person in the relationship to allow each one to be dependent on the other for some aspects of the relationships.

Juvenile era: The third growth and development period. Covers age 6-9 years approximately. Major tasks are entering school, learning about roles, establishing a pal or chum relationship and beginning to produce assigned materials.

Labelling or Stereotyping: Describing and reacting to another on the basis of a single characteristic of that person.

Preadolescence: The fourth growth and development period. Covers age 9-12 years approximately. Major tasks are becoming more independent and increasing productivity in social and educational tasks.

Projection: When one person assumes the other person has the same thoughts and feelings or is to blame for an unwanted occurrence.

Role: Learned pattern of behavior that is expected by others in the sociocultural setting and carried out by the person who is designated and accepts the designation.

Shame: A sense of self-consciousness.

Situational crises: Hazardous situations that are not easily anticipated and for which the person is inadequately prepared.

Social network: Other people with whom the patient or client interacts.

Unit 7 (Continued)

Unconditional love: Love that is given regardless of the other's ability to please or reward.

Chapter 8 Crisis Assessment and Intervention

Emotional support: Conveying an interested, nonjudgmental concern by remaining physically and emotionally present with the patient.

Withdrawal: Not talking or moving; demonstrating physical or emotional movement away from others.

Chapter 9 Dynamics of Pain

Central pain: Pain without an external stimulus; probably due to an injury to sensory nerves or to a persistent memory that a certain body area was in pain at one time.

Deep pain: Pain that occurs in the inner body structures such as muscles, joints, tendons and fascia.

Fascia: Tissues that connect and support body organs and structures.

Ischemia: Localized tissue anemia due to the obstruction of the inflow of arterial blood. As a result, there is an accumulation of wastes and the release of irritating chemicals from the injured cells.

Phantom pain: An example of central pain sometimes observed in patients who have had an amputation; the patient experiences pain below the point of amputation.

Psychogenic pain: Pain which occurs when the observer can find no evidence of tissue damage but is triggered or intensified by a memory, thought, or feeling.

Referred pain: Pain that has a source in one area but is felt or experienced in another area.

Superficial or cutaneous pain: Pain that arises from the skin or mucous membranes of the body.

Chapter 10 Pain Assessment and Intervention

Contraindications: Conditions which forbid use of a particular treatment.

Intermittent pain: Pain that is not constant, it comes and goes.

Leading questions: Questions that introduce ideas the patient may not have thought of; they may result in incorrect information.

Placebo: An inactive substance which is given to satisfy a demand for medication. It may be a capsule filled with sugar (glucose) or an injection of sterile water.

Placebo effect: Positive reaction of the patient to nearly any attempt of the helping person who conveys an interest in helping.

Side effects: Other effects a drug may have besides the one positive effect for which the drug is prescribed.

Chapter 11 The Grief Process

Acceptance stage of the dying process: The dying person peacefully withdraws from the external environment.

Anger stage of the dying process: The dying person is angry that life is being cut off and may direct anger toward the nurses and doctors.

Anticipatory grief: Grief that occurs prior to the actual loss.

Bargaining stage of the dying process: The dying person makes promises in exchange for extended life.

Brain death: Inadequate oxygenated blood supply to the brain for a few minutes.

Cardiac death: Absence of electrical heart impulses.

Clinical death: Absence of audible heartbeat.

Denial stage of the dying process: The dying person cannot believe he is dying.

Depression stage of death: The dying person comes to realize the enormity of the loss.

Grief: A series of internal emotional states in reaction to a loss.

Loss: Lack of external or internal environmental supports that help satisfy basic needs.

Mourning: A social process that includes not only internal emotional reactions, but also external behaviors in dealing with death.

Partial death: Ending of phases or aspects of life.

Psychological death: When a person does not know who he is or that he exists.

Social death: Health personnel accept that death is imminent.

Somatic death: Cessation of the body's vital functions.

Chapter 11 (Continued)

Subintentional death: Unconscious participation in hastening one's own death.

Withdrawal: A coping device where the person physically, emotionally, or socially leaves a disturbing situation.

SECTION 3 THE OBSERVATION-PERCEPTION-COMMUNICATION PROCESS

Chapter 13 Observation

Auscultation: Use of the sense of hearing to interpret sounds produced within the body.

Collector observation: Observing records that have been made by members of the health team.

Decubitus ulcer: Skin breakdown due to inadequate nutrition to the ulcerous area.

Dehydration: Condition brought about by inadequate fluid intake or excessive fluid output; indicated by dry, warm skin.

Dentures: False teeth.

Distention, abdominal: Accumulation of gas or fluid in the abdominal cavity.

Edema: Fluid accumulation in surface body tissues.

Gait: Style of walking, e.g., unsteady, shuffling, staggering, limping, or with assistance.

Inspection: Use of the sense of sight to compare the lack of, additions to, size, shape, and movement of various body parts.

Interpersonal observation: Use of various senses to identify, clarify, and verify hunches about the nurse-patient relationship.

Interviewer observation: Sitting down with the patient to ask for specific information from the patient or to focus on the nurse-patient relationship itself.

Jaundice: Yellow skin color indicating liver malfunction.

Observation, nursing: Use of sense of hearing, sight, smell or touch, together with basic knowledge and questioning to identify patient problems.

Palpation: Use of sense of touch to observe size, temperature, swelling or hardness of various body parts.

Participant observation: Engaging in nursing activities and observing the relationship between nurse and patient at the same time.

Peristalsis: The wavelike, muscular movement of the esophagus and intestines which propels contents through the digestive tract.

Pruritus: Itching.

Role playing: Reliving or preplaying an experience in order to expand its meaning and sharpen observational skills.

Sclera: White part of the eye.

Sign: An objective symptom which can be detected through observation, and frequently can even be measured.

Spectator observation: Observing the patient without patient awareness.

Symptom: A subjective or internal distressing occurrence the patient experiences and is usually associated with disturbed body function or illness process.

Vital signs: Indicators of body condition: temperature, pulse, respiration, and blood pressure. Sometimes referred to as "cardinal signs" indicating their vital importance as measurements of body function.

Chapter 14 Perception

Biofeedback: The ability to control certain functions of the autonomic nervous system such as pulse, blood pressure, brain waves and muscle contractions.

Diurnal time: Perception of time based on a 24-hour cycle rather than on minutes and hours.

Focused attention: A protective device that allows humans to focus on important events in their environment.

Habituation: Becoming unaware of the stressful elements of a situation due to familiarity with the situation.

Institutional time: Perception of time based on clock time where time is thought to be wasted and efficiency is important.

Perception: A complex, learned process involving sensory organs, the central nervous system, past and present experiences, and future expectations.

Perceptual set: Preconceived idea of how a situation will be.

Rorschach inkblot test: A psychological diagnostic tool composed of a series of nondescript inkblots.

Sensory deprivation: A condition that can result when too little sensory information is available to a person.

Chapter 14 (Continued)

Sensory overload: A condition that can result when too much sensory information or sensory information that is monotonous is available to a person.

Stereotyped frames of reference: Categorization of people by labels which restrict perception and subsequently, behavior.

Tunnel vision effect: A narrowing and distortion of the perceptual field due to high anxiety.

Chapter 15 Verbal Communication

Communication: The dynamic process of giving and getting information where one person affects at least one other person through verbal or nonverbal messages.

Denotative: One of the agreed-upon meanings by people who use a particular language; usually a meaning found in the dictionary for that language.

Feedback: A correction device in the communication process where the sender receives correction of errors and learns about the results of his or her own statements.

Loose associations: The speaker's response does not seem to follow or to be related to the preceding discussion.

Metacommunication: A message (about another message) that tells the receiver how the sender feels about the receiver, the sender, or the message.

Chapter 16 Nonverbal Communication

Action language: Form of nonverbal communication which includes all movements not used specifically as signals.

Communication context: The setting within which communication occurs.

Double bind: The verbal message does not fit with the nonverbal message. The receiver is confused about which message to respond to.

Flat Affect: Expressionless face, posture or tone of voice.

Inappropriate affect: Tone of voice, facial expression, or posture that does not fit with the situation being experienced.

Nonverbal communication: All communication that is not spoken or written, including sign language, action language, and object language.

Object language: Form of nonverbal communication where people convey messages about themselves by displaying objects on or about them.

Proxemics: The study of how people communicate by their use of space.

Sign language: Forms of nonverbal communication – such as smoke signals, Morse Code, motorist signals, deaf sign language, hitchhiker, and peace signs.

Chapter 17 Interviewing and Communication Skills

Nursing interview: Conversation with a purpose.

Play therapy: Use of play or activities to help children express their thoughts and feelings.

Process recording: Word-for-word record of nonverbal and verbal communication in an ongoing written form. Analysis and restatement are included.

Probing: Delving into subjects because of personal interest or anxiety.

Theme: Major mood or idea of an interview.

Topics: Things discussed during an interview.

Chapter 18 Blocks to Effective Communication

Blocking: Stammering, stuttering, and inability to remember due to conflict.

Communication block: Interference with effective communication due to the nurse's or the patient's anxiety, conflict, stereotyped attitudes, or other thoughts or feelings.

Conflict: Two opposing goals resulting in indecision, vacillation between goals and blocking.

Chapter 19 Nursing Process

Intervention: The actual act of carrying out nursing actions or order.

Nursing action or nursing order: Statement of what is to be achieved for or with the patient, including when and how the action should occur.

Nurse-centered goals or objectives: Statements concerning what the nurse hopes to accomplish.

Nursing diagnosis: A tool of nursing assessment where the patient's needs are considered in all the following areas: interpersonal needs, self-actualization needs, need for oxygen, need for activity and rest, need to avoid injury and repair damage, need for food and fluid, and need to eliminate waste.

Chapter 19 (Continued)

Nursing history: A tool used to assess the patient's interpersonal needs and preferences, usual patterns of daily living, self-actualization needs, response to hospitalization, expectations about and attitudes toward hospitalization.

Nursing goals or objectives: Statements that describe the result or change in patient behavior that will restore homeostasis.

Nursing process: A way of thinking and acting in a purposeful way which includes a continual cycle through assessment; setting goals, priorities and actions; intervention; and evaluation.

Patient-centered goals or objectives: Statements indicating what the patient will do to restore or maintain homeostasis.

Patient problem: The end product of a patient's inability to meet one or more needs. Patient problems lead to disturbed homeostasis.

Systematic assessment guide: A tool of nursing assessment; the results change, depending on the patient's degree of health or illness.

Chapter 20   Nursing Care Plans

Kardex: A holder that contains a card for each patient with space for written objectives, special needs and preferences; for patient problems and nursing interventions; and for medical orders.

Nursing care plans: Records that summarize information necessary to provide nursing care for patients and families.

Nursing rounds: Evaluation visits to patients usually conducted by the head nurse, team leader, or nurse clinician.

Team leader: The coordinator of health personnel or nursing personnel who care for a specific group of patients.

Team report: Conferences attended by team members and usually called by the team leader; the purpose is to share information about each of the patients in their care.

SECTION 4   COPING WITH ILLNESS

Chapter 21   The Hospital and the Institution

Ambivalent feelings: Having at least two opposite feelings about a person or situation; mixed feelings.

Depersonalization effect: Procedures which treat the patient like an object rather than a person; examples include referring to the patient by diagnosis, stripping him of his clothes and social roles, and keeping him waiting without explanation.

Formal rules for behavior: Written or spoken rules for behavior such as a hospital philosophy.

"Good" or overcooperative patient role: One way patients deal with the effects of hospitalization. This role includes concern about pleasing the nurse as primary and patient needs as secondary patient goals.

Hierarchical communication structure: The flow of communication is primarily one way, from the top to the bottom of the hierarchy. This type of structure makes it more difficult for the patient to have his needs and wants heard and acted upon.

Horizontal or free-flowing communication structure: Every staff member has access to nearly every other staff member in a fluid and diverse communication system.

Informal rules for behavior: Understood or tolerated behavior; what actually occurs in the setting.

Magical thinking: Expecting others to mind read or magically know what one wants or needs without telling the other person.

Mixed messages: Two different and oppositional messages are conveyed in one communication.

Negative sanctions: Punishment placed on those who do not act as expected.

Norms: Behavioral limits of expected behavior.

Positive sanctions: Reward for those who do act as expected.

Regression: A four-part patient attempt to cope with illness including increased need to control the external environment, a focus on basic needs, resentment or anger, and increased dependency.

Social system: A group of people who continually interact and have developed shared expectations, norms, and values.

Staff: Hospital personnel.

Values: Ideas about expected behavior.

Chapter 22 The Therapeutic Environment

Primary nurse approach: One nurse is primarily responsible for the care of one or more patients throughout the entire hospital stay.

Therapeutic community: An approach used primarily on mental health units where the entire staff and patient population make joint decisions about patient care.

Therapeutic environment: An environment which assists people to meet basic needs, and also to grow and increase their potential for more effective and satisfying life or death processes.

Chapter 23 Mind-Body Relationships

Avoidance: A homeostatic device where the person avoids an upsetting situation.

Depression: Condition of withdrawal from physical activities and contacts.

Holistic approach to patient care: An attempt to understand the whole patient, including the interrelationships of physiological, psychological, social, and cultural processes.

Neurosis: Isolation of the impaired emotional aspect of a situation.

Onset: Beginning.

Pathogenic: Disease-producing.

Precipitating factors: Situations which seem to bring on a disturbed condition.

Predisposition: Tendency.

Psychosomatic or psychophysiological disorders: Disorders where both psychological and physiological principles can be applied in their study and treatment.

Rationalization and intellectualization: Two homeostatic devices where the person attempts to explain away an occurrence.

Schizophrenia: Condition manifested by withdrawal from contact with reality.

Somatization: A process where the person converts feelings into body sensations or symptoms.

Somatopsychology: The study and treatment of physical handicaps and disabilities, and their effect on emotional processes.

Chapter 24 Stages of Illness and the Sick Role

Convalescent stage: The return to health that requires passage through certain tasks.

Malingerer: Term sometimes used to describe the patient who considers himself to be ill while health personnel do not.

Secondary gain: Satisfaction, approval, or attention resulting from conspicuous symptoms.

Sick role: A dependent state where the patient is not expected to be a useful or productive member of society.

Chapter 25 Coping Devices

Auditory hallucination: Projection of one's own unacceptable thoughts or feelings onto the environment by "hearing voices."

Compensation: Process by which a person excels in one area to overcome or substitute for a real or imagined weakness in another area.

Conversion: Transforming feelings into a physical disability or symptom.

Coping devices: Thoughts, feelings, and behaviors that help people to deal with stress.

Countertransference: The nurse unconsciously attributes to the patient characteristics that really belong to a significant person in the nurse's life.

Delusion: A false, fixed thought developed as a way to deal with a seemingly unexplainable occurrence.

Delusion of grandeur: Thinking one is an important, great person to cope with feelings of insecurity.

Delusion of persecution: Projecting one's own angry feelings onto other people as a way to protect against intimacy.

Denial: Acting as if the current or past situation is not occurring, or did not occur.

Depersonalization: Having unreal feelings about one's own body.

Displacement: Shifting or placing feelings about an object or person to another object or person.

Identification: Imitating another's behavior.

Intellectualization: Using technical terms when asked to state feelings.

Chapter 25 (Continued)

Projection: Attributing one's own unacceptable thoughts or feelings to others.

Rationalization: Using an excuse to justify behavior while disguising an unconscious motive.

Reaction formation: Developing an attitude or action directly opposite to the actual wish or desire.

Regression: Going back to earlier interest, modes of satisfaction, and problems.

Repression or dissociation: Putting traumatic situations automatically out of conscious awareness.

Sublimation: Redirecting an unacceptable tendency and substituting an acceptable tendency.

Suppression: A conscious decision not to act.

Transference: A second meaning of identification used when the patient attributes characteristics to the therapist or nurse that really belong to significant other people in the patient's life.

Chapter 26 Body Image and Self-Concept

Anticipatory guidance: A preventive nursing intervention in potential crisis situations where people are prepared to cope with upcoming situations through discussion and problem solving prior to the actual situation.

Body image: The mental picture a person develops of his physical or biological self.

Climacteric: Physiological and psychological reactions experienced by the middle-aged adult.

Draw-a-person test: A test used to assess the body image difficulties of young children.

Phantom limb: Body part sensations which are experienced after amputation, possibly as an adaptive maneuver.

Quickening: First movement of the fetus felt by the mother.

Self-concept: The total collection of feelings a person has about herself, including the spiritual, moral, and social self.

SECTION 5 THE LEARNING PROCESS

Chapter 27 Nursing Conferences

In-service education: Supervised learning experiences gained on the job.

Postconference: A group discussion among nursing instructor and nursing students that follows the clinical nursing laboratory experience.

Preconference: A gathering of nursing instructor and nursing students to discuss and plan the clinical nursing laboratory experience.

Chapter 28 Learning Through Teaching

Analysis: Breaking a situation down into its component parts.

Behavioral modification: Process where the patient's behavior is changed or modified in relation to positive or negative responses by the helping person.

Negative reinforcement: Nonresponse to or disapproval that follows a specific patient behavior.

Positive reinforcement: Concern, interest, or approval that follows a specific patient behavior.

Pretest: A test given prior to a learning experience to determine how much the learner already knows.

Reinforcers: Consequences of behavior that strengthen or decrease the behavior.

Role model: Demonstrating through action how others can act effectively.

Self-paced learning: Learning that occurs at the rate most comfortable for the learner.

Synthesis: Putting all the component parts of a situation together to arrive at a new fact or conclusion.

Validation: A communication skill used by the nurse where the nurse checks with the patient to assure they agree on the meaning of a situation.

Chapter 29 Group Process and Learning

Apathy: A group process that can occur when goals are unclearly defined, there is interest in other goals, or fear of the goal or a group member, feelings of powerlessness or conflict.

Chapter 29 (Continued)

Authority figures: People who are thought to be especially powerful. People who are unable to change their belief that all authority figures have the same power over them that their parents did will continue to challenge or fear authority figures.

Cohesiveness: A measure of how attractive the group is to its members. In a highly cohesive group, all members are involved in the group's activities.

Group content: The topics that are discussed in a group or the themes that emerge.

Group decision making: A group process that includes the following steps if it is to be effective: clear statement of the problem, statement of alternate solutions, continued summary and refocus on the problem, testing out the solutions, choosing an appropriate decision.

Group phases of development: The three phases all groups pass through (if there is no impediment to proceeding to the working phase) are: orientation, working, and termination.

Group process: The ebb and flow of group interaction; group process is studied by asking, "What is happening now" and "What is making it happen?"

Leadership: An interpersonal process that helps the group move toward its goals, improve interpersonal relationships, and make the skills of the individual available to the group.

Maintenance functions: Part of the necessary group functions; focus is on improving and maintaining interpersonal relationships.

Monopolizing: A group process where the group allows one member to do all or most of the talking.

Norms: Attitudes or expectations shared by the group.

Orientation phase of group: The first phase where there is concern about being accepted by others, initial distrust of other group members, demands to be told what to do in the group and how to do it, (often) high anxiety levels, some anger, and the giving and getting of information to form group norms.

Peer pressure: Influence by members of one's own group to behave in a certain manner.

Scapegoating: A group process where one member is singled out and agrees to be the target of group hostility.

Task functions: Part of the necessary group functions; focus is on accomplishing group goals.

Termination or separation phase (group): The final phase of group development characterized by looking to the future and attempting to loosen ties within the group. Sadness, anger, rejection of the group, guilt, and satisfaction or relief are some common feelings of group members at this time.

Testing behavior (group): A communication often found in the orientation phase of a group where one or more group members attempt to see what the limits of behavior are for this group.

Transference (group): A group member transfers thoughts and feelings originally held toward his own family member(s) onto group members.

Working phase (group): The second stage in group development which not all groups enter. In this phase, norms are set, group members take more responsibility for what happens in the group, conversation is more spontaneous, and feelings may be expressed more directly.

Chapter 30 Learning in Groups

Closed group: Group members are not added when members leave the group.

Group contract: A verbal or written agreement entered into by the group leader and the group members.

Open group: Group members are added when members leave the group or when the leader decides (sometimes with group permission) to add other participants.

Warm-up activities (group): Communication exercises used to decrease initial anxiety about being in the group.

SUGGESTED READINGS

SECTION 1 HEALTH CARE RELATIONSHIPS

Chapter 1 The Health Team and Nursing Roles

Buchan, J. "Problems of Interdisciplinary Communication." *Canadian Journal of Public Health* 62:227, May-June 1971.

Epstein, C. "Breaking the Barriers to Communication on the Health Team." *Nursing '74* 4:65-68, September 1974.

Germaine, A. "What Makes Team Nursing Tick?" *Journal of Nursing Administration* 1:46-49, July-August 1971.

Hoekelman, Robert A. "Nurse-Physician Relationships." *American Journal of Nursing* 75, 7:1150-1153, 1975.

Kennedy, E. *In Critical Condition — The Crisis in American Health Care.* New York: Simon and Schuster, 1972.

Kohnke, Mary F.; Zimmern, Ann; and Greenridge, Jocelyn A. "Advocacy." *Independent Nurse Practitioner.* New York: Trainex, 1974.

Kosik, S.H. "Patient Advocacy or Fighting the System." *American Journal of Nursing* 72:694-98, 1972.

Kron, T. "Team Nursing — How Viable is it Today?" *Journal of Nursing Administration* 1:19-22, November-December 1971.

Levin, P., and Berne, E. "Games Nurses Play." *American Journal of Nursing* 72:483-87, 1972.

Morris, Karen, and Foerster, J. "Team Work: Nurse and Chaplain." *American Journal of Nursing* 72, 12:2197-99, 1972.

Seiler, K. "The Team Conference." *Supervisor Nurse* 5:64-65, September 1974.

Sheenan, D. "The Game of the Name." *Nursing Outlook* 20:440-44, July 1972.

Stein, Leonard. "The Doctor-Nurse Game." *American Journal of Nursing* 68, 1:101-05, 1968.

Thomstad, Beatrice et al. "Changing the Rules of the Doctor-Nurse Game." *Nursing Outlook* 23, 7:422-27, 1975.

Chapter 2 The Patient and Family

Bowden, Marjorie L., and Feller, Irving. "Family Reactions to a Severe Burn." *American Journal of Nursing* 73, 2:317-19, 1973.

Byers, Mary L. "Grief Work of a Mother of a Child Born with Defects." *ANA Clinical Conference # 3 – Exploring Progress in Maternal and Child Health*, 1965.

Canady, M.E. "SSPE – Helping the Family Cope." *American Journal of Nursing* 72:94-96, 1972.

Fitzpatrick, Patricia. "Parental Reactions to a Visually Handicapped Child." *The Psychiatric Nurse as a Family Therapist.* Edited by Shirley Smoyak. New York: John Wiley, 1975.

Freiberg, K.H. "How Parents React When Their Child is Hospitalized." *American Journal of Nursing* 72:1270-73, 1972.

Hall, Joanne E., and Weaver, Barbara R. *Nursing of Families in Crisis.* Philadelphia: Lippincott, 1974.

Hopkins, Joan. "The Nurse and the Abused Child." *Nursing Clinics of North America*, December 1970.

Jackson, Don D. "The Study of the Family." *Family Process* 4:1-20, 1965.

Kovacs, Liberty. "A Therapeutic Relationship with a Patient and Family." *Perspectives in Psychiatric Care* 4:11-21, March 1966.

Messer, Alfred. *The Individual in his Family.* Springfield, Illinois: Charles C. Thomas, 1970.

Noland, Robert L. *Counseling Parents of the Ill and the Handicapped.* Springfield, Illinois: Charles C. Thomas, 1971.

Portman, R. "Who Cares for the Relatives." *Nursing Times* 70:1125, July 18, 1974.

Roberts, H. "Talking to Relatives." *Nursing Times* 67:860-61, 1971.

Ryan, M.A. "Helping the Family Cope with Cardiac Arrest." *Nursing '74* 4:80-81, August 1974.

Schulz, David. *The Changing Family.* Englewood Cliffs, New Jersey: Prentice-Hall, 1972.

Chapter 2 (Continued)

Sedgwick, R. "The Family as a System: a Network of Relationships." *Journal of Psychiatric Nursing* 12:17-20, March–April 1974.

Sobol, Evelyn, and Robischon, Paulette. *Family Nursing: A Study Guide.* St. Louis: C.V. Mosby, 1970.

VanderMeer, Josephine. "Disciplinary Practices in a Family with a History of Child Abuse." *The Psychiatric Nurse as a Family Therapist.* Edited by Shirley Smoyak. New York: John Wiley, 1975.

Wrightsman, Lawrence S. *Social Psychology in the Seventies.* Monterey, California: Brooks/Cole Publishing Co., 1972.

Chapter 3   Structuring the Nurse-Patient Relationship

Baumgartner, Margaret. "Empathy." in *Behavioral Concepts in Nursing.* Edited by Carolyn Carlson. Philadelphia: Lippincott, 1970.

Dillon, Kathryn M. "A Patient-Structured Relationship." *Perspectives in Psychiatric Care* 9, 4:167-172, 1971.

Dodge, Joan S. "What Patients Should be Told: Patients and Nurse's Beliefs." *American Journal of Nursing* 72:1852-1854, October 1972.

Ehmann, Virginia E. "Empathy: Its Origin, Characteristics and Process." *Perspectives in Psychiatric Care* 9, 2:72-80, 1971.

Epstein, Charlotte. *Effective Interaction in Contemporary Nursing.* Englewood Cliffs, New Jersey: Prentice-Hall, 1974.

Evans, Frances M.C. *Psychosocial Nursing.* New York: Macmillan, 1971.

Hale, Shirley L., and Richardson, Julia H. "Terminating the Nurse-Patient Relationship." *American Journal of Nursing*, September 1963.

Jurgensen, Kathleen. "Limit Setting for Hospitalized Adolescent Psychiatric Patients." *Perspectives in Psychiatric Care* 9, 4:173-183, 1971.

Mercer, Lianne S., and O'Connor, Patricia. *Fundamental Skills in the Nurse-Patient Relationship: A Programmed Text.* 2d. ed. Philadelphia: Saunders, 1974.

Nehran, Jeanette, and Gilliam, Naomi R. "Separation Anxiety." *American Journal of Nursing*, January 1965.

Peplau, Hildegard E. *Interpersonal Relations in Nursing.* New York: Putnam, 1952.

Stankiewicz, Barbara S. "Termination in the Student-Patient Relationship." *Perspectives in Psychiatric Care* 7, 1:39-45, 1969.

Ujhely, Gertrud. *Determinants of the Nurse-Patient Relationship.* New York: Springer, 1968.

Chapter 4 Anxiety in the Nurse-Patient Relationship

Anxiety — Recognition and Intervention. *American Journal of Nursing* 65: 129-153, September 1965.

Burkhardt, Marti. "Response to Anxiety." *American Journal of Nursing* 69:2153-2154, October 1969.

Cohen, R. "Anxiety in a Jewish Patient." *Journal of Psychiatric Nursing and Mental Health Services* 9:5, November-December 1971.

Coopersmith, S. *The Antecedents of Self-esteem.* San Francisco: Freeman, 1967.

Manaser, Janice C., and Werner, Anita. *Instruments for Study of Nurse-Patient Interaction.* New York: Macmillan, 1964.

Mitchell, R. "Anxiety: Part One." *Nursing Times* 70:991-993, June 27, 1974.

_____. "Anxiety: Part Two." *Nursing Times* 70:1030-1032, July 4, 1974.

Peplau, Hildegard E. "Unexplained Discomfort." *Interpersonal Relations in Nursing.* New York: G.P. Putnam and Sons, 1952.

Shafer, D. "The Symptom Complex of Anxiety: Its Interplay with Fear." *Medical Insight* 3:16, April 1971.

Stephens, K.S. "A Toddler's Separation Anxiety." *American Journal of Nursing* 73:1553-1555, September 1973.

Tubbs, A. "Nursing Intervention to Shorten Anxiety-ridden Transition Periods." *Nursing Outlook* 18:27, July 1970.

Wear, E.T. "Separation Anxiety Reconsidered: Nursing Implications." *Maternal-Child Nursing Journal* 3:9-18, Spring 1974.

Chapter 5 The Nurse-Patient Relationship in Mental Illness

Burgess, Ann C., and Lazare, Aaron. *Psychiatric Nursing in the Hospital and Community.* Englewood Cliffs, New Jersey: Prentice-Hall, Inc., 1973.

Clark, Carolyn C. *Recording and Evaluating Nurse-Patient Interactions: Using the Process Recording Guide.* New York: Trainex, 1975.

_____. "A Social System Approach to Short-term Psychiatric Care." *Perspectives in Psychiatric Care* 10, 4:178-82, 1972.

Donner, Gail. "Treatment of a Delusional Patient." *American Journal of Nursing* 69, 12:2642-49, 1969.

Duran, Fernando, and Errion, Gerald D. "Perpetuation of Chronicity in Mental Illness." *American Journal of Nursing* 70, 8:1707-09, 1970.

Ferneau, Ernest W. "What Student Nurses Think About Alcoholic Patients and Alcoholism." *Nursing Outlook* 15, 10:40-41, 1967.

Chapter 5 (Continued)

Field, William. "Watch Your Message." *American Journal of Nursing* 72, 7:1278-80, 1972,

Goldsborough, Judith D. "On Becoming Nonjudgmental." *American Journal of Nursing* 70, 11:2340-43, 1970.

Klerman, Gerald. "Mental Health and the Urban Crisis." *American Journal of Orthopsychiatry* 39, 5:818-26, 1969.

Phinney, Richard P. "The Student of Nursing and the Schizophrenic Patient," *American Journal of Nursing* 70, 4:790-92, 1970.

Riley, Mildred. "Nursing Interview for Psychiatric Patients." *Nursing Outlook* 16, 10:54-57, 1968.

Schwartz, Morris S., and Shockley, Emmy L. *The Nurse and the Mental Patient.* New York: John Wiley, 1956.

SECTION 2 HEALTH-ILLNESS RELATIONSHIPS

Chapter 6 Stability

Beeson, Gerald. "The Health-Illness Spectrum," *American Journal of Public Health* 57, 11:1901-1904, 1967.

Berkowitz, Phillip and Nancy. "The Jewish Patient in the Hospital," *American Journal of Nursing* 67, 11:2335-2337, 1967.

Brinton, D. "Health Center Milieu: Interaction of Nurses and Low Income Families." *Nursing Research* 21, 1:46-52, 1972.

Burnside, Irene. "Clocks and Calendars." *American Journal of Nursing* 70, 1:117-119, 1970.

Campbell, Teresa, and Chung, Betty. "Health Care of Chinese in America." *Nursing Outlook* 21, 4:245-249, 1973.

Coelho, George V. et al eds. *Coping and Adaptation.* New York: Basic Books, 1974.

Dubos, Rene. *Man Adapting.* New Haven: Yale University Press, 1965.

Dunn, Halbert. *High Level Wellness.* Virginia: R.W. Bearry, Ltd., 1961.

Grahm, Saxon. "Studies of Behavior Change to Enhance Public Health." *American Journal of Public Health* 63, 4:327-334, 1973.

Jaco, E. Gartley, ed. *Patients, Physicians and Illness.* 2d ed. New York: The Free Press, 1972.

Jones, K. et al. *Dimensions: A Changing Concept of Health.* San Francisco: Canfield Press, 1972.

Kepler, Milton. "The Religious Factor in Pediatric Care." *Clinical Pediatrics* 9, 3:128-130, 1970.

Leonard, Sister Margaret Ann, and Joyce, Sister Carol Ann. "Two Worlds United." *American Journal of Nursing* 71, 6:1152-1155, 1971.

Levine, M. "Adaptation and Assessment: A Rationale for Nursing Intervention." *American Journal of Nursing* 66, 11:2450-2453, 1966.

Luce, Gay Gaer. *Biological Rhythms in Psychiatry and Medicine.* United States Department of Health, Education and Welfare Public Health Service Publication #2088, 1970.

Luckmann, Joan, and Sorenson, Karen C. "What Patients' Actions Tell you About Their Feelings, Fears and Needs.", *Nursing '75* 5, 2:54-61, February 1975.

Maslow, Abraham H. *Motivation and Personality.* 2d ed. New York: Harper and Row, 1970.

Murray, Ruth, and Zentner, Judith. *Nursing Assessment and Health Promotion Through the Life Span.* Englewood Cliffs, New Jersey: Prentice-Hall, 1975.

Paynich, M. "Cultural Barriers to Nurse Communication." *American Journal of Nursing* 64, 2:87-90, 1964.

Read, Donald, A. *The Concept of Health.* 2d ed. Boston: Holbrook Press, 1973.

Rubel, Arthur. "Concepts of Disease in Mexican-American Culture." *American Anthropologist* 62:795-814, 1960.

Weiss, M. Olga. "Cultural Shock." *Nursing Outlook* 19, 1:40-43, 1971.

Wu, Ruth. *Behavior and Illness.* Englewood Cliffs, New Jersey: Prentice-Hall, 1973.

Chapter 7 Crisis

Abram, Henry et al. "Suicidal Behavior in Dialysis Patients." *American Journal of Psychiatry* 127:1190-1204, March 1971.

Aguilera, Donna C. et al eds. *Crisis Intervention: Theory and Methodology.* St. Louis: C.V. Mosby, 1970.

Baca, Josephine. "Some Health Beliefs of the Spanish Speaking." *American Journal of Nursing* 69, 10:2172-2176, 1969.

Caplan, Gerald. *Support Systems and Community Mental Health.* New York: Behavioral Publications, 1974.

Chambers, Carolyn. "Nurse Leadership During Crisis Situations on a Psychiatric Ward." *Perspectives in Psychiatric Care* 5, 1:29-35, January–February 1967.

Coelho, George V. et al eds. *Coping and Adaptation.* New York: Basic Books, 1974.

Chapter 7 (Continued)

Donner, Gail J. "Parenthood as a Crisis: A Role for the Psychiatric Nurse." *Perspectives in Psychiatric Care* 10, 2:84-87, 1972.

Erikson, Erik H. *Childhood and Society*. 2d. ed. New York: W.W. Norton, 1963.

Gorton, John V. *Behavioral Components of Patient Care*. New York: Macmillan, 1970.

Grace, Helen K., ed. "Symposium on Crisis Intervention." *Nursing Clinics of North America* 9, 1:1-96, March 1974.

Leininger, Madeleine. *Nursing and Anthropology: Two Worlds to Blend*. New York: Wiley, 1970.

Levine, Sidney, and Kahana, Ralph J., eds. *Psychodynamic Studies on Aging: Creativity, Reminiscing, and Dying*. New York: International Universities Press, 1967.

Maloney, Elizabeth M. "The Subjective and Objective Definition of Crisis." *Perspectives in Psychiatric Care* 9, 6:257-268, 1971.

Parad, Howard J., ed. *Crisis Intervention: Selected Readings*. New York: Family Service Association, 1965.

Sullivan, Harry Stack. *The Interpersonal Theory of Psychiatry*. New York: W.W. Norton, 1953.

White, Robert W. "Competence and Psychosexual Stages of Development." *Nebraska Symposium on Motivation*. University of Nebraska Press, 1960.

Chapter 8 Crisis Assessment and Intervention

Aguilera, Donna. "Crisis: Moment of Truth." *Journal of Psychiatric Nursing and Mental Health Services* 9:23, May-June 1971.

_____ . et. al. *Crisis Intervention*. St. Louis: C.V. Mosby, 1970.

Bodie, Marilyn K. "When a Patient Threatens Suicide." *Perspectives in Psychiatric Care* 6, 2:76-79, 1968.

Burnside, Irene. "Crisis Intervention with Geriatric Hospitalized Patients." *Journal of Psychiatric Nursing and Mental Health Services* 8:17, March-April 1970.

Clemmons, P. "The Role of the Nurse in Suicidal Prevention." *Journal of Psychiatric Nursing* 9:27, January-February 1971.

Deibel, A. "Suicide in the Aged." *Journal of Psychiatric Nursing* 9:39, May-June 1971.

Frost, M. "Counselling the Suicidal Patient." *Nursing Mirror* 139:74-75, July 5, 1974.

King, Joan M. "The Initial Interview: Basis for Assessment in Crisis Intervention." *Perspectives in Psychiatric Care* 9, 6:247-256, 1971.

Maloney, Elizabeth. "The Subjective and Objective Definition of Crisis." *Perspectives in Psychiatric Care* 9, 6:257-268, 1971.

Parad, Howard J., ed. *Crisis Intervention: Selected Readings.* New York: Family Service Association, 1965.

Peplau, Hildegard. "Communication in Crisis Intervention." *Psychiatric Forum* 2:1, Winter 1971.

Poulos, J. "Why is Johnny Dead? The Growing Problem of Suicide Among Troubled Adolescents." *Bedside Nurse* 3, 3:27, December 1970.

Seiden, Richard H. "Suicide: Preventable Death." *Public Affairs Report* 15, 4:1-6. Berkeley: University of California Press, August 1974.

Stein, L. "The Doctor-Nurse Game." *Archives of General Psychiatry* 16: 699-703, 1967.

Williams, Florence. "Intervention in Maturational Crisis." *Perspectives in Psychiatric Care* 9, 6:240-256, 1971.

Chapter 9 Dynamics of Pain

Billars, Karen S. "You Have Pain? I Think this will Help." *American Journal of Nursing* 70:2143-2145, October 1970.

Copp, Laurel A. "The Spectrum of Suffering." *American Journal of Nursing* 74, 3:491-495, March 1974.

Copple, D. "What Can a Nurse do to Relieve Pain Without Resorting to Drugs?" *Nursing Times* 68:584, May 11, 1972.

Drakontides, Anna B. "Drugs to Treat Pain." *American Journal of Nursing* 74, 3:508-513, March 1974.

"Emotional and Psychological Aspects of Pain." slide-tape instruction by Trainaide, Glendale, California, 91201.

Lishman, T. "The Psychology of Pain." *Nursing Times* 66:1577-1578, December 10, 1970.

Mastrovito, Rene C. "Psychogenic Pain." *American Journal of Nursing* 74, 3:514-519, March 1974.

McBride, Mary Angela. "Pain and Effective Nursing Practice." *American Nurses' Association Clinical Sessions*, 1967.

McCaffery, Margo. *Nursing Management of the Patient with Pain.* Philadelphia: Lippincott, October 1972.

McLachlan, Eileen. "Recognizing Pain." *American Journal of Nursing* 74, 3:496-497, March 1974.

Chapter 9 (Continued)

Moss, Fay T. "The Effect of a Nursing Intervention on Pain Relief." *American Nurses Association Clinical Sessions*, 1967.

Murray, J.B. "Psychology of the Pain Experience." *Journal of Psychology* 78: 193–206, July 1971.

Noonan, Karen A. *Emotional Adjustment to Illness.* Albany, N.Y.: Delmar, 1975.

"Pain" Parts I and II *American Journal of Nursing* 66:1085–1108 and 1345–1368, 1966. Programmed instruction units on pain assessment and intervention.

Chapter 10 Pain Assessment and Intervention

Copp, Laurel A. "The Spectrum of Suffering." *American Journal of Nursing* 74, 3:491–495, March 1974.

Crowley, Dorothy. *Pain and Its Alleviation.* Los Angeles: School of Nursing, 1967.

Fordyce, Wilbert et al. "Some Implications of Learning in Problems of Chronic Pain." *Journal of Chronic Disease* 21:179–190, 1968.

Karmel, M. *Thank you, Dr. Lamaze: A Mother's Experiences in Painless Childbirth.* Philadelphia: Lippincott, 1959.

LeBow, Michael D. "Behavior Problems Frequently Encountered by Nurses: Chronic Pain." *Behavior Modification: A Significant Method in Nursing Practice.* Englewood Cliffs, New Jersey: Prentice-Hall, 1973.

Mastravito, Rene C. "Psychogenic Pain." *American Journal of Nursing* 74, 3:514–519, March 1974.

McLachlan, Eileen. "Recognizing Pain." *American Journal of Nursing* 74, 3:496–497, March 1974.

Moss, Fay. "The Effect of a Nursing Intervention on Pain Relief." *American Nurses' Association Clinical Sessions*, 1967.

Petrie, A. *Individuality in Pain and Suffering.* Chicago: University of Chicago Press, 1967.

Shontz, Franklin C. "Suffering, Loss, Misfortune." *The Psychological Aspects of Physical Illness and Disability.* New York: Macmillan, 1975.

Sternbach, R.A. *Pain: A Psychophysiological Analysis.* New York: Academic Press, Inc., 1968.

Wiley, L. "Intractable Pain: How Nursing Care Can Help." *Nursing '74* 4:54–59, September 1974.

Chapter 11 The Grief Process

Agee, James. *A Death in the Family.* New York: Avon, 1959.

Benoliel, Jeanne Quint. *The Nurse and the Dying Patient.* New York: Macmillan, 1973.

Brim, Orville et al eds. *The Dying Patient.* New York: Russel Sage, 1970.

Burgess, Ann C. and Lazare, Aaron. *Psychiatric Nursing in the Hospital and Community.* Englewood Cliffs, New Jersey: Prentice-Hall, 1973.

DuCasse, C.J. *The Belief in a Life After Death.* Springfield, Illinois: Charles C. Thomas, 1961.

Elder, Ruth."Dying in the U.S.A." *Nursing Digest* 2, 5:2-11, May 1974.

Evans, Frances M.C. "The Problem of Loss." *Psychosocial Nursing.* New York: Macmillan, 1971.

Fond, K. "Dealing with Death and Dying Through Family-Centered Care." *Nursing Clinics of North America* 7:53, March 1972.

Forbidden Games (Jeux Interdits) Film by Robert Dorfman on how children view death, 1952.

Glaser, Barney G., and Strauss Anselm L. *Awareness of Dying.* Chicago: Aldine, 1965.

Gray, Ruth V. "Grief." *Nursing '74* 4:25-27, January 1974.

Hanlon, Archie J. "Notes of a Dying Professor." *Nursing Digest* 2, 5:36-42, May 1974.

Harrell, Helen C. "To Lose a Breast." *American Journal of Nursing* 72:676-677, April 1972.

Kavanaugh, Robert E. "Facing Death." *Nursing '74* 4:35-42, May 1974.

Kubler-Ross, Elisabeth. *On Death and Dying.* New York: Macmillan, 1969.

_____ . "What is it like to be dying?" *American Journal of Nursing* 71:54, January 1971.

Lester, David et al. "The Attitudes of Nursing Students and Faculty Toward Death and Dying." *Nursing Research* 23:50-53, January-February 1974.

Mannes, Marya. *Last Rites.* New York: Morrow, 1973.

Mitford, Jessica. *The American Way of Death.* New York: Simon and Schuster, 1963.

Murray, Ruth, and Zentner, Judith. *Nursing Concepts for Health Promotion.* Englewood Cliffs, New Jersey: Prentice-Hall, 1975.

Schoenberg, Bernard et al eds. *Psychosocial Aspects of Terminal Care.* New York: Columbia University Press, 1972.

_____ . *Anticipatory Grief.* New York: Columbia University Press, 1974.

Shneidman, Edwin S. *Deaths of Man.* New York: Penguin, 1974.

Solzhenitsyn, Alexander. *Cancer Ward.* New York: Farrar, Strauss and Giroux, Inc., 1969.

Speer, Gertrude M. "Learning About Death." *Perspectives in Psychiatric Care* 12, 2:70-73, 1974.

"Understanding Death." A series of 4 film strips for children, teachers, and parents. Available from Highly Specialized Promotions, 20 Schermerhorn St., Brooklyn, N.Y. 11201.

Watson, Joellen. "Death Revisited." *Perspectives in Psychiatric Care* 7, 2:73, 1974.

Watt, A. "Helping Children to Mourn." Part 1 *Medical Insight* 3:28, July 1971; Part II *Medical Insight* 3:56, August 1971.

Weisman, Avery. *On Dying and Denying.* New York: Behavioral Publications, 1972.

Chapter 12 Grief Assessment and Intervention

Barrocas, Albert. "The Dying Patient — A Team Affair." *Nursing Digest* 2, 5:62–66, May 1974.

Benoliel, Jeanne Quint. "Assessments of Loss and Grief." *Journal of Thanatology* 1:182, 1971.

Burnside, Irene Mortenson. "Grief Work in the Aged Patient." *Nursing Forum* 8, 4:416-427, 1969.

Doyle, Nancy. *The Dying Person and the Family.* Public Affairs Pamphlet #485, 1972. 381 Park Avenue South, New York, New York, 10016.

Epstein, Charlotte. *Nursing the Dying Patient.* Englewood Cliffs, New Jersey: Prentice-Hall, 1975.

Friedman, S.B. et al. *Childhood Leukemia — A Pamphlet for Parents.* Washington D.C.: U.S. Government Printing Office, 1969.

Grollman, Earl A. *Explaining Death to Children.* Boston: Beacon Press, 1967.

Hodge, J.R. "Help Your Patient to Mourn Better." *Medical Times* 99:53, 1971.

Karon, J., and Vernick, J. "An Approach to Emotional Support of Fatally Ill Children." *Clinical Pediatrics* 7:274, 1968.

Koop, C.E. "The Seriously Ill or Dying Child: Supporting the Patient and the Family." *Pediatric Clinics of North America* 16:555, 1969.

Kopf, Rita C., and McFadden, Elizabeth L. "Nursing Intervention in the Crisis of Newborn Illness." *Nursing Digest* 5, 2:43-48, May 1974.

Kubler-Ross, E. "Coping Patterns of Patients Who Knew Their Diagnosis." *Catastrophic Illness in the Seventies.* New York; Cancer Care, 1971.

Kubler-Ross, E. *Death: The Final Stage of Growth,* Englewood Cliffs, New Jersey: Prentice-Hall, 1975.

Noonan, Karen Ann. "The Dying Patient." *Emotional Adjustment to Illness.* Albany, N.Y.: Delmar, 1975.

Olson, Emily. "Effect of Nurse-Patient Interaction on a Terminal Patient." *American Nurses Association Clinical Sessions,* 1968.

Petrillo, Madeline, and Sarger, Sirgay. *Emotional Care of Hospitalized Children.* Philadelphia: Lippincott, 1972.

Ramshorn, Mary T. "Selected Tasks for the Dying Patient and Family Members." *Anticipatory Grief.* Edited by Bernard Schoenberg et al. New York: Columbia University Press, 1974.

Silverman, P. et al eds. *Helping Each Other in Widowhood.* New York: Health Sciences, 1974.

The Dying Patient: A Documentary and Analysis on the Psychodynamics of Dying. 16 mm black and white film. 1 hour. University of California, Irvine, Irvine Office of Medical Education, Irvine, California, 92664.

Toch, Rudolf. "Management of Parental Anticipatory Grief." *Anticipatory Grief.* Edited by Bernard Schoenberg et al. New York: Columbia University Press, 1974.

Ujhely, Gertrud. "Grief and Depression: Implications for Preventative and Therapeutic Nursing Care." *Nursing Forum* 5, 2:23-25, 1966.

Vernick, J., and Karon, M. "Who's Afraid of Death on a Leukemia Ward?" *American Journal of Disease of Children* 109:393, 1965.

Verwoerdt, A. *Communication with the Fatally Ill.* Springfield, Illinois: Charles C. Thomas, 1966.

Watt, A. "Helping Children to Mourn." Part I *Medical Insight* 3:28, July 1971. Part II *Medical Insight* 3:56, August 1971.

SECTION 3 THE OBSERVATION-PERCEPTION-COMMUNICATION PROCESS

Chapter 13 Observation

Byers, Virginia B. *Nursing Observation.* 2d ed. Edited by Anna Kuba (Foundation of Nursing Ser). Dubuque, Iowa: Wm. C. Brown Company, 1973.

Chesler, M. and Fox, R. *Role-Playing Methods in the Classroom.* Chicago: Science Research Associates, 1966.

Dix, D.M. "Role Playing in Nursing Education in the Psychiatric Field." *Group Psychotherapy* 15:231-235, 1967.

Chapter 13 (Continued)

Levit, G. "Learning Through Role Playing." *Adult Leadership* 2:9-16, October 1953.

MacBryde, Cyril M., and Blacklow, Robert Stanley. eds. *Signs and Symptoms: Applied Pathologic, Physiological and Clinical Interpretation.* 5th ed. Philadelphia: Lippincott, 1970.

Mercer, Lianne, and O'Connor, Patricia. *Fundamental Skills in the Nurse-Patient Relationship.* 2d. ed. Philadelphia: Saunders, 1974.

Peplau, Hildegard E. *Interpersonal Relations in Nursing.* New York: Putnam, 1952.

Role Playing in Human Relations Training. Film. University of Califorinia Extension, Media Center. Berkeley, California, Rental $7.00. 25 minutes.

Seedor, Marie M. *The Physical Assessment: A Programmed Unit for Nurses.* New York: Teachers College Press, 1974.

Underwood, P. "Communication Through Role Playing." *American Journal of Nursing* 71, 6:1184-1186, 1971.

Chapter 14 Perception

Bullough, Bonnie, "Where Should Isolation Stop?" *American Journal of Nursing* 62:86-89, October 1962.

Carlson, Sylvia. "Effect of Sensory Input on Geriatric Patients." *American Nurses' Association Clinical Sessions.* New York: Appleton-Century-Crofts, 1968.

Chambers, Carolyn. "Senility or Sensory Deprivation?" *American Nurses' Association Clinical Sessions.* New York: Appleton-Century-Crofts, 1967.

Chodil, Judith. "The Concept of Sensory Deprivation." *Nursing Clinics of North America* 5:453+, September 1970.

Ellis, Rosemary. "Unusual Sensory Disturbances after Cardiac Surgery." *American Journal of Nursing* 72, 11:2021-2025, November 1972.

Fahy, Ellen T. et al. "Environmental Stress: The Isolated Patient." *American Nurses' Association Clinical Sessions.* New York: Appleton-Century-Crofts, 1967.

Karlins, Marvin, and Andrews, Lewis M. *Biofeedback.* New York: Warner Paper, 1973.

Knicely, Kathryn H. "The World of Distorted Perception." *American Journal of Nursing* 67, 5:999-1002, May 1967.

Luce, Gay Gaer. *Body Time.* New York: Bantam, 1971.

Noonan, Karen Ann. *Emotional Adjustment to Illness.* Albany, N.Y.: Delmar, 1975.

Ornstein, Robert E. *The Psychology of Consciousness.* New York: Viking, 1972.

Rabalais, Janice T. "Dangers of Accepting Stereotypes: A Boy Taught Me About Nonacceptance." *Nursing '75* 5, 2:43-44, February 1975:.

Vernon, M.D. *The Psychology of Perception.* Baltimore: Penguin Books, 1962.

Chapter 15 Verbal Communication

Bigham, Gloria D. "To Communicate with Negro Patients." *American Journal of Nursing.* 64, 9:113, 1964.

Clark, Constancia. "Communication, A Good Measurement of Adjustment, Ability to Get Along." *Hospital Topics.* 43:104, April 1964.

Crosley, Wilbur D. "Communication in Successful Supervision." *American Operating Room Nurse* 8:50, October 1968.

Hall, Edward T. *The Silent Language.* Garden City, New York: Anchor, 1973.

Hays, J., and Larson, K. *Interacting with Patients.* New York: Macmillan, 1963.

Hofling, Charles K. and Leininger, Madeleine M. "Communication in the Nurse-Patient Relationship." *Basic Psychiatric Concepts in Nursing* 2d. ed., Philadelphia: Lippincott, 1969.

"Keys to Effective Communication." 8 filmstrips. Garden Grove, California: Trainex, 1973.

Kron, Thora. *Communication in Nursing.* Philadelphia: W.B. Saunders, 1967.

Mercer, Lianne S. and O'Connor, Patricia. *Fundamental Skills in the Nurse-Patient Relationship: A Programmed Text.* 2d. ed., 1974.

Muencke, M. "Overcoming the Language Barrier." *Nursing Outlook* 18, 4:53-54, 1970.

Muller, Theresa. "Dynamics of Communication in Nursing." *American Journal of Nursing* 63, 1:9-16, 1963.

Ruesch, Jergen. *Disturbed Communication.* New York: W.W. Norton, 1957.

Satir, Virginia. "Communication Theory." *Conjoint Family Therapy.* Palo Alto: Science and Behavior Books, 1964.

Skipper, James K. and others, "What Communication Means to Patients." *American Journal of Nursing,* 64, 4:101, 1964.

Underwood, Patricia. "Communication Through Role Playing." *American Journal of Nursing* 71, 1184-1186, 1971.

Veninga, Robert. "Communications: A Patient's Eye View." *American Journal of Nursing* 73, 2:320-322, 1973.

Chapter 16   Nonverbal Communication

Ackerhalt, Judy. "The Concept of Waiting: Supporting the Patient Awaiting Diagnosis." *ANA Regional Conference # 2, Exploring Progress in Medical-Surgical Nursing.* 1966.

Barnett, K. "A Theoretical Construct of the Concepts of Touch as They Relate to Nursing." *Nursing Research* 21:102-110, March/April 1972.

Bender, R.E. "Communicating with the Deaf." *American Journal of Nursing* 66, 4:757-760, 1966.

Cashar, Leah, and Dixson, Barbara. "The Therapeutic Use of Touch." *Journal of Psychiatric Nursing* 5, 5:442-451, 1967.

Fox, Madeleine. "Talking with Patients who Can't Answer." *American Journal of Nursing* 71:1146, June 1971.

Hall, Edward T. *The Hidden Dimension.* Garden City, New York: Anchor Press/Doubleday, 1969.

_____ . *The Silent Language.* Garden City, New York: Anchor Press/Doubleday, 1973.

Hare, A., and Bales, R. "Seating Position and Small Group Interaction." *Sociometry* 26:480-486, 1963.

Izzard, C. *The Face of Emotion.* New York: Appleton-Century-Crofts, 1971.

Leininger, Madeleine M. *Nursing and Anthropology: Two Worlds to Blend* New York: John Wiley, 1970.

Milliken, Mary E. "Observing Nonverbal Behavior." *Understanding Human Behavior* Albany, N.Y.: Delmar, 1974.

"Nonverbal Barriers to Communication." Filmstrip PC-295, Garden Grove, California: Trainex, 1973.

Paynich, Mary. "Cultural Barriers to Nurse Communication." *American Journal of Nursing* 64, 2:87-90, 1964.

Ruesch, Jurgen, and Kees, Weldon. *Nonverbal Communication: Notes on the Visual Perception of Human Relations.* University of California Press, 1956.

Scheflen, A. "The Significance of Posture in Communication Systems." *Psychiatry* 27:316-321, 1964.

Simmons, Janet A. "Nonverbal Behavior." *The Nurse-Patient Relationship in Psychiatric Nursing.* Philadelphia: W.B. Saunders, 1969.

Simon, Sidney B. et al. *Values Clarification.* New York: Hart, 1972.

Ujhely, Gertrud. "When Adult Patients Cry." *Nursing Clinics of North America* 2, 4:725-735, December 1967.

Underwood, Patricia. "Communication Through Role Playing." *American Journal of Nursing* 71, 6:1184-1186, 1971.

Wicker, I.B. "Cultural Barriers to Employee Communications in the Hospital." *Supervisor Nurse* 2:32, July 1971.

Chapter 17 Interviewing and Communication Skills

Bermosk, Loretta. "Interviewing: A Key to Therapeutic Communication in Nursing Practice." *Nursing Clinics of North America* 1, 2:205-214, 1966.

Bird, Brian. *Talking with Patients.* Philadelphia: J.B. Lippincott, 1965.

Clark, Carolyn Chambers. *The Process Recording Guide: Recording and Evaluating Nurse-Patient Interactions.* programmed booklet, audio tape and workbook, Garden Grove, California: Trainex Press, 1975.

_____. "Counteracting Staff Apathy and Hopelessness on a Psychiatric Ward." *Journal of Psychiatric Nursing* 13, 3:3-5, 1975.

Davis, Ann J. "The Skills of Communication." *American Journal of Nursing* 63, 1:66-70, 1963.

Demesaites, Mary. "A Good Sound." *American Journal of Nursing* 61, 4:104-106, 1961.

Dye, Mary C. "Clarifying Patients' Communications." *American Journal of Nursing* 63, 8:56-59, 1963.

Haggerty, Virginia. "Listening: An Experiment in Nursing." *Nursing Forum* 10, 4:382-391, 1971.

Hardiman, M. "Interviewing? or Social Chitchat?" *American Journal of Nursing* 71, 7:1379+, 1971.

Hays, Joyce, and Larson, Kenneth. *Interacting with Patients.* New York: Macmillian, 1963.

Hays, Joyce, and Myers, Jansey B. "Learning in the Nurse-Patient Relationship." *Perspectives in Psychiatric Care* 2, 3:20-29, 1964.

Juzwiak, M. "How Skilled Interviewing Helps Patients and Nurses." *RN* 29, 8:33, 1966.

Kelso, Margaret T. and Barton, David. "The Nursing Questionnaire as a Facilitator of Psychological Care on Medical and Surgical Wards." *Perspectives in Psychiatric Care* 10, 3:123-127, 1972.

King, Joan M. "The Initial Interview: Assessment of the Patient and His Difficulties." *Perspectives in Psychiatric Care* 9, 6:247-256, 1967.

Manaser, Janice C., and Werner, Anita M. *Instruments for Study of Nurse-Patient Interaction.* New York: Macmillan, 1964.

Manthey, M. "A Guide for Interviewing." *American Journal of Nursing* 67, 10:2088-2090, 1967.

Meadow, Lloyd, and Gass, Gertrude. "Problems of the Novice Interviewer." *American Journal of Nursing* 63, 2:97-99, 1963.

Muencke, M. "Overcoming the Language Barrier." *Nursing Outlook* 18, 4:53-54, 1970.

Murphy, Donna, and Dineen, Eleanor. "Nursing by Telephone." *American Journal of Nursing* 75, 7:1137-1139, 1975.

Chapter 17 (Continued)

Murray, Jeanne. "Self-Knowledge and the Nursing Interview." *Nursing Forum* 2, 1:69-79, 1963.

Ortiz, J., and Blyth, Z. "Play Therapy: An Individual Prescription." *Journal of Psychiatric Nursing* 8:30, November/December 1970.

Peplau, Hildegard E. "Talking with Patients." *American Journal of Nursing* 70, 7:964-966, 1970.

Petrillo, Madeleine, and Sarger, Sirgay. *Emotional Care of Hospitalized Children.* Philadelphia: Lippincott, 1972.

Rodger, B. "Therapeutic Communication and Posthypnotic Suggestion." *American Journal of Nursing* 72, 4:714-717, 1972.

Taylor, M. "The Process Recording: Aid to Interviewing." *Canadian Nurse* 64, 10:49, 1968.

Loesch, Larry and Nancy. "What do you say after you say 'MM-hm?" *American Journal of Nursing* 75, 5:807-809, 1975.

Wilson, L. "Listening." *Behavioral Concepts and Nursing Intervention.* Edited by Carolyn E. Carlson. Philadelphia: Lippincott, 1970.

Chapter 18 Blocks to Effective Communication

Brooks, Patricia. "Masturbation." *American Journal of Nursing* 64, 4:820–823 1967.

Burton, Genevieve. *Personal, Impersonal and Interpersonal Relations.* 3d. ed. New York: Springer, 1970.

Dodge, Joan S. "Nurses' Sense of Adequacy and Attitudes Toward Keeping Patients Informed." *Journal of Health and Human Behavior* 2, 3:213-216, 1961.

Epstein, Charlotte. *Effective Interaction in Contemporary Nursing.* Englewood Cliffs, New Jersey: Prentice-Hall, 1974.

Gibney, Helen A. "Masturbation: An Invitation for an Interpersonal Relationship." *Perspectives in Psychiatric Care* 10, 3:128-134, 1972.

Hall, Edward T. *The Silent Language.* Garden City, New York; Anchor Press/Doubleday, 1973.

Hardiman, M. "Interviewing? or Social Chitchat?" *American Journal of Nursing* 71, 7:1379+, 1971.

Hays, Joyce, and Larson, Kenneth. *Interacting with Patients.* New York: Macmillan, 1963.

Hewitt, Helen, and Resnecker, Betty. "Major Blocks to Communicating with Patients." *American Journal of Nursing* 64, 7:101-103, July 1964.

Loesch Larry and Nancy. "What do you say after you say 'MM-hm?" *American Journal of Nursing* 75, 5:807-809, 1975.

Meadow, Lloyd, and Gass, Gertrude. "Problems of the Novice Interviewer." *American Journal of Nursing* 63, 2:97-99, 1963.

"Nonverbal Barriers to Communication." Filmstrip PC-295, Garden Grove, California: Trainex, 1973.

Paynich, Mary. "Cultural Barriers to Nurse Communication." *American Journal of Nursing* 64, 2:87-90, 1964.

Peplau, Hildegard E. *Interpersonal Relations in Nursing.* New York: G.P. Putnam, 1952.

Rabalais, Janice T. "Dangers of Accepting Stereotypes: A Boy Taught Me About Nonacceptance." *Nursing '75* 5, 2:43-44, February 1975.

Ruesch, Jurgen. *Disturbed Communication.* New York: W.W. Norton, 1957.

Thomas, May et al. "Anger: A Tool for Developing Self-Awareness." *American Journal of Nursing* 70:2586+, December 1970.

Ujhely, Gertrud. "The Uses of and Abuses of the So-called Non-Directive Technique in Nursing." *American Nurses' Association Clinical Sessions.* 1967.

Chapter 19 Nursing Process

Ansley, Betty. "Patient-Oriented Recording: A Better System for Ambulatory Settings." *Nursing '75* 5, 8:52-53, August 1975.

Bloom, Judith et al. "Problem-Oriented Charting." *American Journal of Nursing* 71:2144-2148, November 1971.

Carlson, Sylvia. "A Practical Approach to the Nursing Process." *American Journal of Nursing* 72, 9:1589-1591, 1972.

Carrieri, Virginia K., and Sitzman, Judith. "Components of the Nursing Process." *Nursing Clinics of North America* 6, 1:115-124, March 1971.

Chambers, Wilda. "Nursing Diagnosis." *American Journal of Nursing* 62, 1:102-104, 1962.

Levine, Myra. "Adaptation and Assessment: A Rationale for Nursing Intervention." *American Journal of Nursing* 66, 11:2450-2453, 1966.

Little, Dolores E. and Carnevali, Doris L. "Overview of Processes Used in Planning Patient Care." *Nursing Care Planning.* Philadelphia: J.B. Lippincott, 1969.

Johnson, Mae. *Problem-Solving in Nursing Practice.* Dubuque, Iowa: Wm. C. Brown, 1970.

Knight, Jeanne H. "Applying Nursing Process in the Community." *Nursing Outlook* 22, 11:708-711, November 1974.

Mager, Robert F. *Preparing Instructional Objectives.* Belmont, California: Fearon, 1975.

Chapter 19 (Continued)

Mazur, W.P. *The Problem-Oriented System in the Psychiatric Hospital.* Garden Grove, California: Trainex Press, 1974.

"Overview of the Nursing Process." Slides, cassettes and response book. New York: Harper and Row, 1972.

Smith, Dorothy M. "Writing Objectives as a Nursing Practice Skill." *American Journal of Nursing* 71, 2:319-320, February 1971.

The Nursing Process in Practice, compiled by Mary H. Browning. New York: American Journal of Nursing Company, 1974.

Yarnall, Stephen, and Atwood, Judith. "Problem-Orientated Practice for Nurses and Physicians." *NCNA* 9, 2:215-228, June 1974.

Yura, Helen and Walsh, Mary. *The Nursing Process.* Washington, D.C.: The Catholic University of America Press, 1967.

Zimmerman, Donna S. and Gohrke, Carol. "The Goal-Directed Nursing Approach: It Does Work." *American Journal of Nursing* 70, 2:306-310, February 1970.

Chapter 20 Nursing Care Plans

Cornell, Sudie A., and Brush, Frances. "Systems Approach to Nursing Care Plans." *American Journal of Nursing* 71:1376-1378, July 1971.

Cuica, Rudy L. "Over the Years with the Nursing Care Plan." *Nursing Outlook* 20, 11:706-711, 1972.

Garant, Carol. "A Basis for Care." *American Journal of Nursing* 72:699-701, April 1972.

House, Mary J. "Devising a Care Plan You Can Really Use." *Nursing '75* 5, 7:12-14, July 1975.

Little, Dolores, and Carnevali, Doris. *Nursing Care Planning.* Philadelphia: J.B. Lippincott, 1969.

Mayers, Marlene. *A Systematic Approach to the Nursing Care Plan.* New York: Appleton-Century-Crofts, 1972.

Palisin, Helen E. "Nursing Care Plans are a Snare and a Delusion." *American Journal of Nursing* 71, 1:63-66, 1971.

Tyzenbhouse, Phyllis. "Care Plans for Nursing Home Patients." *Nursing Outlook* 20, 3:169-172, March 1972.

Wagner, Bernice M. "Care Plans: Right, Reasonable, and Reachable." *American Journal of Nursing* 69:986-990, May 1969.

SECTION 4 COPING WITH ILLNESS

Chapter 21 The Hospital and the Institution

Caudill, William. *The Psychiatric Hospital as a Small Society.* Cambridge, Mass.: Harvard University Press, 1958.

Goffman, Erving. *Asylums.* Garden City, New York: Anchor, 1961.

Leininger, Madeleine M. *Nursing and Anthropology: Two Worlds to Blend.* New York: John Wiley, 1970.

Marram, Gwen. "Patients' Evaluation of Their Care: Importance to the Nurse." *Nursing Outlook* 21, 5:322-324, 1973.

Nehring, Virginia, and Geach, Barbara. "Patients' Evaluation of Their Care: Why They Don't Complain." *Nursing Outlook* 21, 5:317-321, 1973.

Parsons, Talcott. *The Social System.* New York: Free Press, Paper, 1964.

Shontz, Franklin C. *The Psychological Aspects of Physical Illness and Disability.* New York: Macmillan, 1975.

Schwartz, Morris S., and Schwartz, Charlotte G. *Social Approaches to Mental Patient Care.* New York: Columbia University Press, 1964.

Tagliacozzo, Daisy L. and Mauksch, Hans O. "The Patient's View of the Patient's Role." *Patients, Physicians and Illness.* 2d. ed. Edited by E. Gartley Jaco. New York: Free Press, 1972.

Chapter 22 The Therapeutic Environment

Almond, R. "The Therapeutic Community." *Scientific American* 224:34, March 1971.

Anderson, Barbara et. al. "Two Experimental Tests of a Patient-Centered Admission Process." *Nursing Research* 14:151-157, Spring 1965.

Atty, Louise M. "Introducing the Newcomer – the Patient and the Staff Nurse – to a Psychiatric Hospital." *Perspectives in Psychiatric Care* 3, 2:25-33, 1965.

Berlinger, Arthur K. "The Two Milieus in Milieu Therapy." *Perspectives in Psychiatric Care* 5, 6:266-271, 1967.

Boucher, Michael L. "Personal Space and Chronicity in the Mental Hospital." *Perspectives in Psychiatric Care* 9, 5:206-210, 1971.

Bradshaw, W. "The Coffee-pot Affair: An Episode in the Life of a Therapeutic Community." *Hospital and Community Psychiatry* 23:33, February 1972.

Brown, Martha, and Fowler, Grace R. *Psychodynamic Nursing* 4th ed. Philadelphia: W.B. Saunders, 1971.

Chapter 22 (Continued)

Clark, Carolyn Chambers. "The Clinical Specialist as a Communication Consultant." *Supervisor Nurse* 4, 4:20-27, April 1973.

_____ . "Counteracting Hopelessness and Apathy on a Psychiatric Ward." *Journal of Psychiatric Nursing* 13, 3:3-6, May/June 1975.

Crisham, Sr. Margaret, and Danielsen, Sharon L. "An Experience with Group Orientation Sessions." *Perspectives in Psychiatric Care* 3, 2:34-41, 1965.

Gardner, K. "Patient Groups in a Therapeutic Community." *American Journal of Nursing* 71:528, March 1971.

Haslam, Patricia. "Noise in Hospitals: Its Effect on the Patient" *Nursing Clinics of North America* 5:715-724, December 1970.

Holmes, M. et al. "Creative Nursing in Day and Night Care Centers." *American Journal of Nursing* 62:86-90, 1962.

Jones, Maxwell. *The Therapeutic Community* New York: Basic Books, 1953.

Jones, Maxwell. *Beyond the Therapeutic Community* New Haven: Yale University Press, 1968.

Lieberman, Morton A. "Psychological Effects of Institutionalization." *Journal of Gerontology* 23, 7:343-353, 1968.

Leone, Dolores, and Zahourek, Rothlyn. "'Aloneness' in the Therapeutic Community." *Perspectives in Psychiatric Care* 12, 2:60-63, 1974.

Malone, Mary F. "The Dilemma of a Professional in a Bureaucracy." *Nursing Forum* 3:36-60, 1964.

Norris, Catherine et al. "A Therapeutic Nursing Routine: Feeding Patients." *Perspectives in Psychiatric Care* 1, 1 and 2:2-23, 1963.

Siegel, Nathaniel. "What is a Therapeutic Community?" *Nursing Outlook* 12:49-51, May 1964.

Sommer, Robert, *Personal Space.* Englewood Cliffs, New Jersey: Prentice-Hall, 1969.

Stanton, Alfred H. and Schwartz, Morris S. *The Mental Hospital: A Study of Institutional Participation in Psychiatric Illness and Treatment.* New York: Basic Books, 1954.

Will, Gwen Tudor. "A Sociopsychiatric Nursing Approach to Intervention in a Problem of Mutual Withdrawal on a Mental Hospital Ward." *Perspectives in Psychiatric Care.* 8, 1:11-35, 1970.

Chapter 23   Mind-Body Relationships

Carnes, G. "Understanding the Cardiac Patient's Behavior." *American Journal of Nursing* 71:1187, June 1971.

Cobb, Beatrix. "Cancer: Psychosocial Factors." *Rehabilitation Practices with the Physically Disabled.* Edited by James F. Garrett and Edna S. Levine. New York: Columbia University Press, 1973.

Cope, O. *Man, Mind and Medicine.* Philadelphia: Lippincott, 1968.

Dlinn, Barney M. et al. "Psychosexual Response to Ileostomy and Colostomy." *American Journal of Psychiatry* 123, 3:374-381, September 1969.

Given, Barbara, and Simmons, Sandra. "Care of a Patient with a Gastric Ulcer." *American Journal of Nursing* 70:1472-1475, July 1970.

Hamilton, M. "Management of Hypertension." *Nursing Mirror* 132:33, January 15, 1971.

Hargreaves, Ann G. "Emotional Problems of Patients with Respiratory Disease." *Nursing Clinics of North America.* vol 3. Philadelphia: W.B. Saunders 1968.

Haslam, Pamela. "Noise in Hospitals: Its Effect on the Patient." *Nursing Clinics of North America* 5:715-724, December 1970.

Holland, Bernard C., and Ward, Richard S. "Homeostasis and Psychosomatic Medicine." *American Handbook of Psychiatry.* vol. 3. Edited by Silvano Arieti. New York: Basic Books, 1966.

Janis, Irving. *Psychological Stress: Psychoanalytic and Behavioral Studies of Surgical Patients.* New York: John Wiley, 1958.

Jenkins, C. David. "Social and Epidemiologic Factors in Psychosomatic Disease." *Mental Health Digest* 5, 2:23-25, February 1973.

Kneisl, Carol Ren, and Ames, Sue Ann. "The Patient with Psychophysiological Dysfunction." *Mental Health Concepts in Medical-Surgical Nursing: A Workbook.* St Louis: C.V. Mosby, 1974.

Lewis, Howard R. and Martha E. *Psychosomatics: How Emotions can Damage Your Health.* New York: Viking, 1972.

Loxley, Alice K. "The Emotional Toll of Crippling Deformity." *American Journal of Nursing* 72:1839-1840, October 1972.

Luce, Gay Gaer. *Biological Rhythms in Psychiatry and Medicine.* Chevy Chase, Maryland: Public Health Service Publication #2088, 1970.

Ludwig, A. "Rheumatoid Arthritis: Psychiatric Aspects." *Medical Insight* 2:14, December 1970.

Maslow, Abraham. *Toward a Psychology of Being.* New York: Van Nostrand Reinhold Company, 1962.

Mayer, Bernard C. "The Psychological Effects of Mutilating Operations." *Medical Insight.* September 1970.

Morgan, William L., and Engel, George L. *The Clinical Approach to the Patient.* Philadelphia: W.B. Saunders, 1970.

Ornstein, Robert E. *The Psychology of Consciousness.* New York: Viking, 1972.

Chapter 23 (Continued)

Prugh, Dane G. "Toward an Understanding of Psychosomatic Concepts in Relation to Illness in Children." *Modern Perspectives in Child Development.* Edited by Albert Solnit and Sally Provence. New York: International Universities Press, 1963.

Puritun, Lynn R., and Nelson, Louella I. "Ulcer Patient: Emotional Emergency." *American Journal of Nursing* 68:1930-1933, September 1968.

Reif, Laura. "Managing Life with a Chronic Disease." *American Journal of Nursing* 73: 261-264, February 1973.

Rynearson, R. "When is Musculoskeletal Pain a Functional Disorder?" *Medical Insight* 3:18, February 1971.

Selye, Hans. *The Stress of Life.* New York: McGraw-Hill, 1956.

Sitzman, Judith M. "Psychosomatic Disorders." *New Dimensions in Mental -Health-Psychiatric Nursing.* 4th ed. Edited by Marion E. Kalkman and Anne J. Davis. New York: McGraw-Hill, 1974.

Spielberger, Charles D., ed. *Anxiety and Behavior.* New York: Academic Press, 1966.

Thomas, Mary Durand. "Anger in Nurse-Patient Interactions." *Nursing Clinics of North America* 2:737-745, 1967.

Twerski, Abraham. "Psychological Considerations on the Coronary Care Unit." *Cardiovascular Nursing.* March-April 1972.

Wolff, B. Berthold. "Arthritis and Rheumatism." *Rehabilitation Practices with the Physically Disabled.* Edited by James F. Garrett and Edna S. Levine. New York: Columbia University Press, 1973.

Wright, Beatrice A. "An Assessment of the Field of Somatopsychology." *Physical Disability – A Psychological Approach.* New York: Harper and Row, 1960.

Chapter 24 Stages of Illness and the Sick Role

Adams, John E., and Lindemann, Erich. "Coping with Longterm Disability." *Coping and Adaptation.* Edited by George Coelho et al. New York: Basic Books, 1974.

Burnes, A.J., and Rosen, S.R. "Social Roles and Adaptation to the Community." *Community Mental Health Journal* 3:153-158, 1967.

Campbell, Teresa, and Chung, Betty. "Health Care of the Chinese in America." *Nursing Outlook* 21, 4:245-249, 1973.

Christman, Luther. "Assisting the Patient to Learn the Patient Role." *Journal of Nursing Education* 6, 2:17-21, 1967.

Frank, Jerome. *Persuasion and Healing.* Baltimore: John Hopkins Press, 1961.

Garrett, James F., and Levine, Edna S., eds. *Rehabilitation Practices with the Physically Disabled.* New York: Columbia University Press, 1973.

Gordon, Gerald. *Role Theory and Illness.* New Haven: College and University Press, 1961.

Grahm, Saxon. "Cancer, Culture, and Social Structure." *Patients, Physicians and Illness.* Edited by E. Gartley Jaco. 2d. ed. New York: The Free Press, 1972.

Jamann, Joann. "Health is a Function of Ecology." *American Journal of Nursing* 71, 5:970-973, 1971.

Kaplan, Howard B. "Studies in Sociophysiology." *Patients, Physicians and Illness.* 2d. ed. Edited by E. Gartley Jaco. New York: Free Press, 1972.

Kasl, Stanislav, and Cobb, Sidney. "Health Behavior, Illness Behavior and Sick Role Behavior." *Archives of Environmental Health* 12:531-541, 1966.

Kasselbaum, Gene G. and Barbara O. "Dimensions of the Sick Role in Chronic Illness." *Journal of Health and Human Behavior* 6, 1:16-27, Spring 1965.

Langford, W.S. "The Child in the Pediatric Hospital: Adaptation to Illness and Hospitalization." *American Journal of Orthopsychiatry* 31:667-684, 1961.

Martin, C. "Marital and Coital Factors in Cervical Cancer." *American Journal of Public Health* 58, 5:803-814, 1967.

McGrath, J., ed. *Social and Psychological Factors in Stress.* New York: Holt, Rhinehart and Winston, 1970.

Mechanic, David. "Response Factors in Illness: The Study of Illness Behavior." *Social Psychiatry* 1:11-20, 1966.

——————————. "The Influence of Mothers on Their Children's Health Attitudes and Behavior." *Pediatrics* 33:444-453, 1964.

Norris, Catherine. "The Work of Getting Well." *American Journal of Nursing* 69, 10:2118-2121, 1969.

Parsons, Talcott. "Social Structure and Dynamic Process: The Case of Modern Medical Practice." *The Social System.* New York: The Free Press (paper), 1964.

——————————. "Definitions of Health and Illness in the Light of American Values and Social Structure." *Patients, Physicians and Illness.* 2d. ed. Edited by E. Gartley Jaco. New York: Free Press, 1972.

Phillips, L. *Human Adaptation and Its Failures.* New York: Academic Press, 1968.

Reif, Laura. "Managing Life with a Chronic Disease." *American Journal of Nursing* 73:261-264, February 1973.

Chapter 24 (Continued)

Saunders, L. *Cultural Differences and Medical Care.* New York: Russell Sage, 1954.

Schwartz, Morris S. and Charlotte G. *Social Approaches to Mental Patient Care.* New York: Columbia University Press, 1964.

Selye, Hans. "The Stress Syndrome." *American Journal of Nursing* 65, 3: 97-99, 1965.

Sweetser, Dorrian Apple. "How Laymen Define Illness." *Journal of Health and Human Behavior* 1:219-225, 1960.

Twaddle, A. "The Concepts of the Sick Role and Illness Behavior." *Advances in Psychosomatic Medicine* 8:162-179, 1972.

White, Robert W. *The Enterprise of Living.* New York: Holt, Rhinehart and Winston, 1972.

Whiting, B., ed. *Six Cultures: Studies of Child Rearing.* New York: Jurley and Sons, 1968.

Wu, Ruth. *Behavior and Illness.* Englewood Cliffs, New Jersey; Prentice-Hall, 1973.

Chapter 25 Coping Devices

Burgess, Ann and Lazare, Aaron. "Feelings, Thoughts, and Behaviors." *Psychiatric Nursing in the Hospital and the Community.* Englewood Cliffs, New Jersey: Prentice-Hall, 1973.

Danskin, David G., and Walters, E. Dale. "Biofeedback and Voluntary Self-Regulation." *Nursing Digest* 1, 7:9-14, September 1973.

Epstein, Charlotte. *Effective Interaction in Contemporary Nursing.* Englewood Cliffs, New Jersey: Prentice-Hall, 1974.

Fort, Joel. *The Pleasure Seekers: The Drug Crisis, Youth and Society.* New York: Bobbs-Merrill Company, 1969.

Kloes, Karen B., and Weinberg, Ann. "Countertransference." *Perspectives in Psychiatric Care.* 6, 4:152-162, 1968.

Lipowski, Z.J. "Physical Illness, the Individual, and the Coping Process." *Psychiatry in Medicine* 1, 4:91-102, 1970.

Messer, Alfred. *The Individual in his Family, an Adaptational Study.* Springfield, Illinois: Charles C. Thomas, 1970.

Peterson, M.H. "Understanding Defense Mechanisms." *American Journal of Nursing* 72:1651, September 1972.

Reif, Laura. "Managing Life with a Chronic Disease." *American Journal of Nursing* 73:261-264, February 1973.

Robinson, Lisa. "The Crying Patient." *Nursing '72* 2:16, December 1972.

Symonds, Percival M. *The Dynamics of Human Adjustment.* New York: Appleton-Century-Crofts, 1946.

Ujhely, Gertrud B. "When Adult Patients Cry." *Nursing Clinics of North America* 2:725-735, 1967.

Chapter 26 Body Image and Self-Concept

Blaesing, Sandra, and Brockhaus, Joyce. "The Development of Body Image in the Child." *Nursing Clinics of North America* 7, 4:597-607, December 1972.

Bosonko, Lydia A. "Immediate Postop Prosthesis." *American Journal of Nursing* 71:280-283, February 1971.

Christopherson, Victor A. "Role Modifications of the Disabled Male." *American Journal of Nursing* 68, 2:290-293, 1968.

Corbeil, Madeleine. "Nursing Process for a Patient with a Body Image Disturbance." *Nursing Clinics of North America* 6, 1:155-163, March 1971.

Craft, Carol. "Body Image and Obesity." *Nursing Clinics of North America* 7, 4:677-685, December 1972.

Dempsey, Mary O. "The Development of Body Image in the Adolescent." *Nursing Clinics of North America* 7, 4:609-615, December 1972.

DiLeo, J.H. *Young Children and Their Drawings.* New York: Springer, 1971.

Fisher, Seymour, and Cleveland, S.E. *Body Image and Personality.* 2d. ed. New York: Dover, 1968.

Fisher, Seymour. "Experiencing Your Body: You Are What You Feel." *Saturday Review.* July 8, 1972.

Fujita, Milton T. "The Impact of Illness or Surgery on the Body Image of the Child." *Nursing Clinics of North America* 7, 4:641-649, December 1972.

Gallagher, Ann M. "Body Image Changes in the Patient with a Colostomy." *Nursing Clinics of North America* 7, 4:669-676, December 1972.

Griffin, Winnie et al. "Group Exercise for Patients with Limited Motion." *American Journal of Nursing* 71:1742-1743, September 1971.

Iffrig, Sister Mary C. "Body Image in Pregnancy." *Nursing Clinics of North America* 7, 4:631-639, December 1972.

Koppitz, Elizabeth M. *Psychological Evaluation of Children's Human Figure Drawings.* New York: Grune and Stratton, 1968.

Laufer, Moses. "The Body Image, the Function of Masturbation and Adolescence." *The Psychoanalytic Study of the Child.* vol. 23. New York: International Universities Press, 1968.

Chapter 26 (Continued)

Leonard, Beverly J. "Body Image Changes in Chronic Illness." *Nursing Clinics of North America* 7, 4:687-695, December 1972.

Mayer, Bernard C. "The Psychological Effects of Mutilating Operations." *Medical Insight.* p. 82, September 1970.

McDaniels, J. *Physical Disability and Human Behavior.* New York: Pergamon Press, 1969.

Murray, Ruth L. "Principles of Nursing Intervention for the Adult Patient with Body Image Changes." *Nursing Clinics of North America* 7, 4:697-707, December 1972.

Murray, Ruth L. "Body Image Development in Adulthood." *Nursing Clinics of North America* 7, 4:617-629, December 1972.

Norris, Catherine M. "The Professional Nurse and Body Image." *Behavioral Concepts in Nursing Intervention.* Edited by Carolyn E. Carlson, Philadelphia: J.B. Lippincott, 1970.

Quint, Jeanne C. "The Impact of Mastectomy." *American Journal of Nursing* 63:88-92, November 1963.

Rubin, Reva. "Body Image and Self Esteem." *Nursing Outlook* 16:20-23, 1968.

Schwab, John, and Harmeling, J. "Body Image and Mental Illness." *Psychosomatic Medicine* 30:51, 1968.

Shontz, Franklin C. "Structure and Functions of Body Experience." *The Psychological Aspects of Physical Illness and Disability.* New York: Macmillan, 1975.

Smith, Catherine A. "Body Image Changes After Myocardial Infarction." *Nursing Clinics of North America* 7, 4:663-668, December 1972.

Stunkard, A., and Mendelson, M. "Obesity and the Body Image." *American Journal of Psychiatry* 123:10, April 1967.

Sullivan, Harry S. *The Interpersonal Theory of Psychiatry.* New York: W.W. Norton, 1953.

Ullman, Montague. "Disorders of Body Image After Stroke." *American Journal of Nursing* 64, 10:89-91, 1964.

Zion, L. "Body Concept as it Relates to Self Concept." *Research Quarterly* 4:490-495, 1965.

SECTION 5 THE LEARNING PROCESS

Chapter 27 Nursing Conferences

Alman, Beatrice. "Patients Participate in Nursing Care Conferences." *American Journal of Nursing* 67, 11:2331-2334, November 1967.

Matheney, Ruth V. "Pre and Post Conferences for Students." *American Journal of Nursing* 69:286-289, February 1969.

Mauksch, Ingeborg C. "Let's Listen to the Students." *Nursing Outlook*, 20: 103-107, February 1972.

Mullen, Joseph A. "The Development of Programs for New Employees." *The Supervisor Nurse* 2:3-37, September 1971.

Seiler, K. "The Team Conference." *Supervisor Nurse* 5:64-65, September 1974.

Chapter 28 Learning Through Teaching

Aiken, Linda H. "Patient Problems are Problems in Learning." *American Journal of Nursing* 70:1916-1918, September 1970.

Berni, Rosemarian, and Fordyce, Wilbert. *Behavior Modification and the Nursing Process*. St. Louis: C.V. Mosby, 1973.

Dloughy, Alico et al. "What Patients Want to Know About Their Diagnostic Tests." *Nursing Outlook* 11:265-267, April 1963.

Haferkorn, Virginia. "Assessing Individual Learning Needs as a Basic for Patient Teaching." *Nursing Clinics of North America* 6, 1:199-209, March 1971.

Harms, M. "Teaching-Learning Process." *Nursing Outlook* 14:54-57, 1966.

Hays, Joyce, and Myers, Janesy B. "Learning in the Nurse-Patient Relationship." *Perspectives in Psychiatric Care* 2, 3:20-29, 1964.

Healy, Kathryn M. "Does Preoperative Instruction Make a Difference?" *American Journal of Nursing* 68:62-67, January 1968.

Koberg, Don, and Bagnall, Jim. *The Universal Traveler: A Soft Systems Guide to Creativity, Problem Solving and the Process of Reaching Goals.* Los Altos, California: Wm. Kaufman, 1972.

Laird, Mona. "Techniques for Teaching Pre- and Postoperative Patients." *American Journal of Nursing* 75, 8:1338-1340.

LeBow, Michael. *Behavior Modification: A Significant Method in Nursing Practice*. Englewood Cliffs, New Jersey: Prentice-Hall, 1973.

Loomis, Maxine. *Interpersonal Change: A Behavioral Approach to Nursing Practice*. New York: McGraw-Hill, 1974.

Mager, Robert F. *Preparing Instructional Objectives*. Belmont, California: Fearon, 1962.

Murphy, J.C. "Setting the Stage for Teaching Ancillary Personnel." *Journal of Nursing Administration* 1:51-54, November/December 1971.

Peplau, Hildegard E. "Process and Concept of Learning." *Some Clinical Approaches to Psychiatric Nursing.* Edited by Shirburd and Margaret Marshall, New York: Macmillan, 1963.

Chapter 28 (Continued)

Redman, Barbara K. *The Process of Patient Teaching in Nursing.* St. Louis: C.V. Mosby, 1968.

Salzer, Joan E. "Classes to Improve Diabetic Self-Care." *American Journal of Nursing* 75, 8:1324-1326.

Smith, Dorothy. "Writing Objectives as a Nursing Practice Skill." *American Journal of Nursing* 71:319-320, February 1971.

Smyth, Kathleen, ed. "Symposium on Patient Teaching." *Nursing Clinics of North America* 6, 4:571-806, December 1971.

Williams, Barbara P. "The Burned Patient's Need for Teaching." *Nursing Clinics of North America* 6:615-639, December 1971.

Chapter 29 Group Process and Learning

Brown, Frances G. "Therapeutic Group Discussions." *American Journal of Nursing* 58:836-839, 1958.

Burnside, Irene M. "Group Work Among the Aged." *Nursing Outlook* June 1969.

Cartwright, Dorwin, and Zander, Alvin. eds. *Group Dynamics: Research and Theory.* 3d. ed. New York: Harper and Row, 1968.

Glasser, Paul et al. eds. *Individual Change Through Small Groups.* New York: The Free Press, 1974.

Gorman, Alfred. *The Leader in the Group.* New York: Teachers College Press, 1963.

Hare, Paul, et al., eds. *Small Groups: Studies in Social Interaction.* rev. ed. New York: Alfred A. Knopf, 1965.

Hartlage, Lawrence C. "Mobilizing Group Forces to Modify Behavior of Long-Term Patients," *Perspectives in Psychiatric Care* 2, 3:34-38, 1964.

Hilbarger, Victoria E. et al. "Nurses Use Group Process." *American Journal of Nursing,* 55:334, 1955.

Lieberman, Robert. "A Behavioral Approach to Group Dynamics." *Behavior Therapy* 1:141-175, May 1970.

Marram, Gwen D. *The Group Approach in Nursing Practice.* St. Louis: C.V. Mosby, 1973.

Miles, Matthew B. *Learning to Work in Groups.* New York: Teachers College Press, 1959.

Norris, Catherine M. et al. "A Therapeutic Nursing Routine: Feeding Patients." *Perspectives in Psychiatric Care* 1, 1 and 2:3-23, 1962.

Pullinger, Walter F. "Remotivation." *American Journal of Nursing* 60:683-685, 1960.

Ramshorn, Mary. "The Group as a Therapeutic Tool." *Perspectives in Psychiatric Care,* 8, 3:104-105, 1970.

Sommers, Robert. "Working Effectively with Groups." *American Journal of Nursing,* 60:223-226, 1960.

Werner, Jean A. "Relating Group Theory to Nursing Practice." *Perspectives in Psychiatric Care* 8, 6 :249-261, 1970.

Chapter 30 Learning in Groups

Bell, Ruth W. "Activity as a Tool in Group Therapy." *Perspectives in Psychiatric Nursing* 8, 2:84-91, 1970.

Blythe, Z. "Group Treatment for Handicapped Children." *Journal of Psychiatric Care* 7:172-173, 1969.

Browne, Louise J., and Ritter, Jennie I. "Reality Therapy for the Geriatric Psychiatric Patient." *Perspectives in Psychiatric Care* 10, 3:135-139, 1972.

Burnside, Irene M. "Loss: A Constant Theme in Group Work with the Aged." *Hospital and Community Psychiatry* 21:173-177, 1970.

Clark, Carolyn Chambers. "The Process of Establishing Inpatient, Short-Term Groups." *Group Process* 6:1-11, 1974.

Cochran, M.L., and Yeaworth, R.C. "Ward Meeting for Teen-Age Mothers." *American Journal of Nursing* 67:1044-1047, 1967.

Cooper, I. "Group Sessions for New Mothers. . .The Brownsville Section of Brooklyn." *Nursing Outlook* 22:251, April 1974.

Eddy, Frances L. et al. "Group Work on a Long-Term Psychiatric Service as Conducted by Nurses and Aides." *Perspectives in Psychiatric Care* 6, 1: 9-15, 1968.

Etters, Lloyd, E. "Adolescent Retardates in a Therapy Group." *American Journal of Nursing* 75, 7:1174-1175, 1975.

Gardner, K. "Patient Groups in a Therapeutic Community." *American Journal of Nursing* 71:528-531, 1971.

Gump, Paul, and Sutton-Smith, Brian. "Therapeutic Play Techniques." *American Journal of Orthopsychiatry* 24:755-760, 1955.

Hargreaves, Anne G. "The Group Culture and Nursing Practice." *American Journal of Nursing* 67, 9:1840-1846, 1967.

Heller, U. "Handicapped Patients Talk Together." *American Journal of Nursing* 70:332-335, 1970.

McGrew, W., and Jensen, J. "A Technique for Facilitating Therapeutic Group Interaction." *Journal of Psychiatric Nursing* 10:18, July/August 1972.

Jongeward, Dorothy, and James, Muriel. *Winning with People: Group Exercises in Transactional Analysis.* Reading, Massachusetts: Addison-Wesley, 1973.

Chapter 30 (Continued)

Loomis, Maxine E., and Podenhoff, J.T. "Working with Informal Patient Groups." *American Journal of Nursing* 70:1939-1944, 1970.

Marram, Gwen D. *The Group Approach in Nursing Practice.* St. Louis: C.V. Mosby, 1973.

Mezzanotte, E.J. "Group Instruction in Preparation for Surgery." *American Journal of Nursing* 70:89-91, 1970.

Miles, Matthew B. *Learning to Work in Groups.* New York: Teachers College Press, 1959.

Rosini, L.A. et al. "Group Meetings in a Pediatric Intensive Care Unit." *Pediatrics* 53:371-374, March 1974.

Scarpitti, Frank R. and Stephenson, Richard M. "The Use of the Small Group in the Rehabilitation of Delinquents." *Federal Probation* 30:45-50, 1966.

Schmuck, Richard and Patricia, *Group Processes in the Classroom* Dubuque, Iowa: Wm. C. Brown, 1971.

Smith, E.D. "Group Conferences for Postpartum Patients." *American Journal of Nursing.* 71:112-113, 1971.

Swanson, Mary. "A Check List for Group Leaders." *Perspectives in Psychiatric Care* 7, 3:120-126, 1969.

Ward, Judy Trowbridge. "The Sounds of Silence: Group Psychotherapy with Nonverbal Patients." *Perspectives in Psychiatric Care* 7, 1:13-19, 1974.

Wittes, Glorianne, and Radin, Norma. "Two Approaches to Group Work with Parents in a Compensatory Pre-School Program." *Social Work* 16, 1:42-50, 1971.

Yeaworth, R. "Learning Through Group Experience." *Nursing Outlook* 18: 29-32, 1970.

ACKNOWLEDGMENTS

The author gratefully acknowledges the assistance of the many persons who contributed to the development of this text.

The college staff from Bergen Community College, Paramus, New Jersey.
  Dr. Sidney Silverman, President
  Mr. George Stickel, Photographer
  Ms. Judy Spiegel, Nursing Department
  Ms. Alice MacDonald, Nursing Laboratory
  Mr. Robert Kirchherr, Library and Learning Resources
Christian Sanatorium, Wykoff, New Jersey for providing a clinical setting for photographs
Carole A. Shea and Maura E. Shea for assistance with photography
Dr. Jean Arnold, assistant coordinator, Regents External Degree in Nursing, New York; formerly, instructor of nursing and coordinator of continuing education programs for nurses at Bergen Community College, Paramus, New Jersey, for consultation on chapters 19 and 20.
The college faculty and students from Rockland Community College, Suffern, New York, who assisted with pretesting some of the instructional material in this edition.

The staff at Delmar Publishers
  Director of Publications – Alan N. Knofla
  Source Editor – Angela R. Emmi
  Editorial Assistants – Ruth Saur and Hazel Kozakiewicz
  Director of Manufacturing and Production – Fred Sharer
  Illustrators – George Dowse, Tony Canabush, Tanya Little, John Orozco
  Production Specialists – Sharon Lynch, Lee St. Onge, Jean LeMorta, Patti Manuli, Margaret Mutka, Betty Michelfelder, Debbie Monty

INDEX